Pediatric Orthopedics

Pediatric Orthopedics

A Handbook for Primary Care Physicians

Amr Abdelgawad

*Paul L. Foster School of Medicine,
Texas Tech University, Health Sciences Center
El Paso, TX, USA*

Osama Naga

*Children's Pediatric Practice
El Paso, TX, USA*

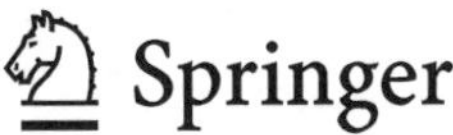

Editors
Amr Abdelgawad, MD
Paul L. Foster School of Medicine
Health Sciences Center
Texas Tech University Health Sciences Center
El Paso, TX
USA

Osama Naga, MD, FAAP
Children's Pediatric Practice
El Paso, TX
USA

ISBN 978-1-4614-7125-7 ISBN 978-1-4614-7126-4 (eBook)
DOI 10.1007/978-1-4614-7126-4
Springer New York Heidelberg Dordrecht London

Library of Congress Control Number: 2013944520

Printed on acid-free paper

Springer is part of Springer Science+Business Media (www.springer.com)

Dedication

To my parents who gave me all the support in my life and never asked for anything in return and to my wife whom without her help I could not have written this book.

Amr Abdelgawad

To my parents, my wife, my daughter, and my friends who supported me to complete the book.

Osama Naga

Preface

"Pediatric Orthopedics: A Handbook for Primary Care Physicians" is designed to be a quick and practical resource for pediatricians, family medicine physicians, residents, nurse practitioners, physician assistants, and medical students caring for pediatric population with musculoskeletal disorders in their busy daily practice. This book is a concise, clinically oriented and readily available resource to study common pediatric musculoskeletal diseases. Great emphasis was given to the natural history of the diseases and indications for referring the child to an orthopedic surgeon. The details of surgical treatment and procedures were not included as this will not be of major benefits to our readers.

This book has a very interesting and easy to follow format. We tried to stay away from long paragraphs and controversial statements. The book is printed in 'pocket' size and is easy to carry around. The information in the book is presented in a simple "bullet" format that allows the reader to understand the topic easily and with minimal effort. More than 300 figures were included in this handbook.

At the end of each chapter, we added "high yield facts" that summarize the important topics. In addition, a table of common orthopedic scenarios that the health care providers may encounter in their daily work is included, to guide them through the next steps in managing children with particular orthopedic presentations.

We are confident that this handbook will assist health care providers with a structured approach to the management of pediatric musculoskeletal conditions, and that they will find it a valuable tool in their daily practice.

Amr Abdelgawad, MD
Osama Naga, MD

Contents

Contributors

Amr Abdelgawad, MD
Orthopedic Department, Paul L. Foster School of Medicine, Texas Tech University Health Sciences Center, El Paso, TX, USA

Walid A. Abdel Ghany, MD, PhD
Ain Shams University Hospitals, Cairo, Egypt

Ayman Bassiony, MD
Orthopedic Department, Ain Shams University, Cairo, Egypt

Angel Garcia, MD
Paul L. Foster School of Medicine, Family and Community Medicine, Texas Tech University Health Sciences Center, El Paso, TX, USA

Courtney Holland, MD
William Beaumont Army Medical Center, El Paso, TX, USA

Enes Kanlic, MD
Texas Tech University Health Sciences Center, El Paso, TX 79905, USA

Michael Lee, MD
Department of Pediatrics, Texas Tech University Health Sciences Center, El Paso, TX, USA

Mahmoud A. Mahran, MD, PhD
Orthopedic Department, Ain Shams University Hospitals, Ramses Street, Abbasseya, Cairo, Egypt

Osama Naga, MD, FAAP
Children's Pediatric Practice, El Paso, TX, USA

Indu Pathak, MD, FAAP
Department of Pediatrics, Paul L. Foster School of Medicine, El Paso Children's Hospital, El Paso, TX, USA

Miguel Pirela-Cruz, MD
Texas Tech University Health Sciences Center, El Paso, USA

Ahmed M. Thabet, MD
Benha University School of Medicine, Orthopedics Department, Benha University Hospitals, Benha, Egypt

Justin M. Wright, MD
CAQ Sports Medicine Paul L. Foster School of Medicine, Family and Community Medicine, Texas Tech University Health Sciences Center, El Paso, TX, USA

Chapter 1

Introduction to Orthopedic Nomenclature

Amr Abdelgawad and Osama Naga

PHYSIS (THE GROWTH PLATE)

- It is a cartilaginous area that is responsible for the longitudinal growth of the bone.
- It appears as a radiolucent area in the radiographs.
- It should not be confused with fractures (physis has specific anatomic location with smooth outline) (Fig. 1.1).

EPIPHYSIS

- It is the proximal or the distal part of the bone (Fig. 1.1).
- The physis separates the epiphysis from the diaphysis.
- Usually articulate with the epiphysis of another bone to form a 'joint.'
- Epiphysis develops by **'secondary ossification center'** (see later).

APOPHYSIS

- Epiphysis which does not articulate with another bone (e.g., iliac crest apophysis, greater trochanter apophysis, calcaneal apophysis, tibial tubercle apophysis) (Fig. 1.2).
- Has a muscle attached to it and exposed to traction from this muscle (e.g., abdominal muscles and gluteal muscles attached to iliac crest).

A. Abdelgawad and O. Naga (eds.), *Pediatric Orthopedics*,
DOI: 10.1007/978-1-4614-7126-4_1,

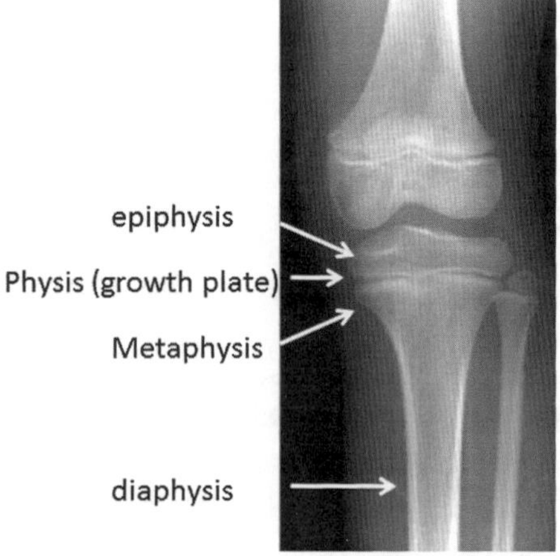

Fig. 1.1 Radiograph of the knee of an 9-year-old child showing anterio-posterior view of the knee. *Arrows* show the epiphysis, physis, metaphysis, and diaphysis

- Can get inflamed "apophysistis" causing pain (e.g., calcaneal apophysitis (Sever's disease), tibial tubercle apophysitis (Osgood Schlatter disease).

DIAPHYSIS (SHAFT)

- It is the midsection part of a long bone (Fig. 1.1).
- It is the middle tubular part of the long bone composed of compact bone (cortical bone) which surrounds a central marrow cavity.
- Diaphysis develops by **'primary ossification center"** (see later).

METAPHYSIS

- The part of the diaphysis which is the adjacent to the physis (Fig. 1.1).

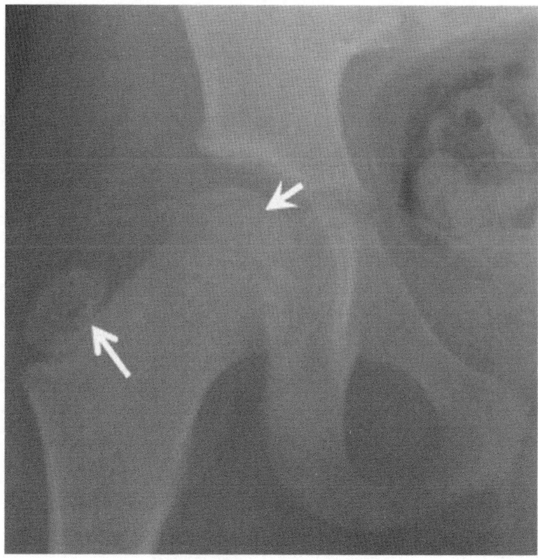

Fig. 1.2 Anatomical nomenclature:proximal femoral epiphysis (*arrow head*) and greater trochanter apophysis (*arrow*). Proximal femoral epiphysis articulate with acetabulum to form the hip joint while the greater trochanter does not articulate with other bone, it has the attachment of the hip abductors muscles

- This is a very active part of the bone with active cell division (cell added from physis are laid in the metaphysis).
- Most of the bone tumors arise in the metaphysis.
- The metaphysis is formed of less dense bone (cancellous bone).
- The circulation in the Metaphysis is sluggish as this is an end-capillary area (the physis is a relatively avascular structure separating the circulation of the metaphysis from the one in the epiphysis) (Fig. 1.3).
    - Hematogenous osteomyelitis usually occurs in the metaphysis. This is because bacteria from remote site will migrate in blood and settle in the metaphysis with its sluggish circulation (see also Chap. 21).

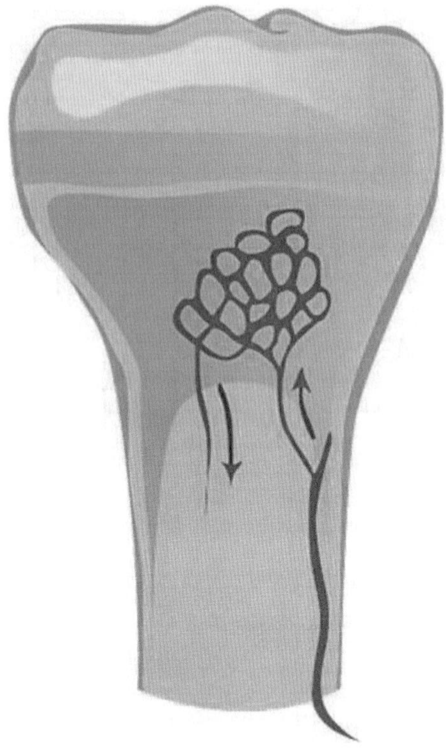

Fig. 1.3 Metaphyseal circulation. The *blood flow* in the metaphysis is slow as it passes from arterial system to venous system. The physis is relatively avascular structure separating the flow in the metaphysis from the epiphysis

PRIMARY CENTER OF OSSIFICATION

- It is the ossification island responsible for changing cartilage tissue to osteoid tissue.
- These develop in the **diaphysis** of all long bones in the **intra uterine life.**

SECONDARY CENTER OF OSSIFICATION

- It differs from the primary center of ossification in that it develops in the **epiphysis after birth** at different ages (except distal femur epiphysis which develops in intrauterine life) (Fig. 1.4).
- The secondary centers of ossification are used to identify the skeletal age of the child. (see identification of bone age in Chap. 2).

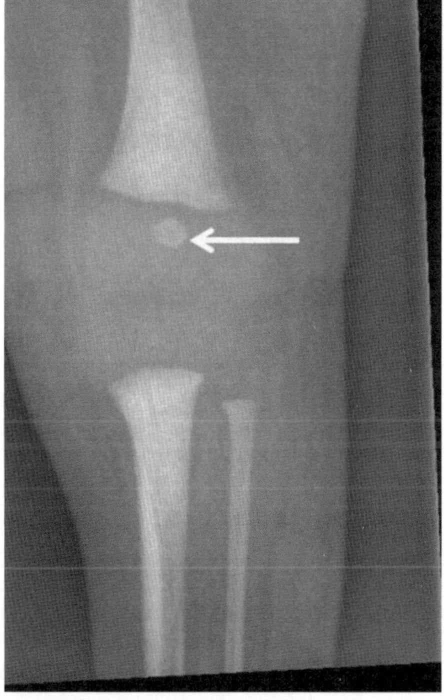

Fig. 1.4 Radiograph of a 3-day-old boy showing the shaft of the femur, tibia, and fibula (primary centers of ossification developing intrauterine). The radiograph also shows the distal femur ossific center which is the only secondary ossific center present at birth (*arrow*).Proximal tibial and fibular epiphyses cannot be seen in the radiograph because they are still cartilaginous

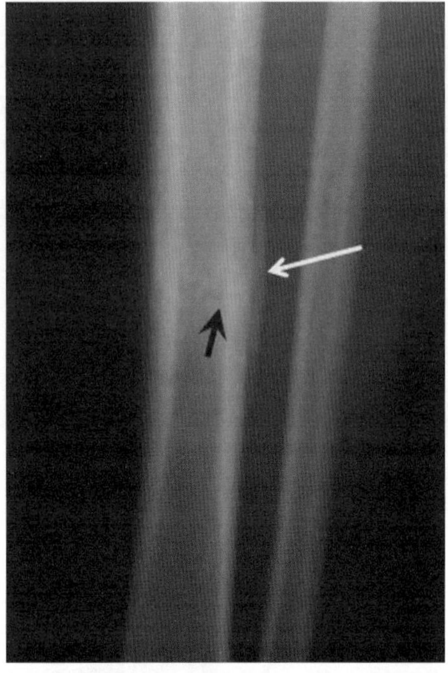

Fig. 1.5 Periosteal new bone formation in case of fracture healing. Plain radiograph of the tibia and fibula anteroposterior view showing periosteal new bone formation (*white arrow*) that happened during fracture healing (*black arrow*)

PERIOSTEUM

- It is a membrane that lines the outer surface of all bones, except at the joints surfaces.
- In children, periosteum is **thick and loosely attached to the bone** (except at the physis where it becomes firmly attached to the bone).
- Raising the periosteum away from the bone surface for any reason (e.g., infections, tumors, trauma) will **cause new periosteal bone formation** (Fig. 1.5).

SOME ANATOMICAL NOMENCLATURE

Proximal:

- The part close to trunk (axial skeleton) of the body.

Distal:

- The part further away from the trunk (axial skeleton) of the body.

Medial:

- The part close to the Medline.

Lateral:

- The part away from the Medline.

DEFORMITIES

Varus Deformity:

- The deformity in which the distal part points medially (Fig. 1.6).

Valgus Deformity:

- The deformity in which the distal part points laterally (Fig. 1.6).

Contracture Deformity:

- The joint is contracted in certain position.
- For example: **flexion contracture** of the knee means the knee is always in flexed position cannot reach **full extension** (Fig. 1.7).

General Joint Examination:

- **Inspection:**

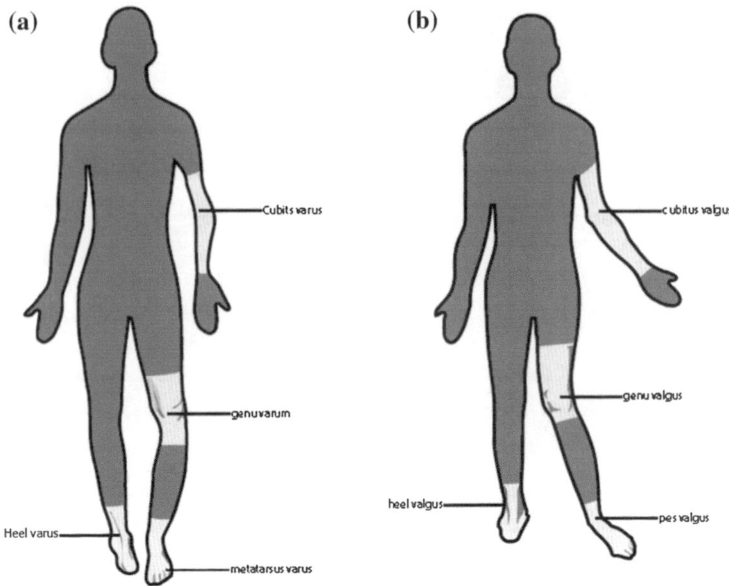

Fig. 1.6 (**a**) varus deformity and (**b**) valgus deformity. In varus deformity, the distal part of the joint is pointing medially and in valgus deformity, the distal part of the joint in pointing laterally

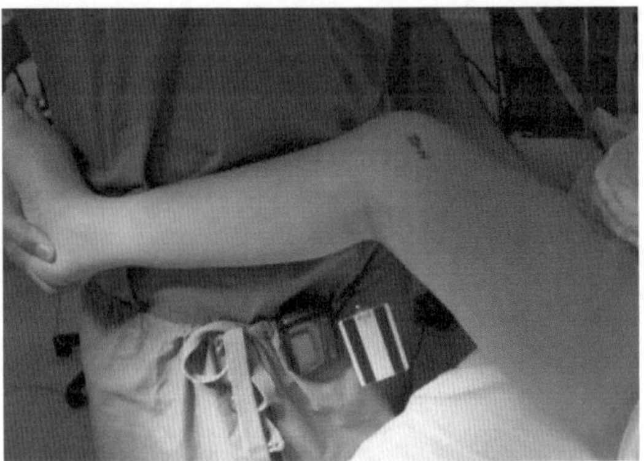

Fig. 1.7 Knee flexion contracture. An 11-year-old girl with spina bifida and 30° flexion contracture of the knee. The knee cannot be extended more than the position in the picture

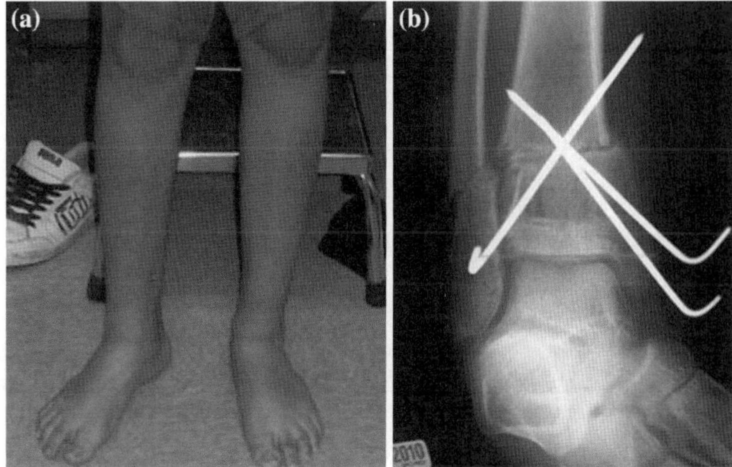

Fig. 1.8 Osteotomy. A 14-year-old boy who had fracture right tibia and fibula treated in cast. (**a**) Patient had malunion in external rotation. The family did not like the shape of the leg. (**b**) Osteotomy of the distal tibia and fibula was done to re-align the extremity in appropriate rotation. The osteotomy was fixed by metal (K-wires)

- Swelling
- Deformity
- Scars of previous surgeries
- Atrophy of the muscles.

■ **Palpation:**

- Anatomical landmark
- Tenderness
- Swelling and effusion.

■ **Movement (active and passive)**

- Assessment of the range of the motion of the joint both active and passive.

■ **Special test (varies according to the examined joint).**

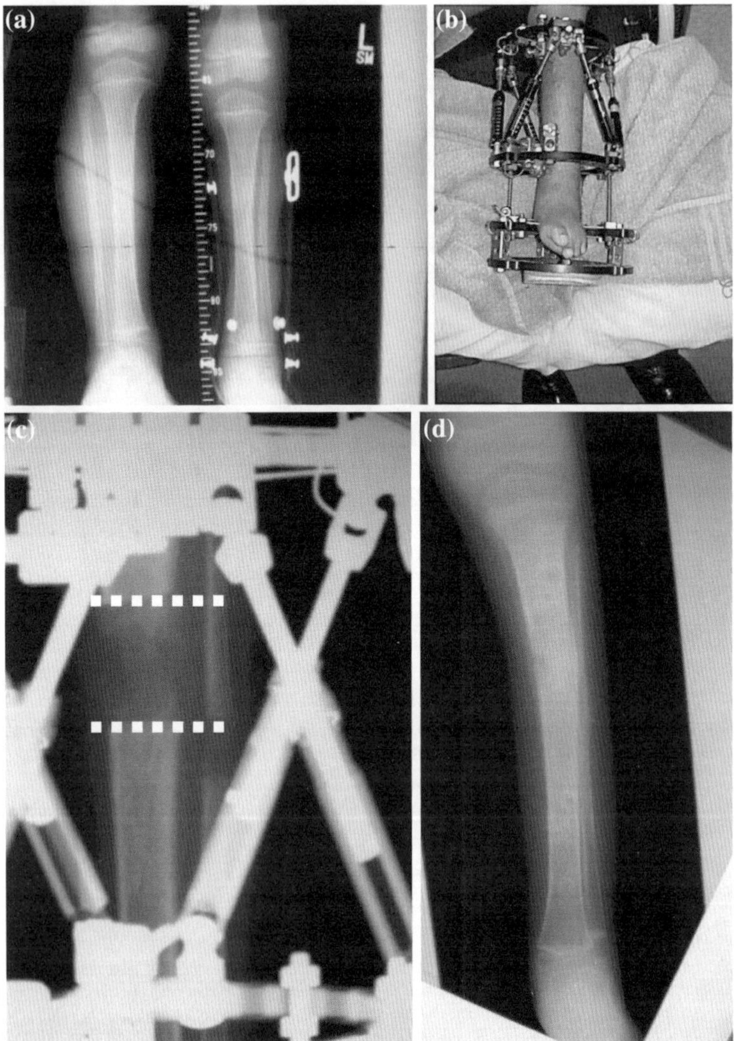

Fig. 1.9 Distraction osteogenesis. (**a**) A 4-year-old girl with limb length discrepancy due to fibular hemimelia (*left side shorter*). (**b**) Lengthening was done by application of external fixator. (**c**) The bone was cut and then the soft callus was stretched to lengthen the bone (distance between two dotted line). The callus is then left to consolidate to hard bone. (**d**) Radiograph taken after removal of the fixator showing the new bone formation and increase length of the bone

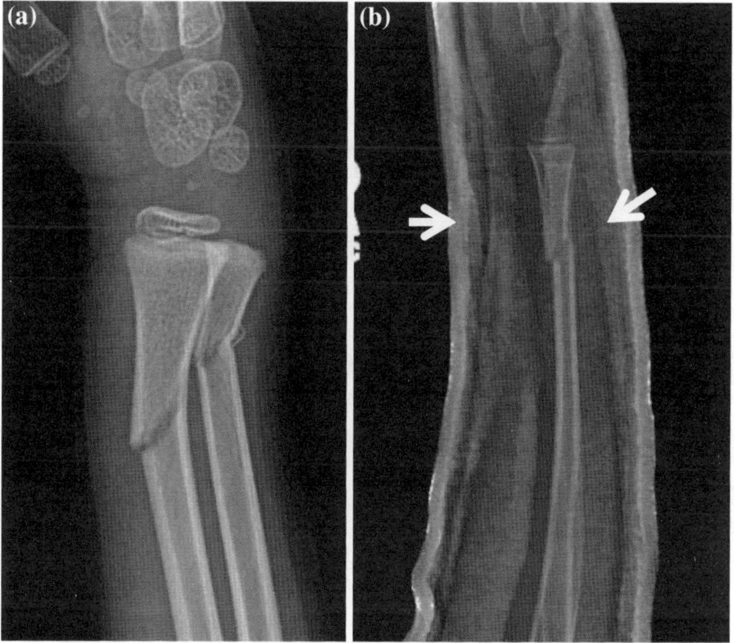

Fig. 1.10 Closed reduction. (**a**) A 6-year-old boy distal radius and ulna fracture with angulation. (**b**) Closed reduction was done by manipulation of the fracture and then sugar tongue splint (*arrows*) was applied to maintain the reduction

ORTHOPEDIC SURGERIES/PROCEDURES

Osteotomy:

- Cutting of the bone. This surgery is used to correct deformity (Fig. 1.8).

Distraction osteogenesis:

- Lengthening of bone by performing osteotomy and then stretching the soft callus tissue which develop at the site of osteotomy 7–10 days after the surgery (Fig. 1.9).

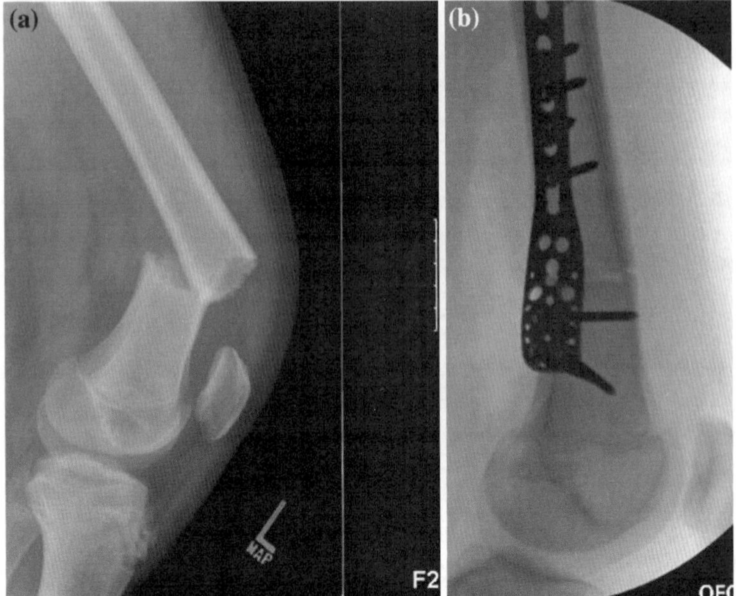

Fig. 1.11 Open reduction internal fixation. (**a**) A 12-year-old boy fell down a hill and fractured distal femur. (**b**) Open reduction internal fixation was done using plate and screws

Closed reduction:

- Reduction of the fracture by manipulation of the extremity without surgical incision (Fig. 1.10).

Open reduction:

- Reduction of the fracture by manipulation of the bone ends directly after performing surgical incision (Fig. 1.11).

Internal fixation:

- Fixation of the fracture or the osteotomy by implant (usually metal) inside the patient body (Fig. 1.11).

Open reduction internal fixation:

- One of the most commonly performed surgeries in orthopedic (Fig. 1.11).

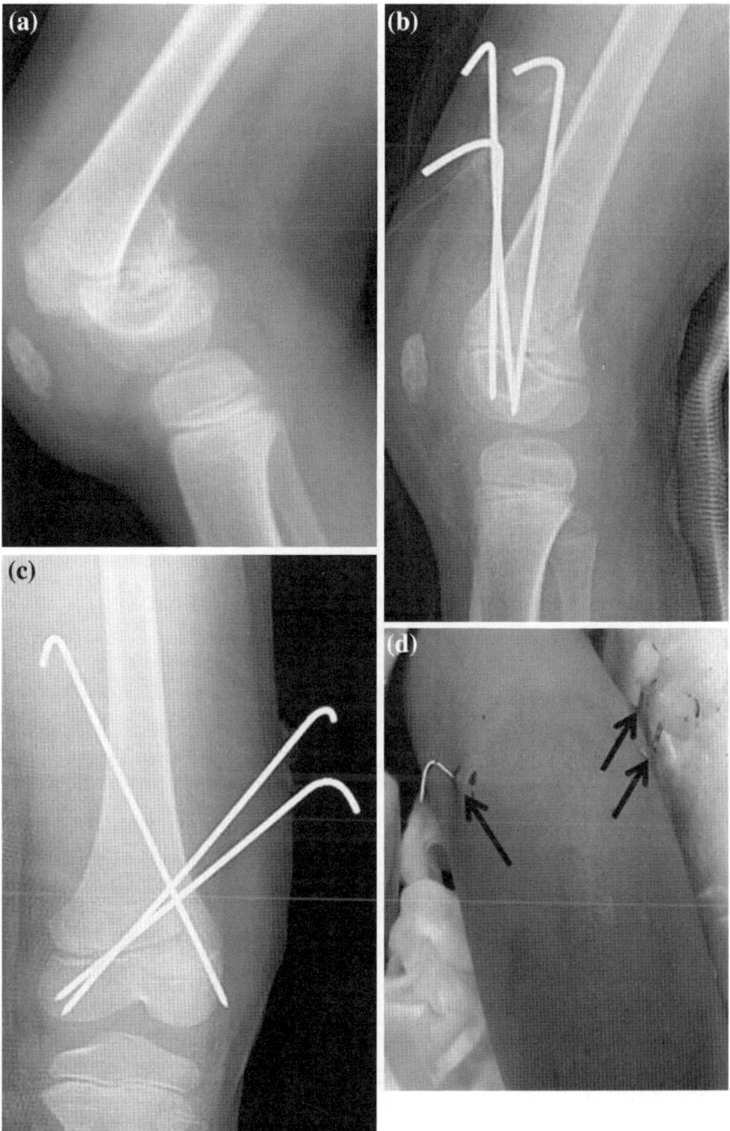

Fig. 1.12 Closed reduction and Percutaneus fixation. (**a**) Salter Harris type II distal femur fracture treated with closed reduction and percutaneous fixation by K-wires (**b**), (**c**). The wires were introduced from the skin without opening by the help of intra-operative fluoroscopy. (**d**) Notice that there is no skin incision around the pin entry points (*arrows*)

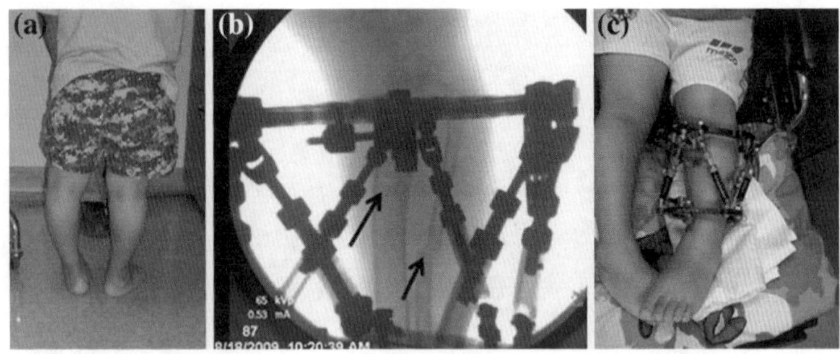

Fig. 1.13 External fixator. (**a**) An 8-year-old child with pseudo-achondroplasia. (**b**) Patient had osteotomy of left tibia and fibula to correct the genu varum (*arrows*). (**c**) External fixator was applied to obtain gradual correction

- The procedure includes open reduction of the fracture ends followed by internal fixation of the fracture.

Closed reduction and Percutaneus fixation:

- The implant used to fix the fracture or the osteotomy is introduced by small opening in the skin (Fig. 1.12).
- Intra-operative fluoroscopy is used to guide the insertion of the implant.

External Fixator:

- A device used to fix the fractures or osteotomies (Fig. 1.13).
- Pins or wires are introduced in the bone and these are connected together from outside by rods.
- Used mainly to corrected deformities or for open fractures.

Cast, splints, and braces:

- See Chap. 18.

REFERENCES

Hopyan S, Alman B. Growth and development. In: Staheli LT, Song KM, editors. Secrets of Pediatric Orthopedic. 3rd ed. Philadelphia: Mosby Elsevier; 2007. p. 9–12.

Sponseller Paul D. Bone, Joint, and Muscle Problems. In: McMillan JA, Feigin RD, DeAngelis C, Jones MD, editors. Oski's Pediatrics: Principles & Practice. 4th ed. Philadelphia: Lippincott Williams & Wilkins; 2006. p. 2471–505.

Chapter 2
Growth and Development and Their Relation to Musculoskeletal Conditions

Ahmed M. Thabet

INTRODUCTION

- Growth and development have close relation with many pediatric orthopedic conditions.
- Orthopedic conditions as cerebral palsy and spina bifida can adversely affect the children normal growth. In most pediatric orthopedic disorders the multi-displinary approach and **especially the co-operation between the pediatrician and the orthopedic surgeons is crucial for successful outcome.**
- Knowing the normal growth and development can affect the surgical planning of lots of musculoskeletal conditions.
- Typical examples of growth disturbances in the musculoskeletal system are limb length discrepancy (LLD), spine deformities, skeletal dysplasia, and paralytic disorders.

BASICS OF NORMAL GROWTH

Children's bones have unique ability to grow. This particular feature of children skeleton differentiates between **children (skeletally immature) and adults (skeletally mature).**

A. Basic definitions:

- **Growth:** increase in total individual body size or increase in size of a particular organ or organ systems
- **Development:** physical changes of maturation that occurs as the child gets older

A. Abdelgawad and O. Naga (eds.), *Pediatric Orthopedics*,
DOI: 10.1007/978-1-4614-7126-4_2,

TABLE 2.1 DEFINITIONS OF ABNORMAL GROWTH AND DEVELOPMENT

Congenital	Anomaly that is present at birth e.g., congenital radial club hand
Deformation	A normally formed structure that is pushed out of shape by mechanical forces
Deformity	A body part altered in shape from normal, outside the normal range
Developmental	A deviation that occurs over time; one that might not be present or apparent at birth e.g., developmental dysplasia of the hip (DDH)
Disruption	A structure undergoing normal development that stops developing or is destroyed or removed
Dysplasia	A tissue that is abnormal or wrongly constructed e.g., Achondroplasia
Malformation	A structure that is wrongly built; failure of embryologic development or differentiation resulting in abnormal or missing structure

B. Abnormal growth and development definitions:

- It is very important to understand the basic definitions reflecting the deviation from normal growth and development.
- Table 2.1 provides these basic definitions about the faults of growth and development (Table 2.1).

C. Structure of the growth plate (Fig. 2.1):

- Reserve zone
- Proliferative zone
- Hypertrophic zone**: is divided into three zones**
  - Maturation zone
  - Degenerative zone
  - Provisional calcification zone.
- The growth plates are responsible for longitudinal growth of the long bones.
- Growth plate can be affected by various pathological processes (e.g., traumatic, neoplastic, infectious, genetic, and nutritional causes).

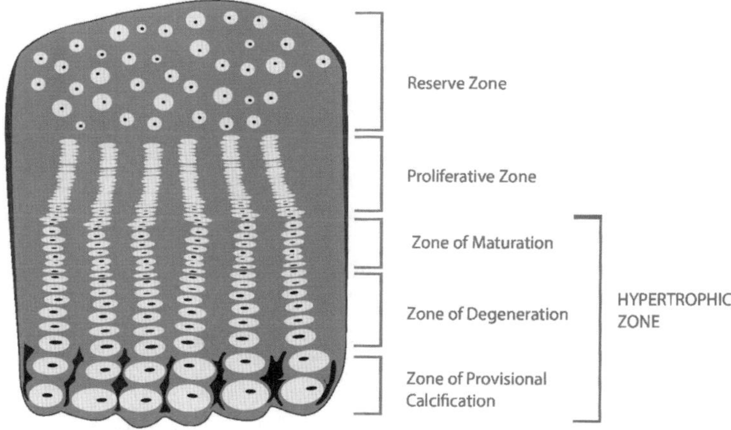

Fig. 2.1 Growth plate histology

- Injuries or infection to growth plate can affect the normal limb development. Limb shortening and/or angular deformities can result from these kinds of injuries (Figs. 16.9/trauma and 16.44/trauma).
- Achondroplasia children have deficiency of fibroblast growth factor receptors (FBGR) which affects the growth plate.

D. Types of growth plates:

There are different types of growth plates. The type of growth plates depends upon the shape of the bone. These include:

- Epiphyseal growth plate: lies at the ends of long bones and provide longitudinal growth.
- Ring epiphyses surround round bones such as the tarsals. These bones grow circumferentially.

E. The contribution of each bone to the overall growth of the extremity:

- The upper limb growth:
  - 40 % proximal humerus

- 40 % distal radius
- 20 % around the elbow

- The lower limb growth:

  - 65 % around the knee
  - 15 % proximal femur
  - 20 % distal tibia

F. Evolution of proportionate body size:

- At birth: the head is 25 % of body size.
- At birth: the upper body segment/lower body segment is 1.7.
- At the age of 10 the ratio between upper and lower body segments is less than 1.
- Children with skeletal dysplasia have abnormalities of these ratios. Measurements of these ratios are very useful in establishing the diagnosis.
- Extremity growth: Girls stop growing around the age of 14 years, and boys around the age of 16 years.
- Spine growth: spine growth continues after puberty. The additional increase in height after puberty is through spine growth.

G. Phases of growth:

1. Fetal phase: in this phase the child grows very fast and limb rotation occurs during this period.

   - Limb rotation: During the seventh week, the upper limb rotates externally and the thumb will be laterally. The lower limb rotates internally and the great toe moves medially).
   - Abnormalities of lower limb rotation can result in tibia internal rotational or external rotational deformities.

2. Early childhood:

   - The child reaches half of his adult height during the 4th year of life.
   - The foot growth reaches half the adult length by the age of 2 years. **The foot matures earlier than the long bones to provide stable base during walking.**

3. Adolescent:

- **The adolescent stage is a phase of rapid growth (peak growth velocity).**
- Most of the limb and spine deformities accelerate during that time e.g.,: adolescent Blount's disease and idiopathic scoliosis (peak growth velocity).
- **The child continues to grow for 3 years after adolescent growth spurt.**
- The spurt in trunk length is greater than the spurt in lower limb growth, so the increase in height in the adolescent growth spurt is more derived from the trunk than the limbs.
- Gender differences in growth become evident during adolescence with proportionally greater growth of the male shoulders and the female pelvis.

ASSESSMENT OF GROWTH POTENTIAL AND ESTIMATION OF DEGREE OF SKELETAL MATURITY

The concept of growth remaining:

- It is very crucial to know the amount of growth remaining for surgical planning and determination of different orthopedic intervention (e.g., spinal fusion for scoliosis or epiphysiodesis for LLD in the growing children).
- The assessment of skeletal maturity can be achieved through clinical and radiological methods.

1. Clinical assessment:

- Using the serial height measurements and Tanner's staging of secondary sexual characters. This can detect the peak growth velocity period (children continue to grow three years after the peak growth)

A. Peak Growth velocity:

- The peak growth velocity is the maximum skeletal growth during adolescent growth spurt.
- The timing of peak growth velocity is estimated by serial (every 6 months) height measurements over time.

- The peak growth velocity is the earliest and best index of adolescent growth spurt. After this peak the growth slows down.
- The peak growth velocity **occurs after closure of triradiate cartilage and before Risser stage 1 and menarche (see Chap. 19**).

B. Tanner staging:

- The assessment of the secondary sexual characters is an important tool in identification of level of skeletal maturity and puberty.
- Tanner's staging uses secondary sexual characters in boys and girls.
- The first physical sign of puberty in boys (which is usually testicular growth), occurs about 1.5 years before the peak height velocity and 3.5 years before attaining final adult height.
- The first physical sign of puberty in girls (which is usually breast budding), occurs about 1 year before peak height velocity. Menarche occurs about 2 years after breast budding, and final height is usually achieved 2.5–3 years after menarche.

C. The height measurement:

Before the age of 5 years, it can measured while the child is lying down which is easier and reliable. After that age it can be measured as standing. It can be subdivided into:

- **Sitting height:**
  - The sitting height is reflecting the trunk growth.
- **Sub-ischial height:**
  - Reflecting the lower limb growth. It can be calculated by subtracting the sitting height from the standing height
- **Arm span:**
  - The span can be measured using tape between the middle fingers of both arms. In 77 % of normal children the arm span is 0–5 cm greater than standing height.

- In certain conditions like Marfan syndrome, the span is greater than standing height by more than 5 cm (see Chap. 4).

2. Radiological assessment:

A. Bone age:

- The bone age is more important that the chronological age in determining the future growth potentials.
- The bone age is the average age at which the bones reach specific maturation stage.
- The average bone age and chronological ages for large group of children should be the same, however for individual child the difference may be up to 1 or 2 years (earlier or delayed bone age).
- The bone age can be studied through hand and elbow radiographs.
- Children with constitutional short stature can have delayed bone age. These children will later on continue to grow and achieve normal final adult height.
- **Radiographs are taken for left hand** and compared with known characteristics of the radiographs for boys and girls hands at certain ages using "Greulich and Pyle Atlas" (Fig. 2.2).

B. The order of ossification centers about the elbow:

- The ossific centers of the elbow are very important in knowing the child's bone age.
- The eponym for remembering these ossification centers is **CRITOE** (the order of appearance is Capitellum, Radial head, Internal (medial) epicondyle, Trochlea, Olecranon, and External (lateral) epicondyle).

  - The ossification centers at the elbow **appear** as the following (**in girls**) (Fig. 2.3):

    - The capitellum appears by about 8 months–1 year.
    - The radial head at about age 3 years.
    - The medial epicondyle at about age 5 years.
    - The trochlea at about age 7 years.
    - The olecranon at about age 9.
    - The lateral epicondyle at about age 11.

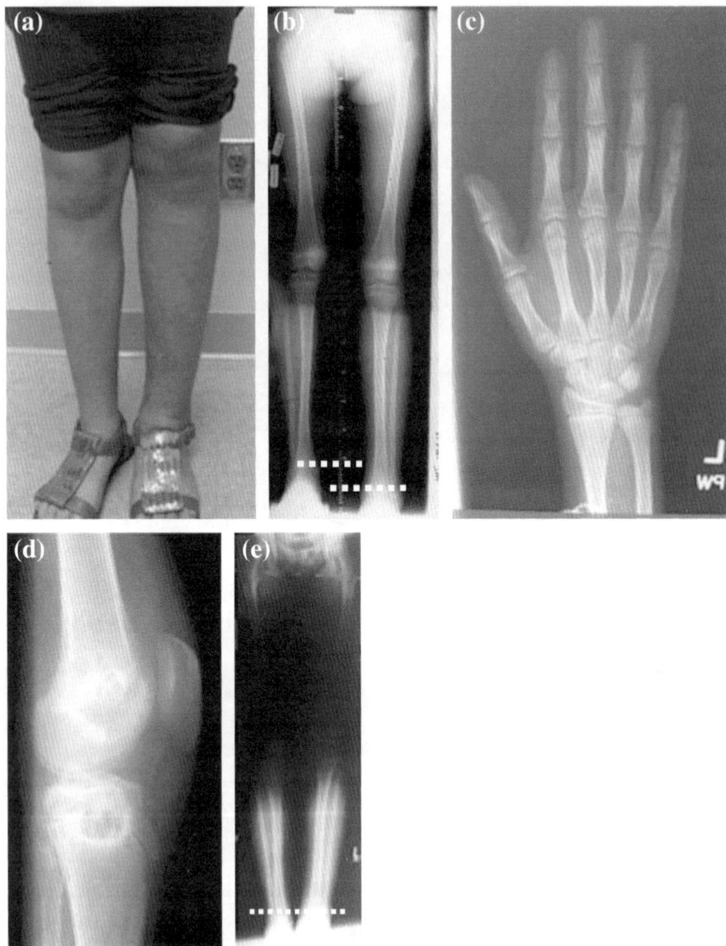

Fig. 2.2 Epiphysiodesis. (**a**) A 13-year-old girl with *left* lower extremity (LE) diffuse hemangioma causing increased blood supply to *left* LE and *left* LE longer than *right* LE by about one inch. One inch block is used underneath the right LE to equalize the length (notice the dotted lines) (**b**). (**c**) Hand radiograph compared to Greulich and Pyle atlas showed bone age of about 12 years and six months. Epiphysiodesis of the distal femur and proximal tibia (**d**). 2 years of follow-up showed equalization of the limb length between *right* and *left* LE (**e**)

- The age of appearance in boys is 1–2 years older than girls (except the capitellum).
- Fusion of the these ossification centers is around the age of 15 years old in girls and 16 years old in boys.

C. Risser's sign and tri-radiate cartilage (**see Chap. 19**):

- The Risser sign is a radiological sign based on the ossification of the iliac apophysis. The sign can be interpreted from the spine radiographs. It is very useful in surgical planning of all spine deformities (Fig. 19.9/spine).
- Closure of the tri-radiate cartilage occurs about one year after the start of adolescent growth spurt and about one and half years before Risser stage 1.

DEVELOPMENTAL MILESTONES

- Gross motor skills: The timing of development of motor milestones is part of routine assessment of the child during office visits. Children with cerebral palsy have delayed development of the motor milestones.
- Examples of the major development of the motor milestones are:
  - Sitting independently at age of 6 months.
  - Walks independently at age of 12 months.
- Gait maturation:
  - Infant's gait is unstable gait and walks with wide base. The walking speed is variable.
  - The infants' unstable gait is due to high center of gravity; under development of their nervous system; low muscle mass to body ratio and immaturity of balance controlling system.
  - As the child continue to grow, the gait becomes more stable and more energy efficient.
  - The gait pattern of children mature to become close to adult walking by the age of 4 years old.

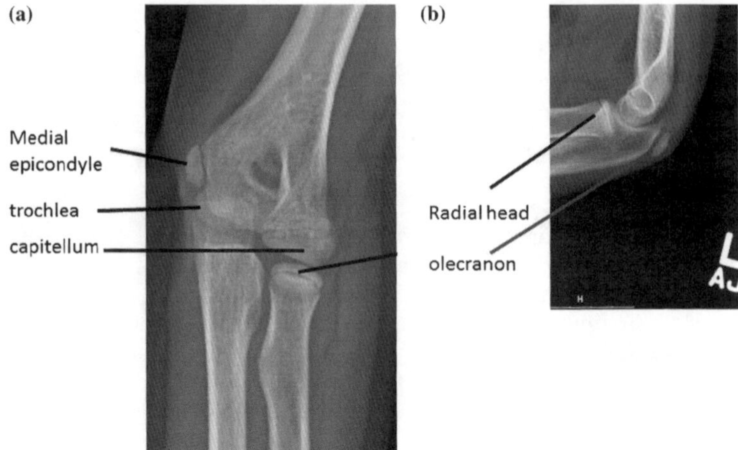

Fig. 2.3 (**a**) Radiograph of the elbow in a 10-year-old girl. (**b**) All ossific centers are formed except lateral epicondyle

GROWTH OF CHILDREN WITH NEUROMUSCULAR DISORDERS

- Children with neuro-muscular disorders like cerebral palsy and spina bifida can have affection of their growth because of their decrease mobility and decreased muscle activity.

PREDICTION OF LIMB LENGTH DISCREPANCY (LLD) AT SKELETAL MATURITY

- The Limb length discrepancy (LLD) in children can be due to congenital, traumatic, tumor, genetic, or infectious causes.
- Prediction of LLD at skeletal maturity is critical for surgical planning. The surgical treatment options are either shortening the long leg by shutting down the growth plate or lengthening the short leg (see below).
- Prediction of LLD at skeletal maturity can be calculated using different methods:

- **Growth remaining method using Green and Anderson charts:**
  - □ The charts for growth remaining of the distal femur and proximal tibia are utilized to predict the LLD at skeletal maturity and timing of closure of the growth plates.
- **Moseley straight line graph:**
  - □ The length of the long side and short side is plotted on the graph on two or more occasion and these are used to draw lines to predict the final LLD.
- **Multiplier method:**
  - □ Using the length of the short and long side, a multiplier can be used to detect the final LLD.

Limb equalizing procedures:

- **Shortening** of long limb can be achieved by closure of growth plate. This procedure is known as epiphysiodesis (Fig. 2.2).
- **Lengthening** of short leg can be done using the principles of distraction osteogenesis as pioneered by Ilizarov (Figs. 16.44/trauma, 4.2/general).
- Distraction osteogenesis means gradual mechanical distraction of immature bone using special devices at the rate of about 1 mm/day. These devices are either external devices (e.g., Ilizarov ring fixator) or using internal devices (e.g., special nails to lengthen the bones).

REFERENCES

Stahli L. Fundamentals of Pediatric Orthopedics. In: Stahli L, editor. Fundamentals of Pediatric Orthopedics. 4th ed. Philadelphia: Lippincott Williams & Wilkins; 2007.

Herring JA. Tachdjian's Pediatric Orthopedics In: Herring JA, editor. Tachdjian's Pediatric Orthopedics. 3rd edition. Phiadelphia: W.B Saunders; 2002.

http://www.posna.org/education/StudyGuide/growth.asp. POSNA Core curriculum.

Dimeglio A. Lovell and Winter's Pediatric Orthopaedics. 6th ed. Philadelphia: Lippincott Williams & Wilkins; 2005.

Chapter 3
Metabolic Conditions

Amr Abdelgawad and Osama Naga

RICKETS

Definition:

- Deficient mineralization of the bone leading to increase in the amount of uncalcified osteoid matrix.

Causes of Rickets:

- Vitamin D deficiency.
  - Nutritional:
    - Remain the most common cause of rickets globally.
    - More common in developing countries.
    - Less common with use of fortified food.
    - Calcium and vitamin D intake are low in infants who are fed vegan diets.
  - Congenital vitamin D deficiency.
  - Secondary vitamin D deficiency.
    - Malabsorption.
    - Increased degradation.
    - Decreased liver 25-hydroxylase.
  - Vitamin D dependent rickets type1.
  - Vitamin D dependent rickets type2.
  - Chronic renal failure.
- Calcium deficiency.
  - Low intake.

A. Abdelgawad and O. Naga (eds.), *Pediatric Orthopedics*,
DOI: 10.1007/978-1-4614-7126-4_3,

- Diet.
- Premature infant.

- Mal-absorption.

- Phosphorus deficiency.

  - Inadequate intake.

    - Premature infants.
    - Aluminum—containing antacid.

  - Renal losses.

    - X-linked hypophosphatemic rickets.
    - Autosomal dominant hypophosphatemic rickets.
    - Autosomal recessive hypophosphatemic rickets.
    - Hereditary hypophosphatemic rickets with hypercalciuria.
    - Fanconi syndrome.
    - Distal renal tubular acidosis.
    - Oculocerebrorenal dystrophy (Lowe syndrome).

- Drugs

  - Anticonvulsant drugs (e.g., phenobarbital, phenytoin) accelerate metabolism of calcidiol, which may lead to vitamin D insufficiency and rickets.

- **Intestinal malabsorption of fat**.
- **Diseases of the liver or kidney may produce a clinical picture similar to nutritional rickets**.

Pathophysiology:

Sources of Vitamin D:

- Vitamin D2 (ergocalciferol) originates from plants.
- Vitamin D3 (Cholecalciferol):

  - Vitamin D3 is produced in the skin via opening of the B-ring of 7-dehydrocholesterol.
  - 7-dehydrocholesterol transformed to previtamin D3 during exposure to the sunlight.

Liver:

- The first hydroxylation occurs at position 25 in the liver, producing calcidiol (25-hydroxycholecalciferol).
  - 25-hydroxyvitamin D is a good indicator of overall vitamin D status and widely used clinically.

Kidney:

- The second hydroxylation step occurs in the kidney at the 1 position.
- It undergoes hydroxylation to the active metabolite calcitriol (1,25-dihydroxycholecalciferol).
- Parathyroid hormone facilitates the 1-hydroxylation step in vitamin D metabolism.

Calcitriol acts at 3 main sites:

- **Intestine:** it promotes absorption of calcium and phosphorus from the intestine.
- **Kidney:** it increases re-absorption of phosphate.
- **Bone:** it releases calcium and phosphate from bone.
  - The net effect of calcitriol is enhancing the mineralization of the bone.

Calcification of osteoid:

- It occurs primarily at the metaphyseal growing ends of bones but also throughout all osteoid tissue in the skeleton.

Changes in the vitamin D deficiency:

- Hypocalcemia or low to normal level of calcium.
- Increase parathyroid hormone level.
- Increase renal phosphorus loss.
- **Hypophosphatemia.**
- Elevation of serum alkaline phosphatase.
- **Decrease calcium deposition in the bone. This will lead to increase in the amount of unmineralized osteoid tissue.**

Clinical Presentation:

- **General symptoms**.

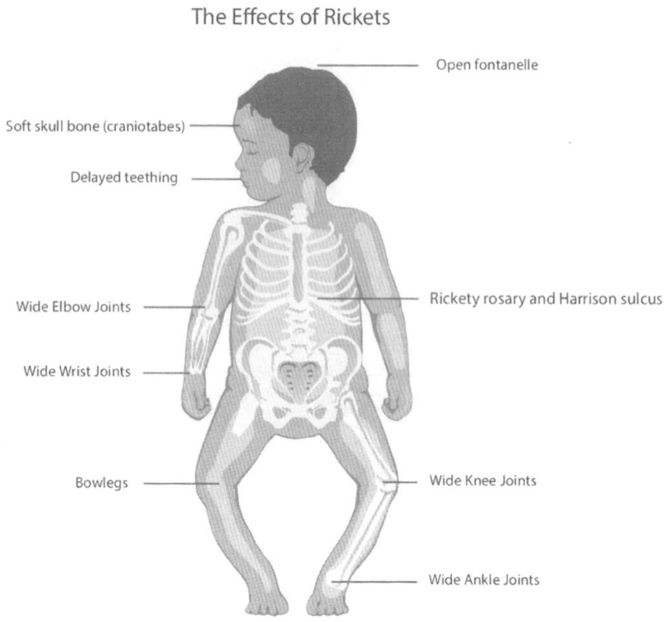

Fig. 3.1 Skeletal manifestation of rickets

- Failure to thrive.
- Muscle weakness.
- Protruding abdomen.
- Delayed teething.

- **Hypocalcemic symptoms**.
  - Tetany.
  - Seizures.
  - Stridor due to laryngeal spasm.

- **Bone manifestations in rickets** (Fig. 3.1):
  - Repeated fractures.
  - Angular deformity of the lower extremity:

- Commonly genu varum, rarely genu valgus (Fig. 3.1).
- Coxa vara.

- Leg pain.
- Broadening of the ends of the bone (wrists and ankles).
- **Rachitic rosary:** It is a knobby chest deformity along the costochondral junction.
- **Harrison sulcus:** Groove at the lower edge of the thoracic cage corresponding to the insertion site of the diaphragm. Pull of the diaphragm on the soft bone will cause this groove.
- Soft skull bone (**Craniotabes**).
- Delayed closure of fontanels.
- Spine.
  - Scoliosis.
  - Kyphosis.
  - Lordosis.

Radiographs (Fig. 3.2):

- **Fraying**: The physis loses its sharp border and look like a brush border.
- **Cupping:** The edge of metaphysis changes from a convex or flat surface to a more concave surface.
- **Widening** of the physis: Increase width of the physis.
- **Osteopenia:** Decrease mineralization of bone will cause decrease density of the bone in the radiographs.
- **Bone deformity**.

Laboratories

In Vitamin D deficiency Rickets:

- Low to normal Ca.
- Low Ph.
- Low 25- hydroxyvitamin D.
- Low or normal 1,25 dihydroxyvitamin D (Calcitriol).
- **High serum Alkaline phosphatase enzyme**.
- Increase PTH.
- Decrease Ca in urine (Table 3.1).

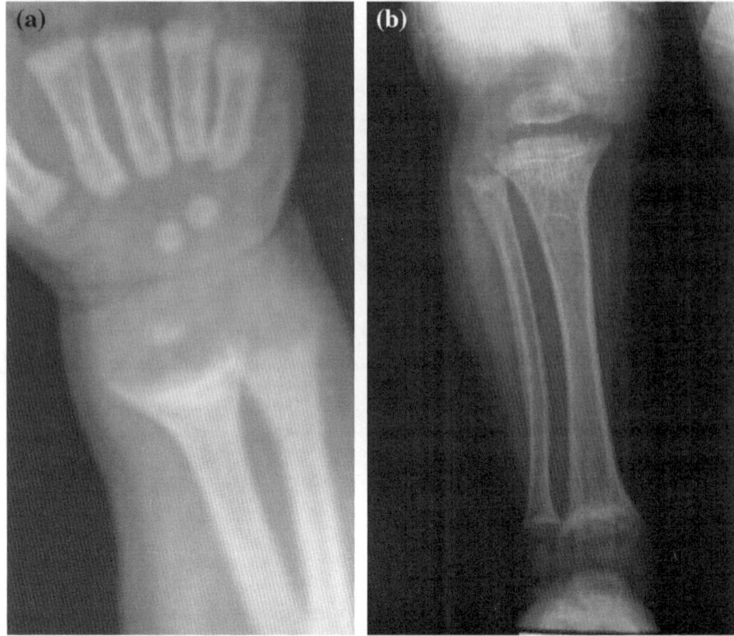

Fig. 3.2 Radiographs of rickets. Radiographs of the wrist (**a**) and leg (**b**) of a 3-year-old boy with nutritional rickets showing the cupping, fraying, and widening of the physis

Table 3.1: Common types of rickets and laboratory values:

Treatment:

Depends on the type and the cause of the rickets.

- **Vitamin D deficiency Rickets**.
- **There are two strategies:**
  - **Single day therapy**
    - Vitamin D with dose range from 300,000 to 600,000 IU are administrated orally or IM as 2–4 doses over 1 day (it is adequate if compliance is questionable).

TABLE 3.1 COMMON TYPES OF RICKETS AND LABORATORY VALUES

Type of rickets	Defect	Ca	ph	PTH	ALP	Calcidiol	Calcitriol	Treatment
Vitamin D deficient	Decreased Vit D intake	nl/low	low	high	high	low	nl/low	Vit D
Vitamin D dependent type I	Calcidiol can't convert to calcitriol	low	low	high	high	nl	low	Calcitriol
Vitamin D dependent type II	End organ resistance to calcitriol	low	low	high	high	nl	high	Calcium
Hypoparathyroidism	Low PTH	low	high	low	nl	nl	nl	Ca and Vit D
Renal rickets	Renal failure	low	high	high	high	nl	low	Calcium/ phosphorous binders
Familial hypophosphatemic	Proximal tubular defect, phosphorous dumped into urine	nl	low	nl	high	nl	low	Phosphorous/ calcitriol
Pseudohypoparathyroidism	PTH resistance	low	high	high	nl	nl	nl	Ca and Vit D

Ca calcium, *Ph* phosphate, *PTH* parathyroid hormone, *ALK* alkaline phosphatase, *nl* normal, *Vit D* vitamin D

- **Alternative method**
  - Oral Vitamin D with doses range from 2,000 to 5,000 IU/day over 2–3 months.
- Both strategies should be followed by daily Vitamin D intake of 400 IU/day if <1 year or 600 IU if >1 year, typically given as multivitamins.
- Children with symptomatic hypocalcemia.
  - Need IV Ca followed by oral Ca which typically tapered over 2–6 weeks in children receiving adequate dietary Ca.
  - Oral Calcitriol (1,25-D, active form) is often helpful in reversing hypocalcemia, until oral Vitamin D is converted to active vitamin D.

Management of skeletal deformities due to rickets.

- Treatment of the underlying medical condition.
- In most cases, the deformity will gradually improve over few months.
- 6 months after adequate treatment, if the deformity is still the same or getting worse, orthopedic referral for correction of the deformity by osteotomy or guided growth correction.

Mucopolysaccharidoses:

Causes:

- All mucopolysaccharidoses are inherited as autosomal recessive disorders with the exception of Hunter syndrome (MPS II), which is inherited as X-linked recessive.

General Manifestations MPS:

- Non musculoskeletal manifestations.
  - Corneal clouding.
  - Organomegaly.
  - Hearing loss.
  - Mental retardation.
- Skeletal manifestations.

- Progressive kyphosis.
- Short stature.
- Hip dysplasia and subluxation.
- Knee and ankle contracture.

Skeletal Manifestations of specific types of MPS:

- Hunter syndrome:
  - Claw hand.
  - Joint stiffness.
- Morquio syndrome:
  - Genu valgum.
  - Odontoid hypoplasia.
  - Ligamentous laxity.
  - Atlantoaxial instability: can lead to severe myelopathy, paralysis, and death from cord compression.

Management of Orthopedic conditions:

- Flexion extension radiograph of the cervical spine for assessment of instability. These should be repeated every 3–5 years.
- Orthopedic referral for management of musculoskeletal manifestation.
- For any surgical interference, great care should be given to the cervical spine to avoid neurological complication during intubation.
- **Management of specific musculoskeletal pathologies:**
  - Hip dysplasia and subluxation: pelvic and hip osteotomy to reduce the hip. If arthritis is advanced, arthroplasty (joint replacement) may be needed.
  - Genu valgum: osteotomy or guided growth (hemiepiphysiodesis).
  - Carpal tunnel syndrome: Carpal tunnel release.
  - Joint contracture: soft tissues release.

- Scoliosis: spinal fusion.
- Atlantoaxial instability: C1–C2 fusion.

OSTEOGENESIS IMERFECTA

Definition:

- It is a defect in collagen type 1 which is an important constituents of bone, ligaments, dentin, and sclera.
- The defect can be qualitative or quantitative reduction in type 1 collagen.
- Mutations in genes encoding type 1 collagen (COL1A1 or COL1A2 genes) accounting for, approximately, 80 % of Osteogenesis imerfecta cases.

Types of Osteogenesis imerfecta

- Classically 4 types of osteogenesis imerfecta have been reported (Silence Classification):
  - Type I: Mild forms.
  - Type II: Extremely severe; is often lethal due to fractures in utero.
  - Type III: Severe.
  - Type IV: Moderate.
    - The above four types are all autosomal dominant.
- More recently new types had been added:
  - Type V, VI:
    - Non collage types (no mutation).
    - Both of these types are clinically similar to type IV.
    - Type V has distinctive histology of 'mesh-like' appearance of bone lamellae.
      - Clinically this type has a triad of:
        - Hypertrophic callus formation.
        - Dense metaphyseal bands.

- ◆ Ossification of the interosseus membranes of the forearm.

- □ Type VI has "fish-scale" histological appearance with Elevated alkaline phosphatase activity.

- Type VII, VIII, IX.
  - □ Autosomal recessive.
  - □ The defect in Collagen Prolyl 3-hydroxylation Complex.
  - □ Types VII, VIII: severe forms of disease, type IX: moderate to severe.

Clinical Presentation:

- ■ **General manifestations**
  - **Blue sclera**.
  - Growth retardation.
  - Easy bruising.
  - Osteoporosis.
  - Presenile hearing loss.
  - Dentinogenesis imerfecta may be present.

- ■ **Skeletal Manifestation**
  - **Repeated fractures**
    - □ Fractures are most common during infancy and childhood and decrease in frequency after skeletal maturity.
    - □ Old fractures can be discovered in infants after radiographs are obtained for reasons other than an assessment of osteogenesis imerfecta.
  - Macrocephaly.
  - Triangular facies.
  - Malocclusion of the jaw.
  - Barrel chest.
  - kyphoscoliosis.
  - Progressive limb deformities.
  - Generalized bone aches.

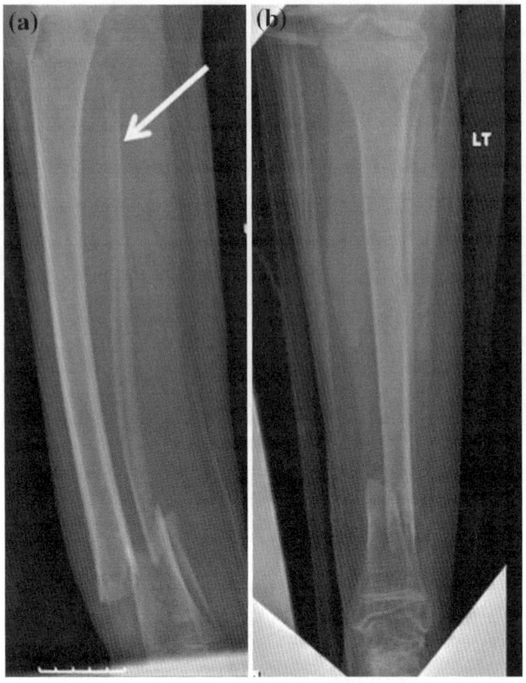

Fig. 3.3 **a**, **b** A 12-year-old with osteogenesis imerfecta. The patient developed fracture tibia and fibula when fell down in his class room. Notice the severe osteopenia of bone (bone density is similar to soft tissue density) and the thin fibula (*arrow*)

Diagnosis

Radiological Features (Fig. 3.3)

- Fractures—Commonly, transverse fractures and those affecting the lower limbs.
- Severe osteopenia.
- Thin fibula (gracilis fibula).
- Bony deformity.
- Excessive callus formation (type V).

Genetic testing:

- Direct sequencing of COL1A1 or COL1A2 genes.

Skin biopsy

- Collagen can be isolated from cultured fibroblasts and assessed for defects, with an accuracy of about 85 %.

Management:

- **Medical treatment:**
  - Bisphosphonate has been used in children with osteogenesis imerfecta.
    - □ Indications include multiple fractures or marked demineralization of the bone.
    - □ Duration of therapy not well established yet.
  - Vitamin D and Calcium supplement.
- **Orthotics**
  - For protection against fracture.
  - Have limited efficacy.
- **Orthopedic interventions:**
  - **Intramedullary rodding:**
    - □ Acts as internal support to the bone (Fig. 3.4).
    - □ Allows the bone to grow in a straight pattern.
  - **Osteotomy:**
    - □ For correction of the deformities of the bone.
    - □ Combined with internal fixation (intramedullary).
  - **Scoliosis:**
    - □ Spinal fusion for advanced scoliosis curves.
    - □ Orthopedic surgeon has to use multiple techniques to enhance the implant fixation in the osteoporotic bone.

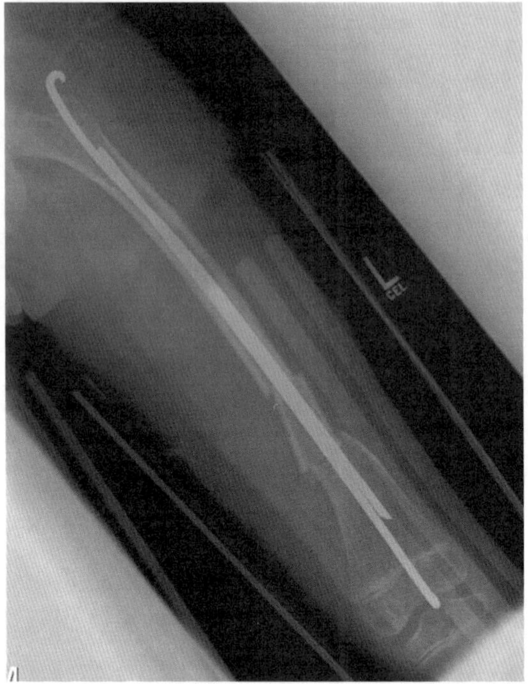

Fig. 3.4 A 10-year-old boy with osteogenesis imerfecta. Osteotomy of the left femur was done and two nails were applied intramedullary to straighten the bone and allow it to grow straight

- **Management of osteogenesis imerfecta in patient with fractures:**

  See Chap. 12.

Musculoskeletal diseases associated with childhood obesity.

Definition of obesity

- Obesity means an excess of fat relative to lean body mass.
- Children with BMI in the 85–95th percentile range for age and gender are considered overweight.
- Children with BMI >95th percentile for age and gender are termed obese.

Causes of obesity

- Non syndromic (exogenous) or polygenic obesity in childhood is poorly understood.
- Syndromic e.g., Prader-Willi syndrome, Albright hereditary osteodystrophy.
- Hormonal e.g., Cushing syndrome, hypothyroidism, polycystic ovary syndrome (PCOS) and growth hormone deficiency.
- Genetic e.g., congenital leptin deficiency or leptin receptor deficiency.

Diseases associated with obesity in children:

Cardiac diseases

- Obese children have an approximately threefold higher risk for hypertension than non-obese children.

Respiratory

- Obstructive sleep apnea syndrome (OSAS).

Gastrointestinal

- Nonalcoholic fatty liver disease is associated with obesity and insulin resistance.
- Obesity is well recognized as a risk factor for the development of cholesterol gallstones in adults and children.

Gynecological

- Polycystic ovary syndrome.

Musculoskeletal disorders associated with obesity

Slipped capital femoral epiphysis (SCFE) (Fig. 3.5).

- SCFE is a hip disorder in adolescents that causes symptoms of hip or knee pain (see Chap. 6).
- SCFE is more likely to occur in boys especially overweight.
- Obesity in early age increase the risk of SCFE.

Infantile tibia vara (Blount disease) (Chap. 7, Fig. 7.11).

- Infantile Blount disease is also related to obesity.

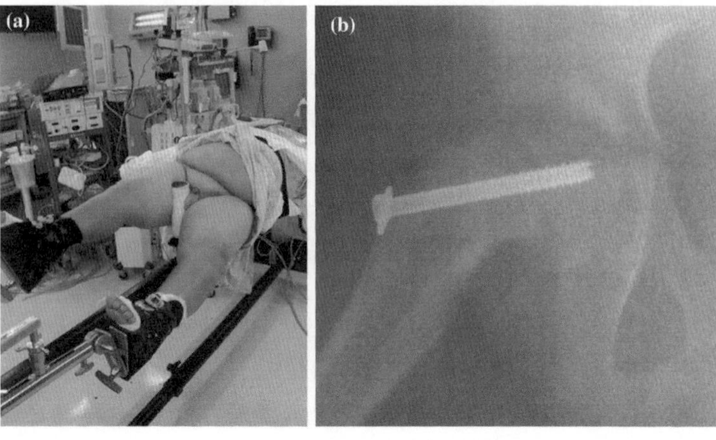

Fig. 3.5 **a** A 14-year-old boy who weighs three hundred fifty pounds. The patient had 3 months history of knee pain. Radiographs of the right knee were normal while radiographs of the hip showed SCFE. **b** Fixation of the physis (In situ pinnin) was done

- Obesity leads to increase mechanical stresses on the medial aspect of the growth plate suppressing the growth from the medial side.
- Growth plate suppression leads to decreased growth and a varus deformity.

Bone density and fractures

- Children and adolescents who are overweight are more likely than their normal-weight counterparts to have fractures.
- Dual-energy X-ray absorptiometry (DXA) shows that overweight children have a greater bone density, but it does not protect them from fractures.

Osteoarthritis

- Abnormal mechanical joint loading that occurs in obesity is a primary cause of osteoarthritis.

Pediatric Osteoporosis

Definition in the pediatric age group:

- Osteoporosis is a decrease in the bone density.
- In pediatric population, the Z-score (which compare the child to matched age and gender) is used.
- Peak density for gender (T-score) is **not** used to in pediatric testing of bone density.

Causes

- **Primary bone disease:**
  - Osteogenesis imerfecta.
  - Idiopathic juvenile osteoporosis.
- **Gastrointestinal disorders**
  - Celiac disease and inflammatory bowel disorders.
  - These conditions interfere with calcium absorption from the intestine and cause vitamin D deficiency.
- **Chronic liver disease**
  - Calcium and vitamin malabsorption, failure of vitamin D activation.
- **Decrease ambulation:**
  - E.g., Cerebral palsy, spina bifida, and muscular dystrophy.
  - Decreased muscle development and impaired ambulation will cause disuse atrophy of the extremity and increased risk of osteoporosis.
- **High-turnover conditions (increase bone resorption)**
  - Hyperparathyroidism.
  - Hyperthyroidism.
- **Trauma and burn injury increase the risk of bone loss due to the following:**

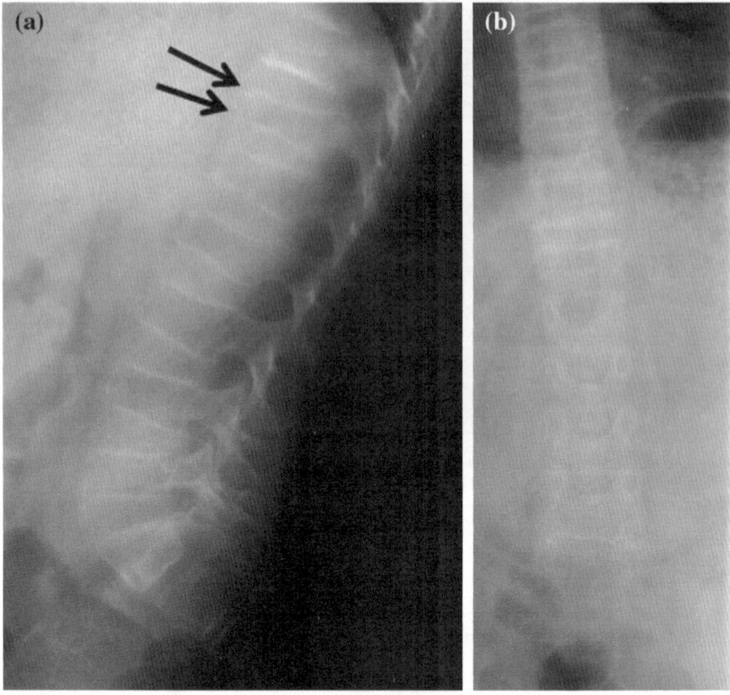

Fig. 3.6 Osteoporosis. A 14-year-old boy with chronic inflammatory bowel syndrome on long-term steroid intake. The patient has steroid-induced osteoporosis, which resulted in compression fractures of the vertebrae with back pain. **a** Notice severe osteopenia and loss of bone density of the vertebra, also notice the compression of the vertebrae (*arrows*). **b** The patient also developed scoliosis deformity due to vertebral body compression fractures

- Immobilization.
- Inflammatory responses leading to production of large quantities of resorptive cytokines.
- High endogenous glucocorticoid production that rapidly accelerate bone loss.

- **Medications**

  - Corticosteroids, chronic long-term steroid use contributes to loss of bone (Fig. 3.6).

- Cyclosporine, and other cytotoxic agents.
- **Anti epileptic medications.**

- **Total parenteral nutrition.**
  - Calcium and phosphorus requirements cannot be met by TPN in any age group, and the infant, especially the very premature infant, presents with hypophosphatemic metabolic bone disease.
- **Nutrition**:
  - Adolescents with anorexia nervosa are at risk for developing osteoporosis caused by inadequate nutrition.
- **Lifestyle**:
  - Increased alcohol intake and smoking among adolescent lead to impaired bone formation.
  - Lack of exercises and physical activity.

Clinical Presentation

- Patients may be asymptomatic or may present with bone pain.
- Children may present with spinal deformities (e.g., kyphosis, kyphoscoliosis).
- Pigeon chest deformity.
- Short stature and long-bone deformities.
- Back pain (from compression fractures) (Fig. 3.6)
- Fractures:
  - Repeated fractures (including vertebral compression fractures).

Diagnosis

- Laboratory studies for underlying disease.

- Urinary deoxypyridinoline, an index of bone resorption, is high in the urine of children who have rapid bone turnover.

Radiology

- **Dual-energy x-ray absorptiometry (DEXA)**
- According to AAP, DEXA is recommended for children with the following conditions (testing should be performed on initial evaluation and before treatment begins).
  - Primary bone disorders such as idiopathic juvenile osteoporosis and osteogenesis imerfecta.
  - Secondary conditions known to increase fracture risk (e.g., chronic inflammatory diseases, immobilization for long periods, endocrine or hematologic diseases, cancer and associated treatments that adversely affect bone).
  - A history of clinically significant fracture, where significance is defined as 1 long-bone leg fracture, $\geq$2 long-bone arm fractures, or vertebral fracture resulting from low trauma (Low trauma is defined as a fall from standing height or less).
- **The AAP** clinical guidelines for DEXA in children and adolescents include the following recommendations for interpretation of results and diagnosis:
  - Pediatric osteoporosis may be diagnosed when there is a clinically significant history of fracture and low bone mass, defined as bone mineral density (BMD) more than 2 standard deviations (SD) below reference data (Z-score).
  - For children with chronic illness or delayed puberty, BMD should be adjusted based on height or should be compared with reference data specific for age, sex, and height.

Treatment

- Management is primarily medical, depending on the underlying condition.
- **Bisphosphonate**:

- E.g., pamidronate, alendronate, and risedronate.
- **Mechanism of action.**
  - It is an antiresorptive agent, they prevent osteoclast attachment to the bone matrix.

- **Anabolic steroids** (e.g., testosterone, oxandrolone) may be helpful in forming new bone.
- **Calcium and Vitamin D recommendations:**
  - Calcium intake of 800 mg/d until age 10 years, 1,200 mg/d during adolescence, and 1,000 mg/d after adolescence.
  - Calcium intake should be increased for women who are pregnant, for women who are lactating (1,200 mg/d).
  - An intake of vitamin D of 400–800 IU/d.
- **Correction of the underlying risk factors:**
  - Correction of the underlying medical condition (malabsorption, hyperparathyroidism).
  - Healthy nutrition, avoiding alcohol and smoking and frequent aerobic exercises.

HIGH YIELD FACTS

- Rickets can cause poor muscle tone, skeletal deformity, and developmental delay.
- Classic radiographic features of rickets are cupping, fraying, widening, and osteopenia.
- Osteogenesis imerfecta has different types with variable degrees of severity. Orthopedic referral is needed to manage the fractures, deformities, and possible intramedullary rodding of long-bone to act as internal spint.
- Osteoporosis can affect pediatric population for variety of causes.

- Bisphosphonate can be used to treat osteoporosis.

CLINICAL SCENARIOS

The presenting patient	The most probable diagnosis and plan of action
3-years-old boy with severe developmental delay brought to the clinic by his mother for referral to physical therapy. The child is not able to walk, had eye surgery 1 year ago for cataract, and he is able to say only few words. On physical examination, the child has broaden wrist, bossing of the forehead, nystagmus, poor muscle tone, and poor reflexes. Laboratory tests shows Na 135, K 3.5, Cl 110, Co2 17, BUN 12, Creatinine is 0.4, glucose is 95, normal Ca, Ph is 2.3, alkaline phosphatase is 1250, Ck 70, urine Ph and Ca were elevated. Brain MRI is positive for white matter abnormality in the periventricular area, what is the most likely diagnosis?	Oculocerebrorenal Dystrophy (Lowe Syndrome) The patient has renal tubular acidosis with hypophosphatemic rickets, high urine Ph and Ca together with ocular and neurological manifestations; they are all consistent with Lowe syndrome Treatment of hypophosphatemic rickets: Vitamin D, oral Ph, and bicarbonate to keep plasma bicarbonate >22
14-years-old male with morbid obesity presents to your clinic with right knee pain, no history of trauma, On Examination, the child has external rotation deformity of the right lower extremity. Right knee examination is unremarkable, however, movement of the right hip cause marked discomfort. What is the differential diagnosis?	SCFE Obtain AP and LAT view of the right hip and right knee

REFERENCES

Chapman T, Sugar N, Done S, Marasigan J, Wambold N, Feldman K. Fractures in infants and toddlers with rickets. Pediatr Radiol. 2010;40(7):1184–9. Epub 2009 Dec 9.

Shah BR, Finberg L. Single-day therapy for nutritional vitamin D-deficiency rickets: a preferred method. J Pediatr. 1994;125:487–90.

Tandon V, Williamson JB, Cowie RA. Spinal problems in mucopolysaccharidosis I (Hurler syndrome). J Bone Joint Surg Br. 1996;78:938–44.

Craig JG, Holsbeeck MV, Zaltz I. The utility of MR in assessing Blount disease. Skeletal Radiol. 2002;31:208–13.

Felson DT, Chaisson CE. Understanding the relationship between body weight and osteoarthritis. Baillieres Clin Rheumatol. 1997;11:671–81.

White KK. Orthopaedic aspects of mucopolysaccharidosis. Rheumatology (Oxford). 2011;50(suppl 5):v26–33.

Shapiro JR, Sponsellor PD. Osteogenesis imerfecta: questions and answers. Curr Opin Pediatr. 2009;21:709–16.

Forlino A, Cabral WA, Barnes AM, Marini JC. New perspectives on osteogenesis imerfecta. Nat Rev Endocrinol. 2011;7:540–57.

Henwood MJ, Binkovitz L. Update on pediatric bone health. J Am Osteopath Assoc. 2009;109:5–12.

Chapter 4
General Conditions Affecting the Bones

Amr Abdelgawad and Osama Naga

DYSPLASIA

Definition:

- Affection of the bony skeleton with deformity and shortness.
- Can affect the epiphysis, the metaphysis, or the diaphysis.
- Can sometimes affect the spine (spondylodysplasia).

Clinical Presentation:

- The affected child is **short disproportionate dwarf** (the distance between the tips of the stretched hands is less than the height).

ACHONDROPLASIA

Definition:

- It is a **mesomelic** dysplasia (i.e. proximal segments (femur and humerus) are affected more than the distal segments (tibia/fibula and radius/ulna).
- **Achondroplasia is the most common type of dysplasia.**

Inheritance:

- This condition is inherited as an autosomal dominant.
- Approximately 80 % of cases are due to new or de novo dominant mutations.

A. Abdelgawad and O. Naga (eds.), *Pediatric Orthopedics*,
DOI: 10.1007/978-1-4614-7126-4_4,

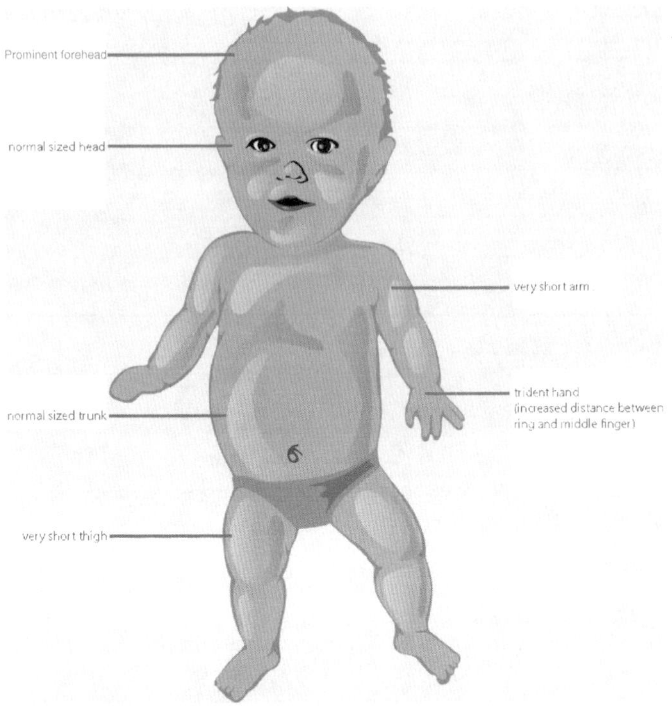

Fig. 4.1 General manifestation of achondroplasia

- **Results from heterozygous mutation of genes encoding: FGFR3 (Fibroblast growth factor receptor 3).**

Clinical Presentation (Fig. 4.1):

- **General manifestations**
  - **The child will be severely short (less than 5th percentile for his age).**
  - **Prenatal diagnosis can be done by measuring the length of the femur by ultrasound.**
  - Delayed milestones; Often do not walk unsupported until 18–24 months.
    - Due to hypotonia, the child will have difficulty in balancing the head on a normal size trunk and short extremities.

- Intelligence is usually normal.
- A relatively long narrow trunk.
- Midfacial hypoplasia.
- Prominent forehead.

- **Skeletal Manifestations**

  - Short limbs (very short upper arms and thighs)
  - Genu varum
  - Trident hand configuration (increased space between third and fourth fingers)
  - lumbar hyperlordosis
  - Lumbar and cervical spinal stenosis.
  - Cervical stenosis may cause compression over the spinal cord leading to cervical myelopathy:

    - Cervical myelopathy can lead to:

      - Quadriparesis
      - Hypotonia,
      - Central and obstructive apnea,
      - Possible sudden death.

    - Lumbar stenosis will lead to:

      - Bilateral leg pain (radiculopathy)
      - Leg weakness

Treatment:

- **Growth hormone treatment**:

  - The availability of somatotropin (recombinant human growth hormone) has revolutionized the treatment of short stature.
  - Growth hormone is currently being used to augment the height of patients with achondroplasia.
  - The greatest acceleration in growth velocity is seen during the first year of treatment and in those with the lowest growth velocities before treatment.
  - A young age at initiation of therapy (1–6 y) is recommended for maximum benefits.

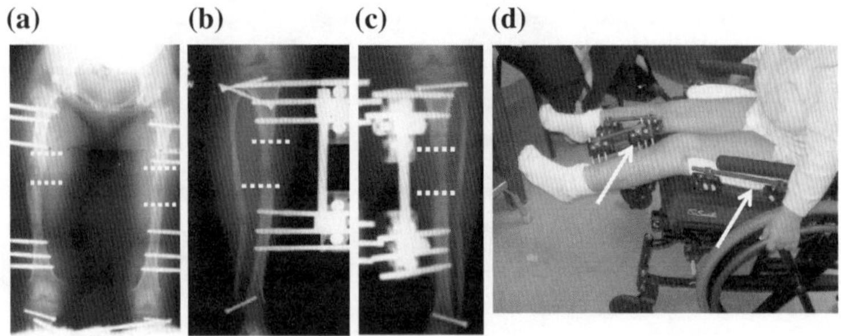

Fig. 4.2 a–d A 15-year-old girl, with achondroplasia had simultaneous lengthening of both femurs and both tibia and fibulas using external fixators (*arrows*). She was lengthened two inches in the thigh and two inches in the leg (*dotted line*)

- Orthopedic referral:
  - Refer to orthopedic surgery if the family is interested in lengthening surgeries.
    - Lengthening surgeries: (Fig. 4.2)
      - These relay on the basis of **'distraction osteogenesis'** (see the Chap.1 of introduction)
  - Severe cases of spinal or lumbar stenosis may require surgical decompression.

NEUROFIBROMATOSIS

Definition:

- Neurofibromatosis (NF) is a multisystem genetic disorder that is associated with cutaneous, neurologic, and musculoskeletal manifestations.

Genetics:

- Autosomal dominant

- Over half of the cases are sporadic representing de novo mutations
- Types of neurofibromatosis
  - NF-1 is a mutation of a gene on long arm chromosome 17 (the most common type)
  - NF-2 is a mutation of a gene on long arm chromosome 22.

Clinical Presentation of NF-1 (Von Recklinghausen's disease)

- Clinical diagnosis requires the presence of at least 2 out 7 criteria to confirm the diagnosis
- Many of these signs do not appear until later childhood or adolescence.
- **Clinical criteria used to diagnose NF1 are as follows:**
  - Six or more café-au-lait spots or hyperpigmented macules greater than or equal to 5 mm in diameter in children younger than 10 years and 15 mm in post-pubertal (Fig. 4.3)
  - Axillary or inguinal freckles
  - Two or more typical neurofibromas or one plexiform neurofibroma
  - Optic nerve glioma
  - Two or more iris hamartomas (Lisch nodules), identified by slit-lamp examination
  - Distinct bony lesions as sphenoid wing dysplasia, scoliosis, or typical long-bone abnormalities (see below)
  - First-degree relative (e.g., mother, father, sister, brother) with NF-1
- **Skeletal manifestation:**
  - Sphenoid bone dysplasia is usually asymptomatic.
  - Anterolateral bowing of the tibia (Fig. 7.27 knee Chap. 7).
  - Congenital pseudarthrosis of the tibia (Fig. 7.27 knee Chap. 7).
    - Usually present within the first two years of life.

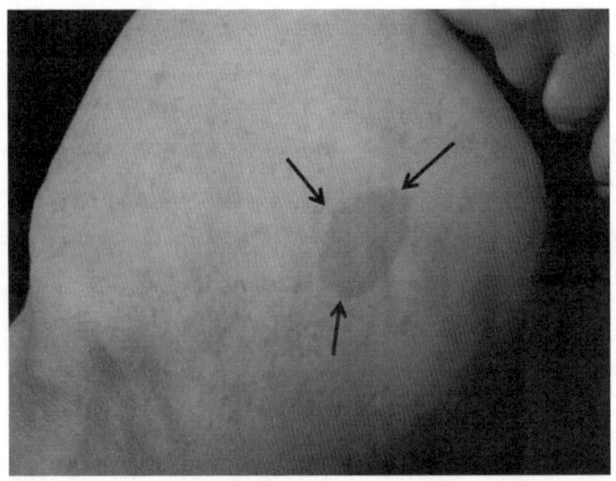

Fig. 4.3 A 16-year-old girl with neurofibromatosis (NF1). Café-au-lait patch can be seen (*arrows*)

- Scoliosis with or without kyphosis may become evident in childhood or adolescent.
  - □ Affects about 30 % of patients with NF1.
  - □ Short segment scoliosis with angular deformity (Fig. 4.4).
  - □ **Dural ectasia**:
    - ○ Widening of the dural sac and the spinal canal causing erosion of the surrounding vertebral bone.
    - ○ It is thought to be due to weakening of the dura which expands with the pressure of cerebrospinal fluid.
    - ○ Will cause **scalloping of the posterior portions of the vertebral bodies and erosion of the pedicles** (Fig. 4.5).
- **Cervical spine instability**
  - □ **flexion–extension views are needed before any endotracheal intubation to assess cervical spine stability.**

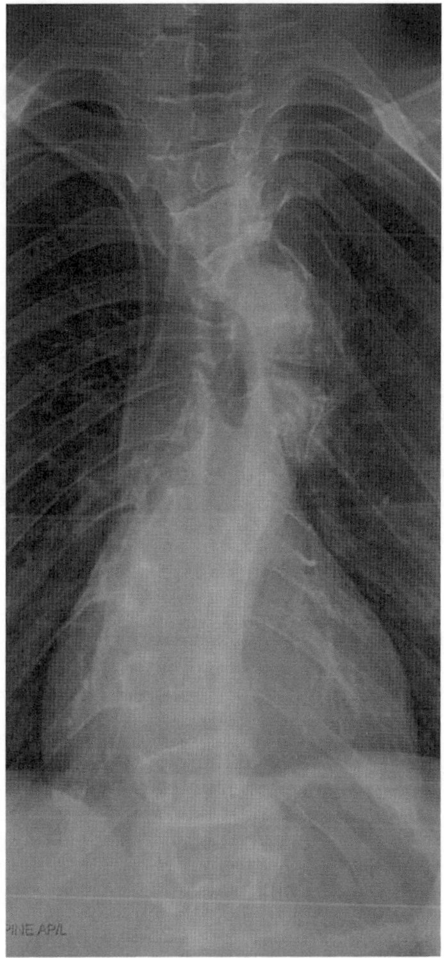

Fig. 4.4 A 16-year old with NF1 and kyphoscoliosis (notice the relatively short segment of scoliosis with acute angular deformity)

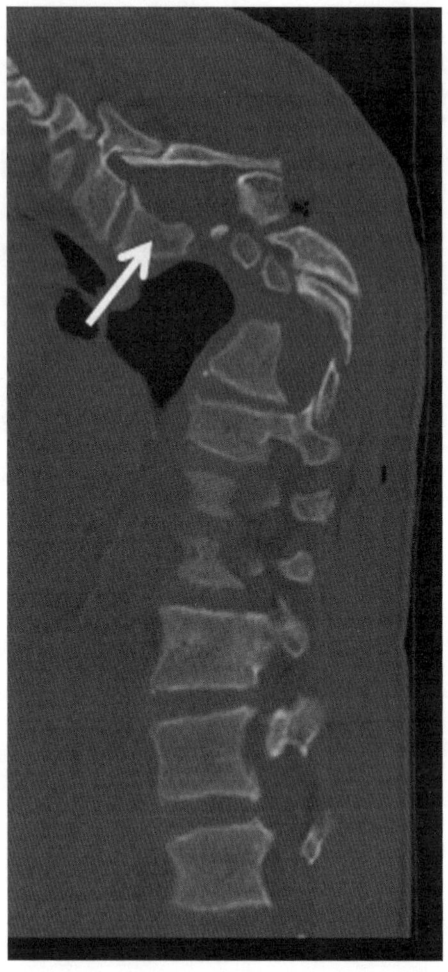

Fig. 4.5 Dural ectasia. A 15-year old with NF1 and kyphosis. CT scan shows widening of the canal and scalloping of posterior vertebral bodies (*arrow*)

Diagnosis

- Genetic testing

- Testing the family members should be done.

- **Orthopedic management of NF1**
  - Anterolateral bowing, congenital pseudoarthrosis of the tibia (see knee chapter, congenital condition affecting the leg):
    - Orthopedic referral.
      - Bracing is indicated for the anterolateral bowing.
      - Avoid contact sports.
  - Scoliosis:
    - Orthopedic referral.
      - Surgery is usually needed as these patients do not respond to bracing treatment.
      - CT or MRI is needed before surgery to assess bony anomalies (deficient posterior parts of the vertebrae) to plan for surgery.

MARFAN SYNDROME

Definition:

- Marfan syndrome (MFS) is a spectrum of disorders caused by a heritable genetic defect of connective tissue that has an autosomal dominant mode of transmission.

Pathology

- The defect in the *FBN1* gene on chromosome 15, which codes for the connective tissue protein fibrillin.
- Abnormalities in fibrillin protein cause anomalies of the musculoskeletal, cardiac, and ocular systems.

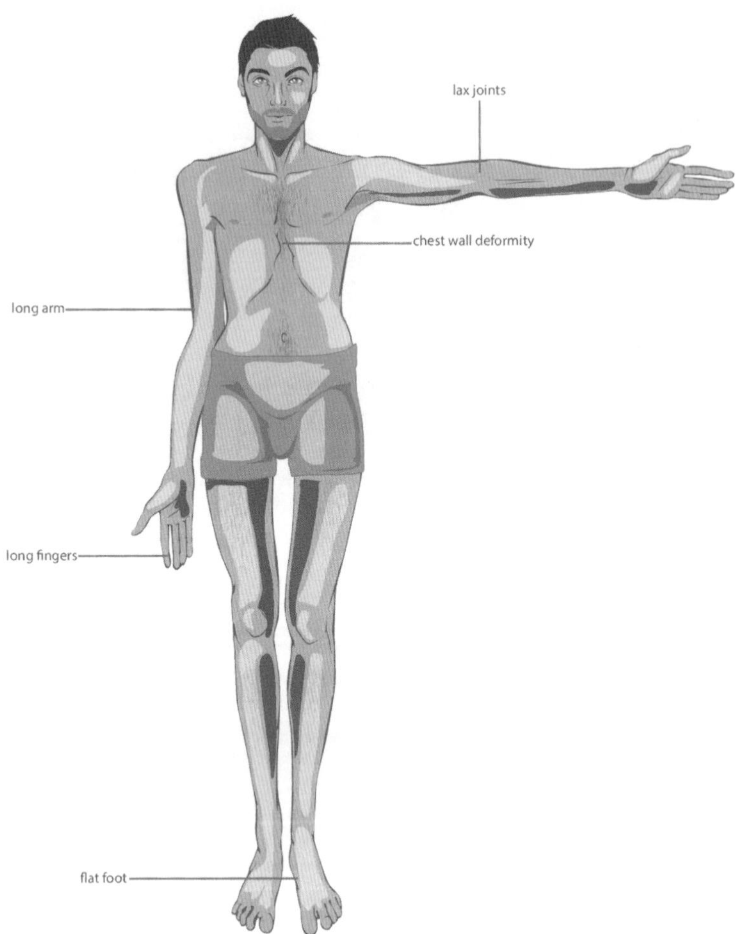

Fig. 4.6 General manifestation of Marfan syndrome

Skeletal Manifestations (Fig. 4.6):

- Pectus carinatum, and pectus excavatum

- **Pectus excavatum** is a chest wall deformity with a concave appearance in the anterior chest wall (the sternum is inward).
- **Pectus carinatum (Pigeon chest)** is a chest wall deformity with protrusion of anterior chest wall (the sternum is outwards).

- Ligamentous laxity of the joints
- Limbs are disproportionately long compared with the trunk (dolichostenomelia)
  - Reduced upper to lower segment ratio (distance from the head to symphysis pubis divided by the distance from symphysis pubis to sole of the foot is less than 0.85)
  - An Increased arm span-to-height ratio (greater than 1.05)
- Arachnodactyly is a common feature:
  - Positive thumb (Steinberg) and wrist sign (Fig. 4.7).
- Joint hypermobility
- Scoliosis:
  - More than half of patients with Marfan have scoliosis.
- Pes planus
  - **Definition:** Flattening of the arch of the foot.
  - Due to laxity of the ligaments of the foot, will not be able to support the arch of the foot.
  - On examination:
    - Hindfoot valgus (outward angulation of the heel).
    - Loss of the arch of the foot.
    - Flexible deformity (restoration of the arch with standing on the tip toes or with dorsiflexion of the big toe).
- Protrusio acetabuli:
  - **Definition:** deepening of the acetabulum in the pelvic region.
  - Due to softening of the pelvic bones, the femoral head pushs the hip joint deep inside the pelvis.

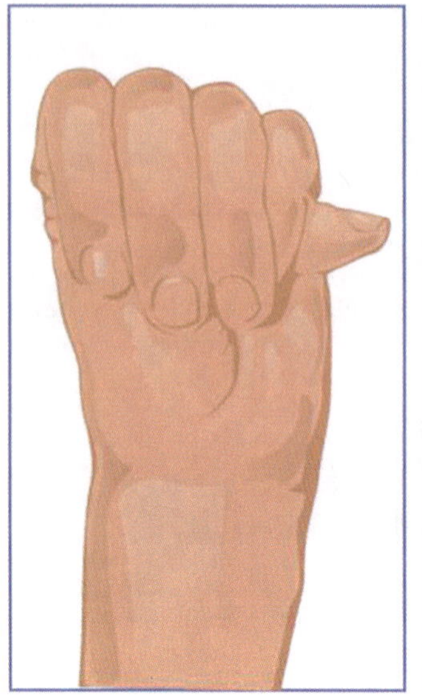
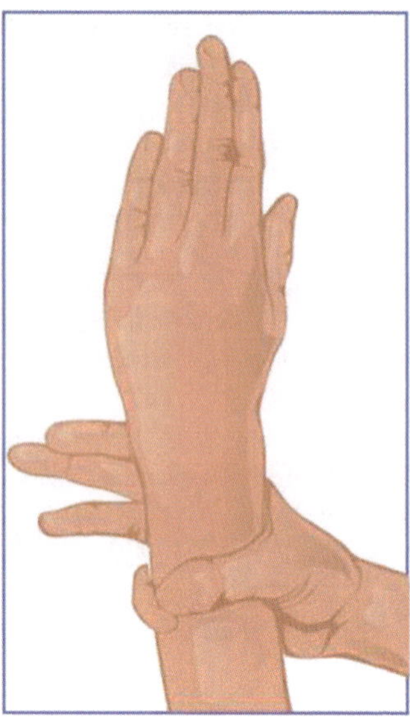

Fig. 4.7 Positive thumb (Steinberg) and wrist in Marfan patients. When the patient make a fist with thumb in the palm, the tip of the thumb protrude from the outer side of the small finger. The patient is able to encircle his wrist with the other hand thumb and small finger

- Clinical manifestations include:
  - Hip joint stiffness
  - Progressive limitation in activity related to joint pain
  - Eventual osteoarthritic change

Management:

Indication for Orthopedic referral:

- **Scoliosis:**
  - Treatment is by brace or surgery.
- **Protrusio acetabuli:**
  - Patient will need surgical interference.

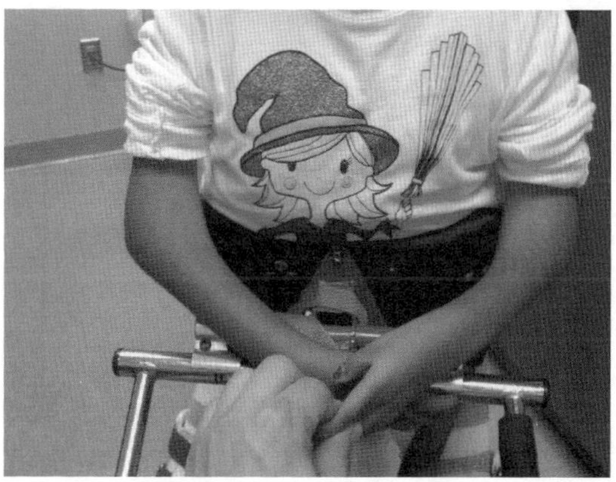

Fig. 4.8 Arthrogryposis. Notice the absence of elbow and wrist creases

- **Pectus repair**
  - Pectus excavatum:
    - Repair of pectus excavatum is performed to improve respiratory mechanics by increasing the space available for lung.
    - Better to be delayed until mid-adolescence to lessen the risk of recurrence.
  - Pectus carinatum,
    - Repair is mainly performed for cosmetic reasons

ARTHROGRYPOSIS

Definition:

- It is a nonprogressive conditions characterized by congenital multiple joint contractures.

Pathophysiology

- Decreased fetal movements or fetal akinesia due to intra-uterine abnormalities e.g.
  - Neurogenic muscle
  - Connective tissue abnormalities
  - Mechanical limitations to movement
  - Maternal disorders
  - Infection, drugs, trauma
- Arthrogryposis is associated with:
  - **Short umbilical cord**
  - Polyhydramnios (some cases may be associated with oligohydramnios)
  - Pulmonary hypoplasia
  - Micrognathia
  - Ocular hypertelorism

Epidemiology

- The frequency is about 1 in 3,000 live births

Age

- Arthrogryposis is detectable at birth or in utero using ultrasonography

Etiology

- The causes of arthrogryposis are varied and not entirely understood but are presumed to be multifactorial.
- Multiple syndromes and pathologies (more than one hundred) are associated with arthrogryposis.
- Arthrogryposis multiplex congenita (AMC) is the most common cause of arthrogryposis.

Clinical Presentation:

- Family history

- Review the history of children with arthrogryposis and other affected family members for possible associated syndromes or pathologies.

- Pregnancy history, e.g.
  - Congenital myotonic dystrophy
  - Myasthenia gravis
  - Maternal infections
  - Exposure to teratogens, e.g. alcohol, and phenytoin

Physical Examination (Fig. 4.8)

- **Skeletal manifestations**
  - Involved extremities:
    - Fusiform or cylindrical in shape.
    - **Absent skin creases** over the joints (knees and elbows).
  - Joint contracture:
    - Very limited range of motion specially the knee and elbow.
    - The knee is usually contracted in **flexion** (which may be associated with skin pterygium (web fold)).
    - The elbow is usually contracted in **extension**. This can affect the patient ability to feed him/her self.
  - Hip dysplasia
  - Scoliosis

- **General manifestation:**
  - Facial deformities
  - Jaw deformities
    - Micrognathia
    - Trismus
  - Sensation is usually intact, although deep tendon reflexes may be diminished or absent
  - Inguinal hernia.

CLINICAL CRITERIA FOR DIAGNOSING ARTHROGRYPOSIS MULTIPLEX CONGENITA(AMC)

- Presence of arthrogrypotic deformity of the limbs.
- Absence of characteristic features of other causes of arthrogryposis (diagnosis of exclusion).
- Lack of visceral involvement.
- Lack of significant dysmorphic features.
- Negative family history.

Imaging Studies

- Radiography to evaluate skeletal and joint abnormalities
- Ultrasonography can help in evaluating the CNS and other viscera for congenital anomalies
- CT scanning can be used to evaluate the CNS and the muscle mass
- Prenatal ultrasonography can be used to assess the following:
  - Decreased fetal movement
  - Abnormal fetal lie
  - Polyhydramnios or oligohydramnios

Management:

- Assess the patient ability to eat, clean him/her self, or write
- Most of the limb deformities can be managed non operative by modification of the instruments to perform activity of daily living e.g. walker, eating utensils, mouse, and keyboard for the computers etc. (Fig. 4.9)
- Orthopedic referral is sometimes needed for management of skeletal deformities:
  - Muscle transfer
  - Osteotomies
  - External fixator for joint contracture.

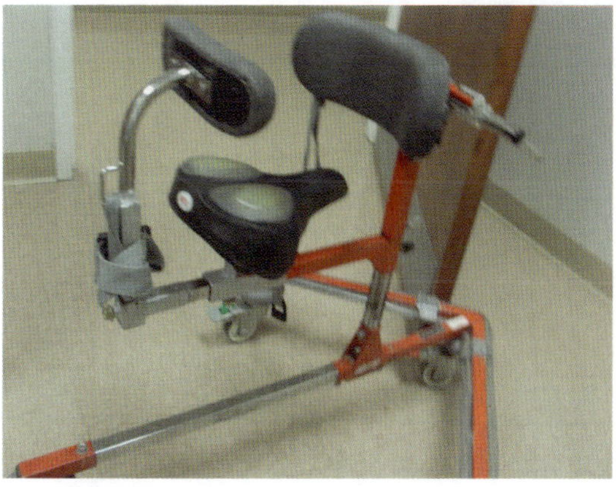

Fig. 4.9 Sitting walker. This walker is designed for arthrogrypotic patient with knee flexion contracture. The child can sit on the chair of the walker and uses her flexed knee to move the walker

- Coordination with plastic surgeons may be needed in cases of knee flexion for management of the skin pterygium posterior to the knee.

LYME DISEASE

- Lyme disease is the most common tick-borne illness in the United States.

Etiology

- Lyme disease is caused by *B burgdorferi* which is transmitted by ixodid tick species–primarily *Ixodes scapularis,* the common deer tick

Clinical Presentation

- History of travel to endemic areas.
- Most patients with Lyme disease do not recall a tick bite.
- The clinical presentation depends on the stage at which the disease is recognized:

- Early disease
- Early disseminated disease
- Late disease

Early disease

- Usually develops 7–14 days after a tick bite
- Erythema migrans (EM) is the most common presentation and is a pathognomonic skin lesion
- It starts at the site of the bite and is a slowly spreading irregular erythematous lesion with a clear center
- Lyme disease in this early stage is a clinical diagnosis, and serologic testing for children with a single EM lesion is generally not recommended because patients may be seronegative early in the course of illness.
- During early disease, with or without the rash, patients may complain of a flulike illness characterized by:
  - Fever
  - Chills
  - **Myalgias**
  - **Arthralgias**
  - Headache
  - Malaise

Early disseminated disease

- Usually develops 3–10 weeks after inoculation.
- Multiple EM lesions are present.
- These are relatively small oval erythematous macules (1–5 cm).
  - Patients with early disseminated disease have general complaints similar to early disease (fever, **myalgias, arthralgias,** malaise, and headache).
- Neurological manifestations:
  - Bell's palsy
  - Aseptic meningitis may develop at this stage
  - Encephalitis is rare
- Carditis may present as complete heart block.

Late disease

- **Arthritis is the hallmark of this stage**
  - Arthritis affects about half of the non treated patients.
  - Develops few months after disease onset.
  - Pathology:
    - Synovitis of the joint.
    - *B burgdorferi* does not produce proteolytic enzymes (in contrast to bacteria septic arthritis), this leads to less damage to the articular cartilage.
  - Usually involve large joints (the knee is involved in 90 % of cases).
  - The joint is warm, swollen, and **limited range of motion.**
    - These findings distinguish arthritis from simple arthralgia (pain only) which is common in early disease.
    - The swelling is usually large with relatively less complain of pain (in contrast to bacterial septic arthritis).
  - Fever is present in about one third of patients with arthritis.
  - Most patients presenting with late disease do not have a history of EM, because the rash typically leads to earlier treatment, which prevents the development of late disease.
  - **Clinical presentation of Lyme arthritis:**
    - **Two common forms:**
      - **Classic arthritis** is characterized by episodic synovitis with involvement of one to four joints lasting less than one week, separated by asymptomatic periods of more than 2 weeks.
      - **The acute pauciarticular form (pseudoseptic)** is defined by continual involvement of one to four joints for less than 4 weeks. This presentation is similar to bacterial septic arthritis.
    - Less commonly the presentation can be **similar to juvenile rheumatology arthritis** (chronic pauciarticular, migratory, and polyarticular)

- **Antibiotic-refractory Lyme arthritis**
    - Patients who do not respond to an initial course of antibiotic therapy and who display objective signs of synovitis (e.g., persistent or recurrent joint swelling).
    - It is thought to be due to immune reaction to the organism.

Diagnosis of Lyme disease:

- The most sensitive and specific test for Lyme disease is identifying the erythema migrans rash.
- For cases without a rash, workup for pediatric Lyme disease may include:
    - Blood studies
    - Serology
        - ELISA test is used to screen patient samples. A positive or indeterminate ELISA test should be followed by confirmatory Western blot assay, which is more specific for *B burgdorferi*
    - Polymerase chain reaction (PCR)
    - Lumbar puncture if indicated
- **Diagnosis of Lyme arthritis:**
    - Recognition of characteristic clinical findings
    - History of exposure in an area in which the disease is endemic.
    - Confirmatory serologic testing.
    - Arthrocentesis.
        - positive PCR for *B burgdorferi* DNA in synovial joint
        - cell count (WBCs) is similar to septic arthritis
    - Differentiation from bacterial septic arthritis:
        - Lyme disease patients has a lower average peripheral WBC, lower percentage of neutrophils in the CBC with differential, less likely to present with a temperature more than 101.5 °F (38.6 °C), and less likely to refuse to bear weight on the affected extremity.

Treatment

- Early disease and isolated bell palsy
    - Oral doxycycline 100 mg PO bid for 21 days (Or)
    - Amoxicillin (for children less than 8 years) for 21 days
- Cardiac and neurologic sequelae
    - Ceftriaxone (75 mg/kg/day) IV max 2 grams for 21 days (Or)
    - Penicillin 300,000 U/kg/day divides every 4 hours IV for 21 days

Management of Lyme arthritis:

- Can be treated by oral (doxycyclin or Amoxicillin) or intravenous antibiotics (Ceftriaxone or Penicillin).
- NSAIDS for pain and swelling.
- After complete course of antibiotic therapy:
    - Most patients should have resolved their symptoms.
    - If the child shows partial improvement: oral antibiotic for 4 more weeks.
    - If no improvement: intravenous antibiotic for 2–4 more weeks.
- **Management of antibiotic-refractory Lyme arthritis**
    - NSAIDS.
    - intra-articular corticosteroids.
    - orthopedic referral for possible surgical interference (synovectomy).

HIGH YIELD FACTS

- Polyhydramnios, short umbilical cord, and fetal akinesia are associated with arthrogryposis.
- Inheritance of Achondroplasia is autosomal dominant trait complete penetrance.
- Approximately 80 % of achondroplasia cases are due to new or de novo dominant mutations.

- Risk of apnea and sudden death in achondroplasia can be due to cervical spinal stenosis.
- Growth hormone is currently being used to augment the height of patients with achondroplasia.
- More than half of patients with Marfan syndrome have scoliosis.
- Lyme disease in its early stage is diagnosed clinically and not requiring Lyme serology to start treatment.
- Arthritis is the hall mark of late Lyme disease.
- Lyme arthritis commonly presents as episodes of acute arthritis or as an attack of acute inflammation of a large joint (knee) similar to bacterial septic arthritis.

CLINICAL SCENARIOS

The presenting patient	The most probable diagnosis and plan of action
▪ A baby died unexpectedly after birth, he was born vaginally after a pregnancy was complicated by reduced fetal movement, polyhydramnios, and a very short umbilical cord, what is the most likely associated condition:	Arthrogryposis
▪ 15-month-old child with achondroplasia, mother is worry that he not walking yet	Reassurance ▪ Most children with achondroplasia will walk by 18–22 month
▪ 3-year-old child with achondroplasia started having episodes of apnea, cyanosis, and respiratory distress, what is the best method to establish the diagnosis	MRI of cervical spine ▪ Central apnea occurs due arterial compression at the cervical level of the foramen magnum

REFERENCES

Bailey JA 2nd. Orthopaedic aspects of achondroplasia. J Bone Joint Surg Am. Oct 1970;52:1285–301.

Nelson MA. Orthopaedic aspects of the chondrodystrophies. The dwarf and his orthopaedic problems. Ann R Coll Surg Engl. Oct 1970;47:185-210.

Tucker T, Schnabel C, Hartmann M, Friedrich RE, Frieling I, Kruse HP. Bone health and fracture rate in individuals with neurofibromatosis 1 (NF1). *J Med Genet*. Apr 2009;46:259–65.

Darin N, Kimber E, Kroksmark AK, Tulinius M. Multiple congenital contractures: birth prevalence, etiology, and outcome. J Pediatr. Jan 2002;140:61–7

Chen H, Immken L, Lachman R. Syndrome of multiple pterygia, camptodactyly, facial anomalies, hypoplastic lungs and heart, cystic hygroma, and skeletal anomalies: delineation of a new entity and review of lethal forms of multiple pterygium syndrome. Am J Med Genet. Apr 1984;17:809–26.

Crawford AH, Schorry EK. Neurofibromatosis. In Staheli LT, Song KM, editors. Secrets of pediatric orthopedic. 3rd ed. Philadelphia: Mosby Elsevier; 2007. P. 237–243.

Feder HM Jr. Lyme disease in children. Infect Dis Clin North Am. Jun 2008;22:315–26.

Smith BG, Cruz AI Jr, Milewski MD, Shapiro ED. Lyme disease and he orthopedic implications of Lyme arthritis. J Am Acad Orthop Surg. 2011 Feb;19:91–100.

Rose CD, Fawcett PT, Eppes SC, Klein JD, Gibney K, Doughty RA: Pediatric Lyme arthritis: Clinical spectrum and outcome. J Pediatr Orthop. 1994;14:238–41.

Chapter 5

Birth Injuries and Orthopedic Manifestations in Newborns

Amr Abdelgawad and Osama Naga

BIRTH INJURIES

Obstetric brachial plexus palsy (OBPP):

Anatomy of the brachial plexus (Fig. 5.1):

- The brachial plexus is formed by the roots of C5, C6, C7, C8, and T1.
- It consists of Roots, Trunks, Divisions, and Cords.

Types of OBPP

- **Erb's Palsy:**
  - Affection of the **upper trunk** (C5,6) of brachial plexus.
  - **The most common type of OBPP**.
- **Total Palsy:**
  - Affection of all roots of the brachial plexus.
  - **Total flaccid limb**
- **Klumpke's Palsy:**
  - Affection of the lower truck of the brachial plexus (C8 and T1).
  - Associated with Horner's syndrome in about one-third of cases.
  - Affects mainly the **hand function**.

A. Abdelgawad and O. Naga (eds.), *Pediatric Orthopedics*,
DOI: 10.1007/978-1-4614-7126-4_5,

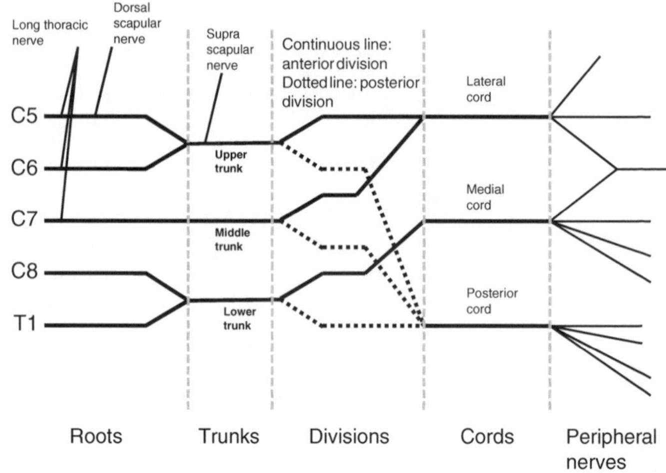

Fig. 5.1 Brachial plexus schematic

Neurological types:

- **Neurapraxia:**
  - Stretching of the nerves
  - Recovery is usually complete with no residual symptoms.
- **Axonotmesis:**
  - Due to nerve fiber (axons) disruption with intact sheath.
  - Recovery is variable but never complete. The child will have functional limitations due to his injury
- **Neurotmesis:**
  - Disruption of both the nerve axons and their surrounding sheath (total sever, avulsion injury)
  - The worst prognosis.

ERB'S PALSY

Definition:

- Nerve palsy of the upper truck (C5 and C6) of the brachial plexus that occurs during labor.

Risk Factors:

- Macrosomia (>4,000 gm).
- Shoulder dystocia
- Assisted labor (Forceps delivery)

Clinical presentation:

- The newborn will keep the limb in the **'waiter tip position'** (Fig. 5.2):
    - Shoulder: adducted, internally rotated
    - Elbow: extended, pronated
    - Wrist: flexed
- Asymmetrical Moro's reflex.
- Horner's syndrome
    - Miosis, Ptosis, Anhydrosis
    - Indicates affection of the sympathetic trunks.
    - Bad prognostic sign as it is usually associated with root avulsion injury

Imaging studies:

- **Chest radiographs:**
    - Elevation of the diaphragm in the affected side:
        - Indicates phrenic nerve injury.
        - Bad prognostic sign as it indicates root avulsion (phrenic nerve originates close to the root origin).

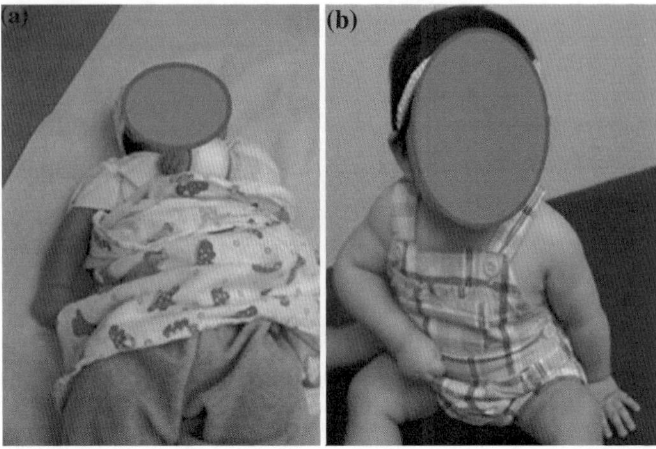

Fig. 5.2 **a** A 1-week-old girl with shoulder dystocia. The child developed Erb's palsy on the *right upper* extremity (note internal rotation of the shoulder, extension and pronation of the elbow, and flexion of the wrist). The *left arm* suffered mid shaft humeral fracture during labor and was treated with sling. **b** A 9-months-old girl with right Erb's Palsy (internal rotation of the shoulder with pronation)

- Clavicle fracture:
  - Can be associated with Erb's palsy (shoulder dystocia).

- **MRI cervical spine:**
  - Pseudomeningocele:
    - Small pockets of CSF protruding out from the meninges at the level of nerve roots.
    - Indicates root avulsion (bad prognostic sign).
  - **MRI is not indicated for the routine diagnosis of Erb's Palsy**.
  - It is indicated only for pre operative planning.

- **Electrophysiological studies:**
  - Used to detect nerve regeneration.

- Not sensitive, causes discomfort for the child and provide information which may not be very useful clinically (electrically re-inervated muscles may not have enough power to move the limb against gravity).

Prognosis:

- **About 80 % of patients with Erb's palsy will show complete recovery within the first 3 months**, 90 % recovers by 12 months.
- The majority of the cases that do not fully recover will show some sort of partial recovery.

Management:

- Rest of the arm for few days followed gentle ROM of the affected shoulder.

Indication for orthopedic referral:

- Absence of full recovery by age of 3 months.
- Presence of signs of root avulsion (Horner syndrome, Phrenic nerve affection) (indication for early referral).
- Total palsy and Klumpke's palsy (always refer to orthopedic)

Fractures during birth:

- Clavicle fracture
- Femur fracture
- Humerus fracture

Clavicle fracture:

- Usually mid shaft clavicular fracture.
- Associated with shoulder dystocia.
- Will heal within 1 week with large callus (warn the family in advance) (Fig. 16.16 in trauma).
- No treatment is needed.

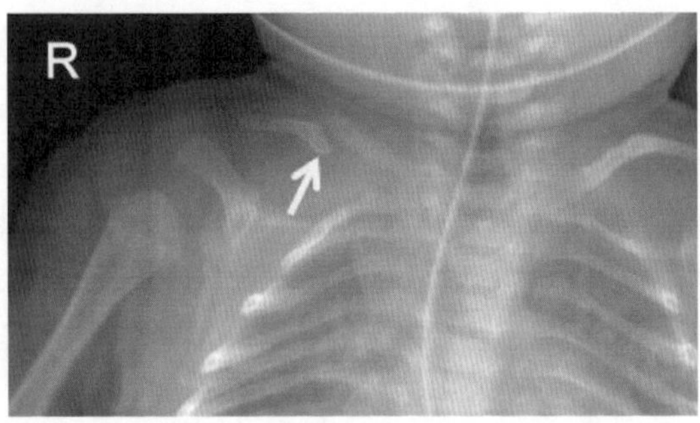

Fig. 5.3 Congenital pseudo-arthrosis of the clavicle (*arrow*). Notice the atrophic ends of clavicle fracture

Differential diagnosis:

Congenital pseudo-arthrosis (false joint) of the clavicle (Fig. 5.3):

- Congenital condition, atraumatic.
- Always on the **right side**.
- Does not heal spontaneously, needs orthopedic referral.
- Surgery is usually done at the age of 2 years.

Femoral fracture:

- Femoral shaft fracture from the excess pulling of the child's thigh.
- **Treatment:**
  - Splinting the limb with padded tongue depressor and compressive wrap.
  - The fracture will heal in about 1–2 weeks.

Humeral fracture:

- Fracture of the humerus due excess pulling on the arm (Fig. 5.4)
- **Treatment:**
  - Same as femoral fracture.

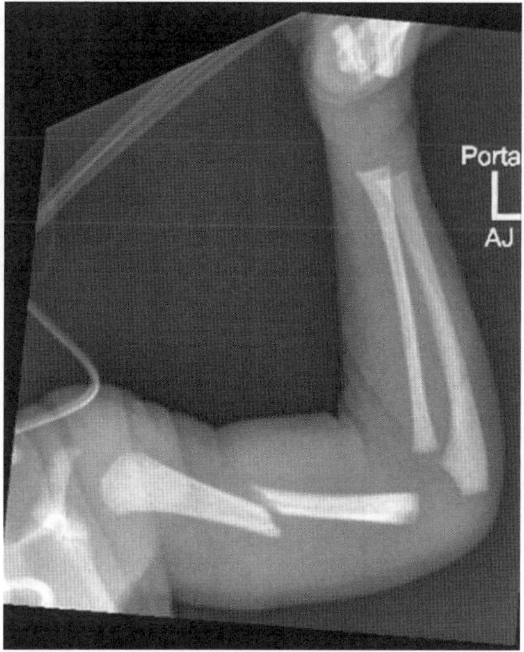

Fig. 5.4 Humerus fracture in a neonate

Differential diagnosis for fracture during birth:

Osteogenesis Imerfecta

Other orthopedic conditions at birth

- Congenital hand and foot deformities (see hand and foot chapters).
- Developmental dysplasia of the hip (see hip chapter)
- Spina bifida (myelomeningocele) (see neurology chapter)
- Dysplasias (see General diseases affecting bone chapter)
- Larsen syndrome:
  - multiple joint dislocations
  - requires orthopedic referral
- Congenital knee dislocation:

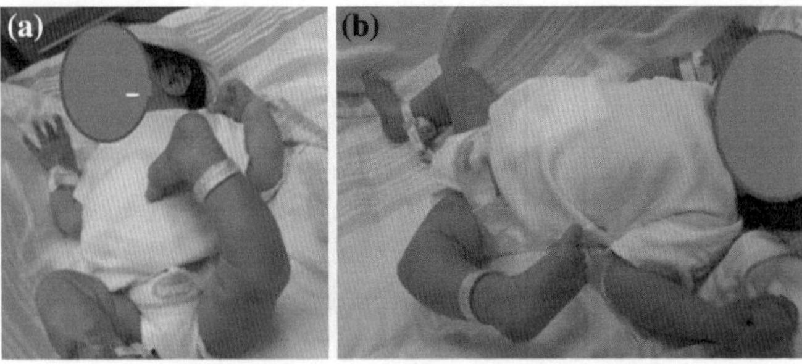

Fig. 5.5 a and **b**. Congenital dislocation of the knee. Newborn girl with *left knee* dislocation. Notice the hyperextension of the *left knee* in which the foot is pointing to the abdomen

- The knee is hyper extended (Fig. 5.5).
- It is related to intra uterine position (breech position in utero).
- the quadriceps muscle is contracted
- orthopedic referral:
  - Closed reduction and splinting.

HIGH YIELD FACTS

- Always examine the clavicles in your routine well baby exam in the newborns.
  - If a newborn with clavicular fracture discharged without diagnosis, the mother will bring the child back with clavicular mass evaluation (Callus)
- Approximately 90 % of patients with neonatal brachial plexus injuries recover by 12 months.
- Up to one third of the cases of Klumpke's paralysis is associated with Horner syndrome.
- Fractures femur and humerus that occur during birth are treated with splint for 1–2 weeks.

CLINICAL SCENARIOS

4 kg newborn with history of difficult delivery present with of inability to move the right shoulder and asymmetric moro reflex. On examination, the child keep the right arm adducted, the right elbow extended. He can grasp the finger when put in the palm. No other abnormity in the child can be detected	Erb's Palsy. Examine the eye and respiratory pattern to rule out Horner syndrome and phrenic nerve injury Rest of the arm in a sling for few days followed gentle ROM exercise. Follow up: • If complete resolution before 3 months, no further action is needed. • If not completely recovered (difference between right and left sides), orthopedic referral.

REFERENCES

Thabet AM, Mackenzie WG. Orthopedics problems of the neonates. In: Gomella T, Cunningham D, Eyal F, editors. Neonatology: Management, procedures, on-call problems, diseases, and drugs. 6th ed. New York: McGraw-Hill; 2009.

Amr Abdelgawad. Shoulder deformity in children with Erb's Palsy. [Dissertation]. Faculty of Medicine, Ain Shams University (2005).

Sankar WN, Weiss J, Skaggs DL. Orthopaedic conditions in the newborn. J Am Acad Orthop Surg. 2009;17(2):112–22.

Chapter 6
The Hip

Amr Abdelgawad and Osama Naga

INTRODUCTION TO THE HIP JOINT ANATOMY

- Hip joint is formed by the acetabulum on one side and the head of the femur on the other side (Fig. 6.1).
- Hip joint is a synovial "ball and socket" joint which allows large range of motion in the 3 planes [flexion–extension, internal rotation-external rotation, adduction (medial deviation)-abduction (lateral deviation)].
- The blood supply to the head of the femur is very scanty and it is related to many pathological conditions of the hip.

Blood supply to the femoral head:

- Most of the blood supply to the femoral head is from the **medial femoral circumflex artery** which provides about 75 % of the blood supply to the head (Fig. 6.2).
- The lateral femoral circumflex artery provides about 25 % of the blood supply to the head.
- The artery of the ligamentum teres, provides blood supply to a small part of the head in the first few years of life only.
- The branches of the medical and lateral femoral circumflex arteries will pierce the capsule, travel along the neck "epiphyseal blood vessels" to supply the head of the femur.
- The blood supply of the femoral head is by "end artery circulation." This means that there is NO anastomosis between the medial and lateral circumflex arteries.
- **Significance:**
  - Injury to the blood supply of the femoral head will result in Avascular necrosis (AVN) of the femoral head.

A. Abdelgawad and O. Naga (eds.), *Pediatric Orthopedics*,
DOI: 10.1007/978-1-4614-7126-4_6,

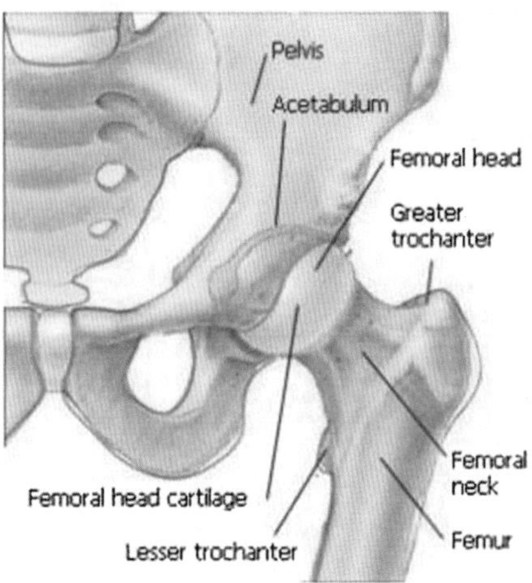

Fig. 6.1 Hip Anatomy. The hip joint is a ball and socket joint which allows large range of motion. The acetabulum constitutes the 'socket' while the femoral head forms the 'ball.' The proximal femur is composed of femoral head, femoral neck, greater trochanter, and lesser trochanter

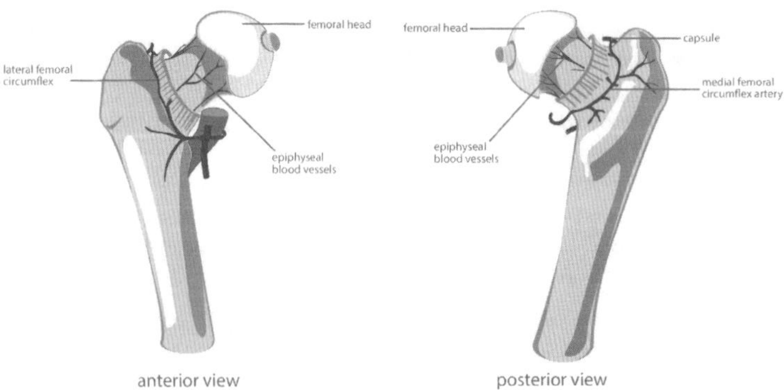

Fig. 6.2 Femoral head blood supply. The lateral and medial (main supply) femoral circumflex arteries give off 'epiphyseal blood vessels' that penetrate the capsule and ascend along the neck to supply the femoral head

- Intracapsular fractures of the neck of the femur can injure the blood vessels on the femoral neck supplying the femoral head.
- Stretching of the vessels at the edge of the epiphysis in cases of Slipped Capital femoral Epiphysis (SCFE) can cause damage to the blood supply of the head of the femur.

Nerve supply to the hip joint.

- The hip joint is supplied by branches of the femoral nerve and the obturator nerve.
- Anterior branch of the obturator nerve supplies both the hip joint and the knee joint.
- **Significance:**
    - Patients with hip pathology (e.g., SCFE) can present with knee pain.
    - In any child presenting with knee pain, hip pathology must be excluded.

EXAMINATION OF THE HIP JOINT

- The child should wear a gown or shorts
- **Inspection:**
    - Atrophy of the gluteal muscles (indicates chronic pathology).
    - Scars (indicate previous surgeries done on the hip region).
    - Deformity.
- **Palpation:**
    - Presence of deep tenderness.
    - The hip joint is a deep joint; swelling and effusion cannot be easily palpated.
- **Movement:**
    - Passive and active Range of Motion (ROM)
    - Compare with the other hip for normal range.

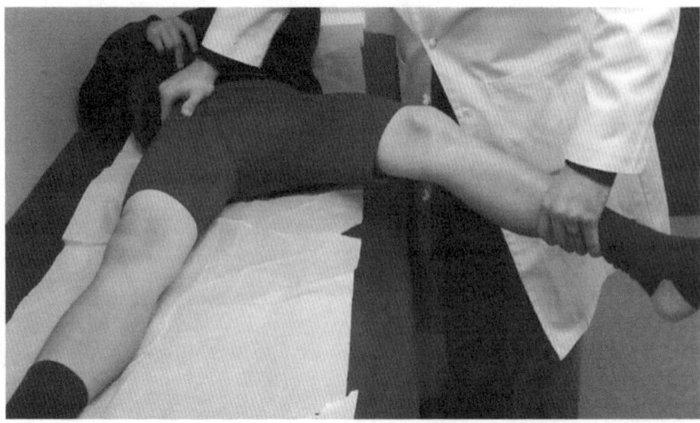

Fig. 6.3 Examination of the hip joint. While assessing the examined hip (*left hip* in this picture), one hand should be applied to the contralateral pelvis to differentiate between hip movement and movement at the lumboscaral joint

- One hand should be put on the contralateral pelvis to be able to differentiate between movement originating from the hip joint and movement from lumbopelvic region (Fig. 6.3).
  - If the hand on the contralateral pelvis starts moving with motion of the hip, this will indicate the end of the ROM of the examined hip and any more movement will be from the lumbopelvis articulation.

- **Special tests:**
  - Assessment of flexion contracture (**Thomas test**) (Fig. 6.4):
    - Flexion contracture is **inability to extend** the hip fully.
    - It can occur with multiple hip pathologies (e.g., Perthes disease).
    - Flexion contracture of the hip joint is hidden by hyperlordosis of the spine.
    - To obliterate hyperlordosis, flex the contralateral hip fully. This will make the flexion contracture become more obvious.

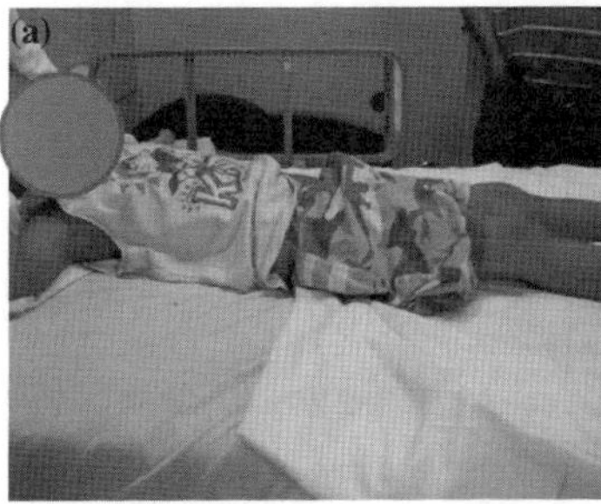

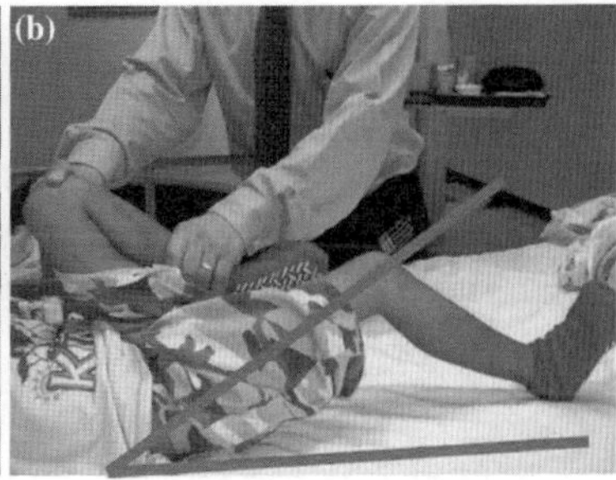

Fig. 6.4 Thomas test to detect flexion contracture. 5-year old with Perthes disease of the right hip. **a** The child when lying on bed does not show any flexion contracture (both legs lying flat on bed) as the child is compensating by lumbar hyperlordosis. **b** The left hip is flexed all the way to obliterate the hyperlordosis, this makes the flexion contracture of the right hip more obvious (the right thigh in no longer on the bed)

- Assessment of the abductor strength (**Trendelenburg test**) (Fig. 6.5):
  - Causes of positive Trendelenburg:
    - Dislocation of the joint (DDH)
    - Short neck (skeletal dysplasia, coxa vara)
    - Muscle weakness (paralysis, nerve injury)

COMMON HIP PATHOLOGIES

DEVELOPMENTAL DYSPLASIA OF THE HIP (DDH)

Definition:

- Dysplasia of the hip that develop during fetal life or in infancy.
- It ranges from dysplasia of the acetabulum (shallow acetabulum) to subluxation of the joint to complete dislocation.
- The old name was "congenital dysplasia of the hip (CDH)." The name has changed to indicate that not all cases are present at birth and that some cases can develop later on during infancy and childhood.

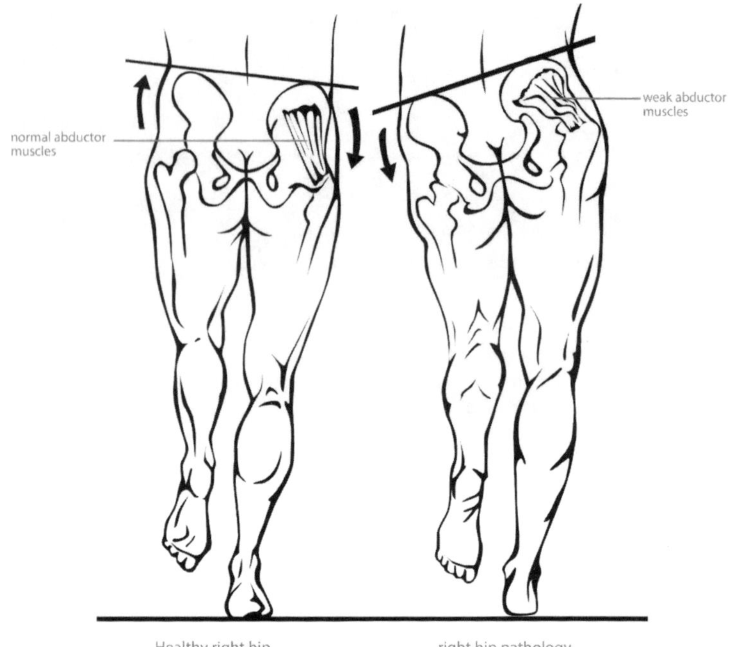

Fig. 6.5 Trendelenburg test. If the patient stands on the healthy side, his abductor muscles will support his weight, the contralateral side will not tilt down. While if the patient stands on the affected side, because of his weak abductor, the pelvis will drop on the other side (Sound Side Sag [SSS]) (positive Trendelenburg sign)

Incidence:

- Incidence of dysplasia is 1 in 100.
- Incidence of dislocation is 1 in 1,000.
- Usually affects the left side.
  - The left hip is forced into adduction against the mother's spine in the left occiput anterior position which is the most common position for the fetus.

Risk factors:

- First-born female.

- Breach presentation.
- Positive family history.
- Any condition that leads to tighter intrauterine space and consequently less room for normal fetal motion.

CLINICAL PRESENTATION

At newborn:

Screening physical examination should be done for **all newborns**. This is done by stressing both hips using Ortolani and Barlow's maneuvers.

Ortolani and Barlow maneuvers (Figs. 6.6, 6.7):

- These tests are done while the patient is supine.
- The child has to be relaxed.
- One side is assessed at a time.
  - If the hip is outside the acetabulum (**dislocated**), positive Ortolani maneuver (**reduction of dislocated hip**) (Fig. 6.6).
  - If the hip is **subluxable**, positive Barlow test (**dislocation of subluxable unstable hip**) (Fig. 6.7).
  - Positive test means **clunk** not **click** (click is a normal finding).
  - **Other signs of Dislocation:**
    - **Limited abduction of the hip.**
    - **Asymmetrical gluteal folds (can be a normal finding).**

ULTRASOUND OF THE HIP

- Because the proximal femur at birth is all cartilaginous, radiographs cannot be used to detect the position of the head of the femur in relation to the acetabulum.
- Ultrasound is used to assess the position of the head of the femur until the age of 4–6 months when the ossific center of the proximal femur starts to develop.
- Dynamic ultrasound:

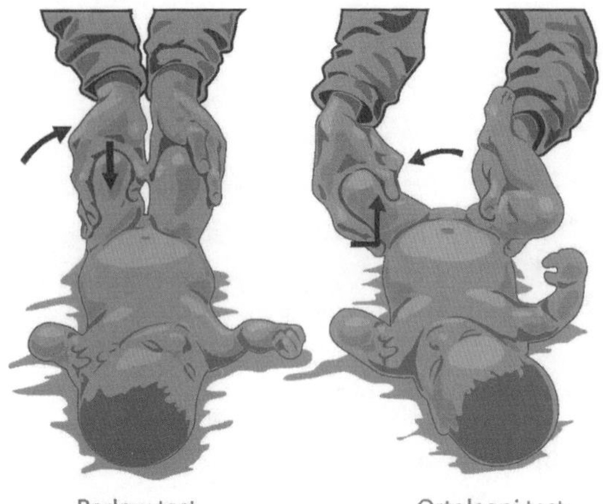

Fig. 6.6 Barlow and Ortolani test: The leg is hold in between the thumb on the medial aspect and the other four fingers on the lateral aspect with the knee of the infant in the palm of the examiner. In Barlow test: the examiner holds the limb adducted and push the hip backwards with his palm to dislocate subluxable hips. Ortolani test: the examiner holds the limb abducted and push the hip forwards (with the four lateral fingers) to reduce dislocated hips

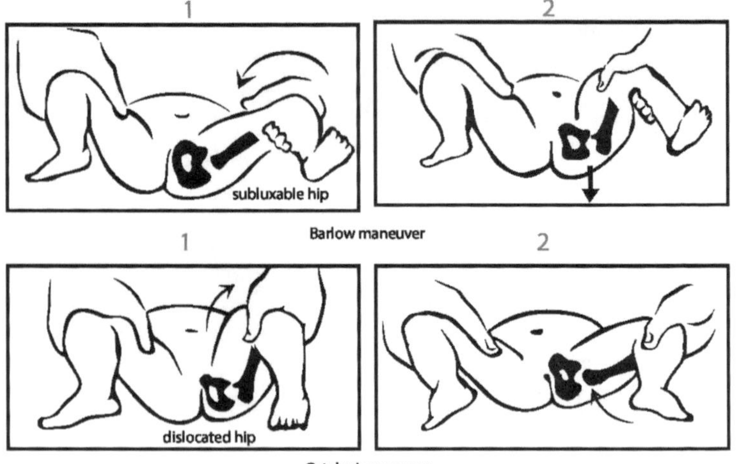

Fig. 6.7 Barlow test: dislocation of subluxable hip. Ortolani test: reduction of a dislocated hip

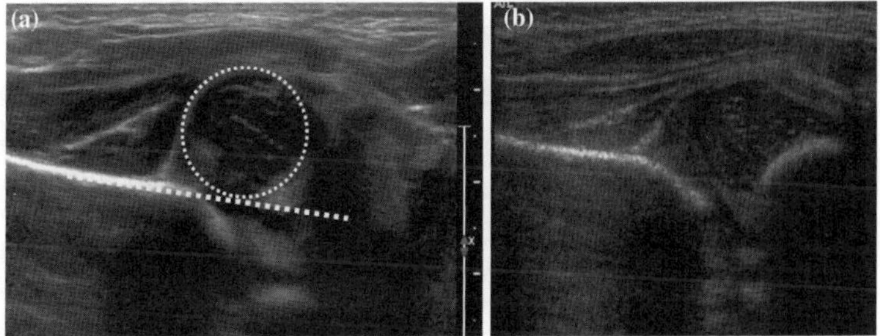

Fig. 6.8 Dynamic ultrasound. Assessment of the hip position by ultrasound during various positions. **a** To the left with hip adduction, the femoral head (dotted circle) lies outside a line along the pelvic bone (dotted line). **b** With hip abduction, partial reduction occurs

- Using ultrasound to assess the stability of the head of the femur in the acetabulum during various movement of the hip joint (Fig. 6.8).

- After the ossific center is formed (around 4–6 months), the ultrasound waves cannot penetrate the ossific center. Plain radiographs are used to assess the hip joint.

INTERPRETATION OF THE ULTRASOUND OF THE HIP

Alpha angle (Fig. 6.9):

- It represents the bony acetabulum.
- Normal is **more** than 55°, this indicates good bony coverage of the head of the femur (deep acetabulum).

Beta angle:

- It represents the cartilaginous acetabulum.
- Beta angle should be **less** than 50° to indicate that the head of the femur is not subluxated (**B**ig **B**eta **B**ad).

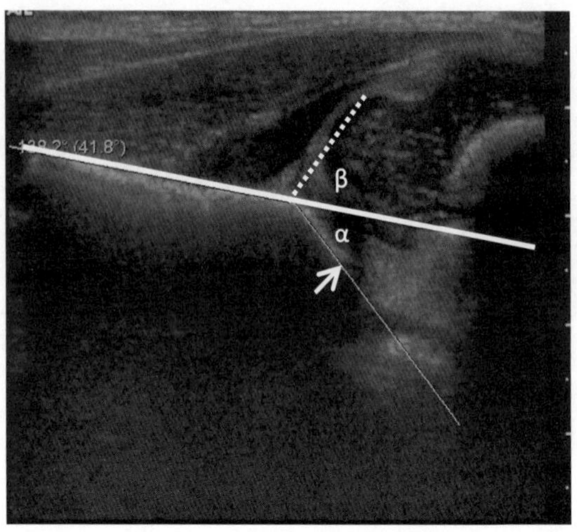

Fig. 6.9 Ultrasound assessment of the hip joint. Alpha angle is the angle between the ileum (thick line) and a line extending from the triradiate (arrow) to the edge of the acetabulum (thin line). Beta angle is the angle between the ilium (thick line) and line extending from the edge of the bony acetabulum to the edge of the labrum (dotted line)

RECOMMENDATION OF THE AMERICAN ACADEMY OF PEDIATRICS (AAP) FOR HIP ASSESSMENT FOR DDH

- All newborns should be screened by physical exam. Routine ultrasound for all newborns is NOT needed.
- If there is a positive Ortolani or Barlow sign (clunk):
  - Orthopedic referral.
  - No need for ultrasound or radiograph.
  - Use of triple diapers is not recommended (will delay more appropriate treatment).
- If there is 'equivocal' (soft click or asymmetry), repeat the exam after 2 weeks.
  - **Follow-up after 2 weeks**:
    - If the results are the same (soft click, asymmetry): Orthopedic referral or ultrasonography.

- If the results became negative: no need for further action.
- If the results became positive Ortolani or Barlow (clunk): Orthopedic referral.

- **Risk factors**.

  If the results of the newborn examination are negative (or equivocally positive), risk factors may be considered.

  - **Female:**
    - Hips should be reevaluated at 2 weeks of age.
  - **Infants with a positive family history of DDH or Breech presentation**
    - For boys, hips should be reevaluated at 2 weeks of age.
    - For females, ultrasound at the age of 6 weeks or radiographs at the age of 4 months should be performed.
    - Consider radiographs for all breech (boys and girls) at the age of 4 months for detection of acetabular development.

- **Periodicity**
  - The hips must be examined at every well-baby visit.
  - If DDH is suspected (by abnormal exam or parental complain for difficult change of diaper) in any visit, one of the following has to be done:
    - Focus exam of the hip with the child relaxed.
    - Orthopedic referral.
    - Imaging study (ultrasound for children less than 4 months or radiographs for children older than 4 months).

TREATMENT AT THE NEONATAL PERIOD

- Orthopedic referral for **Pavlik Harness application** (Fig. 6.10)
  - Pavlik harness works by keeping the hips flexed and abducted.
  - The hips should be flexed between 90 and 100 degrees (controlled by anterior straps).

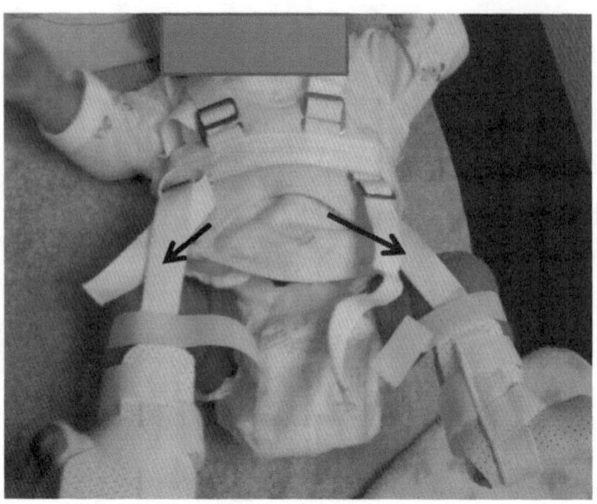

Fig. 6.10 Pavlic harness. Pavlik Harness has two set of straps (two anterior ones to control hip flexion (arrows); and two posterior ones to control hip abduction)

- The hips should be abducted so that with distance between the two knees cannot be less than 3–4 finger breadths (avoid excessive abduction) (controlled by posterior straps).
- Should be left 23 h/day for the duration of "age at application + 2" months (e.g., if the Pavlik harness was applied at the age of 1 month, it should be left for 3 months).

DIAGNOSIS OF MISSED DDH AFTER THE AGE OF SIX MONTHS

- Limited abduction of the affected hip (Fig. 6.11).
- Limb length discrepancy (LLD) ("positive Galeazzi sign") (Fig. 6.11).
- Limping (for unilateral cases) and waddling gait (for bilateral cases):
- Pain is NEVER a symptom of UNTREATED DDH until the development of hip arthritis (usually by the 4th decade of life).
- Radiographs of missed DDH (Fig. 6.12):
  The femoral head is ossified and the following can be seen in the radiographs of dislocated hip:

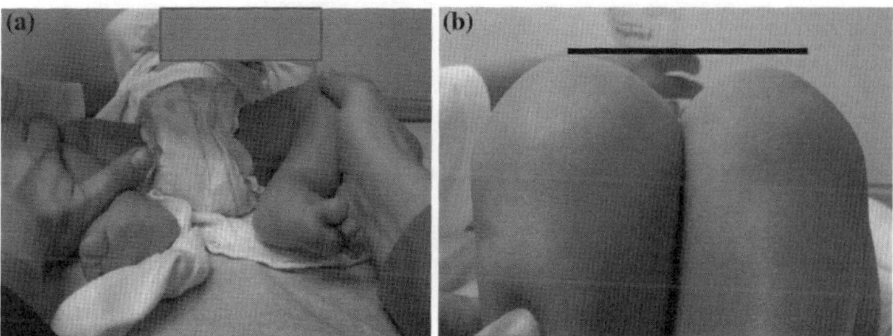

Fig. 6.11 A 10-month-old girl with left hip DDH. (**a**) Notice the limited abduction on the left hip. (**b**) Galeazzi sign:with flexing both leg and putting the feet together, the short side 'left, dislocated' will have the knee at a lower level compared to the right side (**b**), this indicate limb length discrepancy with the dislocated side shorter than the normal side

- Femoral head is out of the acetabulum [in the upper lateral quadrant formed by crossing of Hilgenreiner line and Perkins' line (Fig. 6.12)].
- Broken Shenton's line (imaginary line between the obturator foramen and lower border of the neck of femur).
- Increased acetabular index (normal acetabular index should be less than 24° at age of 24 months).
- Delayed ossification of the femoral head (the affected side is smaller than the normal side).

TREATMENT OF MISSED DDH

Orthopedic referral

- Between 6 and 18 months: closed reduction and casting.
- After 18 months: needs open reduction (with possible osteotomy of the femur or the pelvic bone).
- Any form of treatment for DDH can affect the blood supply to the femoral head resulting in avascular necrosis of the head of femur (AVN) and pain.

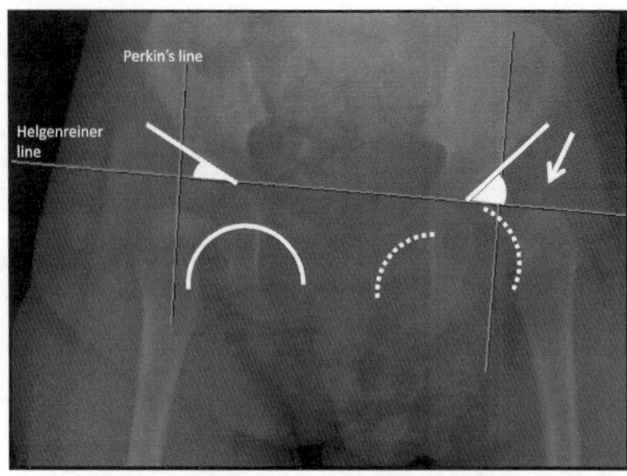

Fig. 6.12 Anteroposterior pelvis radiographs of 14-month-old girl with left hip DDH. The radiograph shows the ossific center on the left side (arrow) smaller than the right side and lying in the upper lateral quadrant of the crossing two lines (Hilgenreiner and Perkins) (the normal right side lies in the lower medial quadrant). The Shenton's line (curved line across the obturator foramen and lower border of the neck) is intact on the right side (continuos curved line) and broken in the left side (curved dotted line). The dislocated side shows increased acetabular index (the angle between the Hilgenreiner line and line from the triradiate to the lateral part of the acetabulum) compared to the right side

LEGG–CALVE–PERTHES DISEASE (LCPD)

Definition:

AVN of the head of the femur in a skeletally immature child

Incidence:

- Boys more affected than girls (4:1)
- More common between the ages of **4–8 years**.
- Can be bilateral (10 %)
    - In bilateral cases, usually the two hips are at different pathological stages (the disease starts in one hip and later on affects the other hip).

Risk factors:

- Protein C and S deficiency.
- V Laiden mutation.
- Steroid intake.
- Lupus anticoagulants.
- Anticardiolipin antibodies.

Clinical picture:

- Hip pain.
  - Related to activity.
  - Can be referred to the thigh and the knee.
- Limping.

Staging and pathology:

- The disease is a self limiting condition.
- The pathological stages are
  - **Necrosis**: necrosis of part of the femoral head.
  - **Revascularization:** new blood vessels invade the necrotic bone. Osteoclasts digest the dead bone causing weakening of the bone structure. This will lead to collapse.
  - **Fragmentation:** the head of the femur will be fragmented due to the weakened structure.
  - **Re-Ossification and remodeling:** Healing process starts with deposition of new bone followed by remodeling of the head of the femur.
- The whole course of the disease can take up to 24 months.

Radiograph:

- AP and frog-leg lateral views are used for diagnosis.
- Radiographic appearance will depend on the stage of the disease. Early on there will be a sub-chondral facture (Fig. 6.13) followed by collapse and fragmentation of the femoral head (Fig. 6.14).

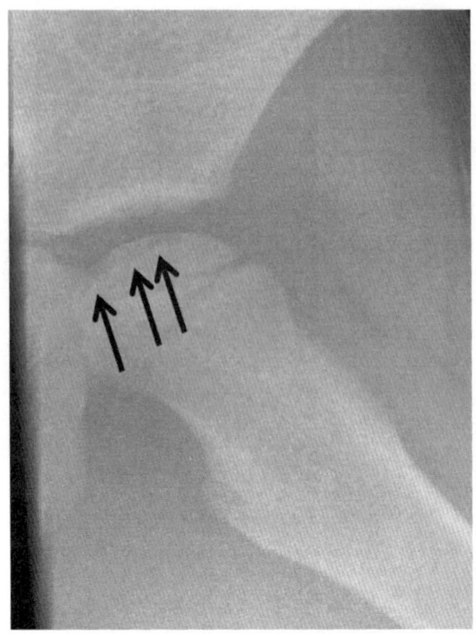

Fig. 6.13 A 5-year-old boy with a 2-month history of left hip pain and limping. Lateral radiographs of the left hip shows the subchondral fracture line (arrows) indicating early stage of Perthes disease

Treatment:

Orthopedic referral:

There is NO universal consensus on the treatment of Perthes disease.

- Patients under the age of 6 years: treatment is usually symptomatic (avoid sports, NSAIDs).
- Patients above the age of 6 years: usually will need some sort of surgical interference (femoral or pelvic osteotomy) to allow the head to heal in better position.

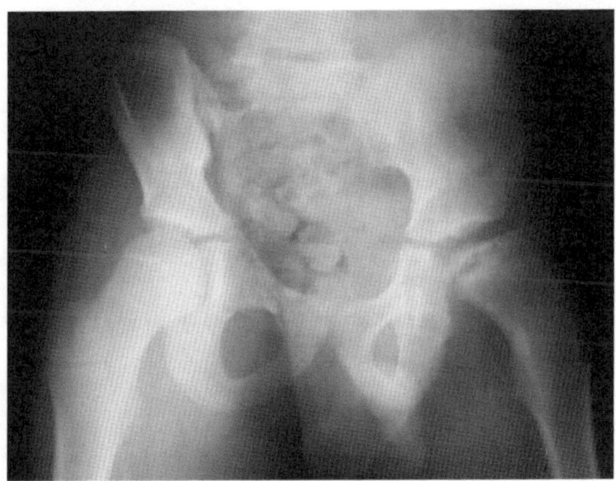

Fig. 6.14 An 8-year-old boy with 1 year history of Perthes disease in the left hip. Radiograph shows collapse of the left hip epiphysis (compare right and left side)

SLIPPED CAPITAL FEMORAL EPIPHYSIS (SCFE)

Definition:

- Displacement of the proximal femoral **metaphysis** in relation to the capital (proximal) femoral **epiphysis**.
- SCFE is misnomer: the capital femoral epiphysis is located inside the acetabulum and does not move or slip, what moves is the metaphysis in relation to epiphysis (Fig. 6.15).

Incidence:

- More common in obese black boys.
- Common around the age of 11-years old in girls and 13-years old in boys.

Etiology:

- Most cases are idiopathic.
- Endocrinopathy:

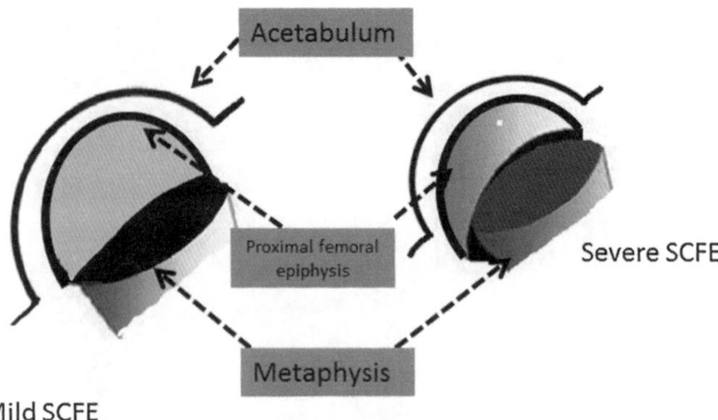

Fig. 6.15 The pathology of SCFE. The proximal femoral epiphysis is contained in the acetabulum and does not move, while the slippage occurs when the metaphysis starts to move in relation to the epiphysis

  - Hypothyroidism: most common endocrine abnormality.
  - Growth hormone deficiency.
  - Hypopituitarism.

- Renal osteodystrophy
  - usually associated with bilateral SCFE.

Symptoms:

- Hip or **knee** pain
  - The pain is referred along the anterior branch of the obturator nerve which innervates both joints.
  - **Any child complaining of knee pain should get plain radiograph on both the hip and knee joints.**
- **External rotation deformity:**
  - The child will have the hip fixed in external rotation position (Fig. 6.16).

Classification of SCFE:

- **Stable SCFE:**

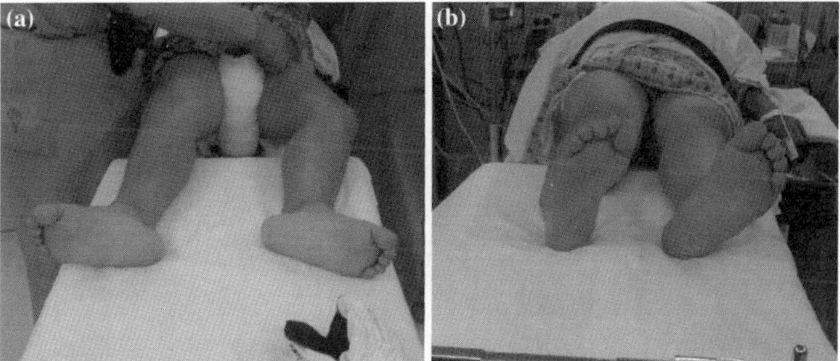

Fig. 6.16 A 14-year-old boy with bilateral SCFE (stable on the right and unstable on left). **a** Patient has bilateral external rotation deformity (notice the position of both feet on the operating table). **b** Gentle reduction was attempted and pinning of both hips was done (notice the improved position of the lower extremity)

- The patient is able to bear weight on the affected extremity with or without crutches.
- Has low incidence of avascular necrosis.

- **Unstable SCFE:**
  - The patient is **unable to bear weight** on the affected extremity with or without crutches.
  - Has a much higher incidence of AVN of the head of the femur (due to the stretch of the blood vessel supplying the head of the femur by the displacement of the metaphysis).

Radiographs:

- AP and lateral view of both hips will be sufficient for diagnosis (Fig. 6.17).
  - For cases of unstable SCFE: cross table lateral is preferred over frog lateral to avoid further displacement of the metaphysis during positioning of the hip.
  - Klein line can be used to assess the relationship of epiphysis to metaphysis (Fig. 6.17).
  - The main deformity will be more obvious in the **lateral view** which will show posterior displacement of proximal femur.

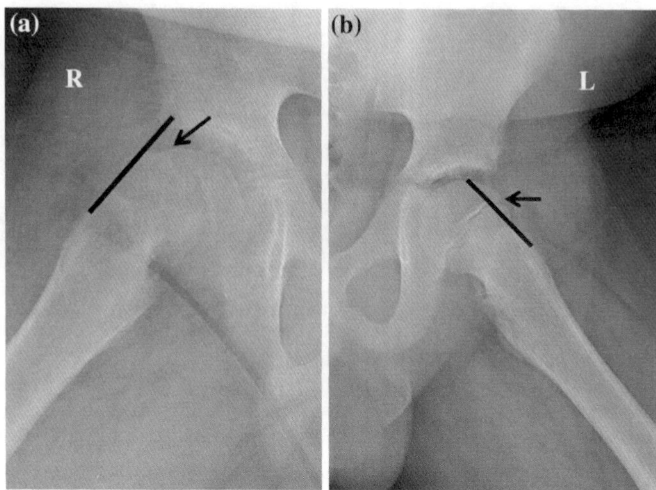

Fig. 6.17 A 13-year-old boy with right hip and knee pain of 2 weeks duration. Radiographs taken for both hips AP and Lateral views. Lateral radiograph of the both hips are presented in this figure. Klein's line (the black line) is drawn along the anterior femoral neck and normally (left hip) should intersect part of the epiphysis of the proximal femur (an arrow is pointing to the anterior edge of the epiphysis). On the right hip (SCFE) the Klein's line does not intersect any part of the epiphysis

- With progression of deformity, the displacement can be seen also in the AP view (inferior displacement of the epiphysis in relation to the proximal femur).
- Crescent sign (the edge of posteriorly displaced epiphysis) (Fig. 6.18).
- Decrease height of the epiphysis in the AP view.

Treatment:

- **Immediate admission to the hospital with urgent orthopedic consultation**.
- Non-weight bearing and bed rest.
- Delay in the treatment can result in stable SCFE becoming an unstable SCFE with further displacement and increase in the possibility of developing AVN (Fig. 6.19).

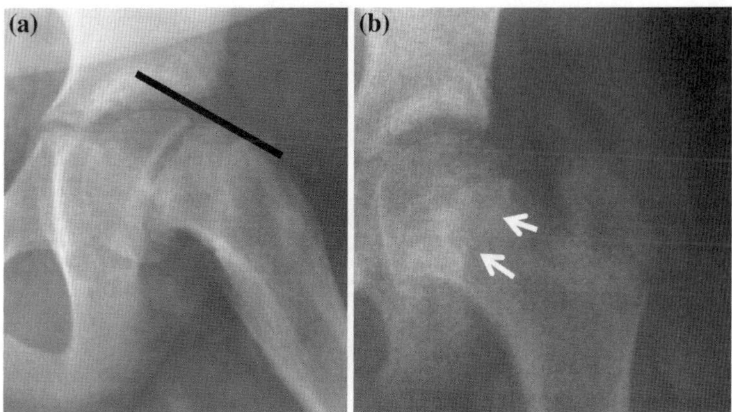

Fig. 6.18 A 12-year-old boy with left knee pain of 2 month duration. Radiograph of the left hip shown in the lateral view (**a**), the Klein's line not intersecting the femoral epiphysis. In the AP view (**b**), the crescent sign (arrows) can be seen

- Treatment is usually by screw fixation of the physis to prevent further progression (in situ fusion) (Fig. 6.20).
- No need for routine hormonal study for each case of SCFE.
  - For atypical cases (less than 10 years old, thin, short stature for age): consider endocrinological studies (see chap. 12).

Affection of the other hip:

- About half of the patients with SCFE with have affection of the contralateral hip.
  - One-third of the patients with bilateral affection will present with bilateral **simultaneous** affection.
  - Two-third of the patients with bilateral affection will present with one hip affection **followed** by the other hip within 1 or 2 years.
- Instruct the family: with first sign of contralateral hip or knee pain, to immediately inform the physician.

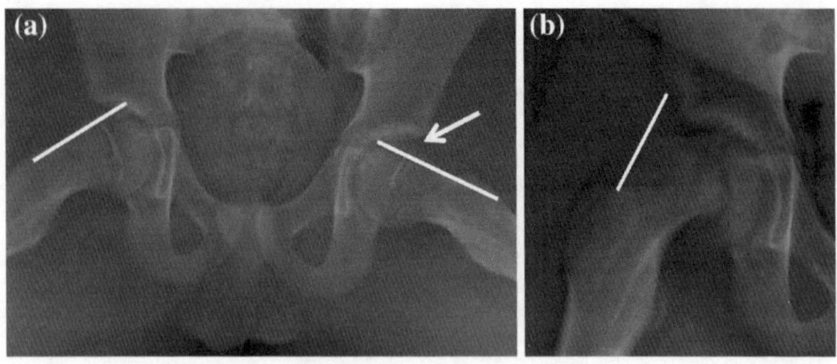

Fig. 6.19 A 13-year-old boy with 2-month history of right knee pain, Radiographs of right hip showed mild slip (stable SCFE) (**a**). The child was sent home after booking him for surgery after 7 days and instructed to be non-weight bearing with crutches. After 4 days, the child twisted while sitting on the floor and developed severe hip pain and was not able to bear weight. Radiographs showed marked increase in the amount of slippage (**b**)

Septic Arthritis and Transient Synovitis of the Hip Joint

- These are two different conditions that sometimes have very similar presentation:
- Differentiation between hip septic arthritis and transient synovitis sometimes is very difficult.

Septic Arthritis of the Hip Joint: (see septic arthritis in Chap. 12)

Clinical presentation:

- General signs of infection (fever, vomiting, ill looking)
- **Refusal to move the hip joint** (the affected joint is fixed in a flexed position).
- Inability to bear weight.
- Hip joint is a deep joint and local signs of inflammation may be hard to detect.

Management:

- Imaging studies:

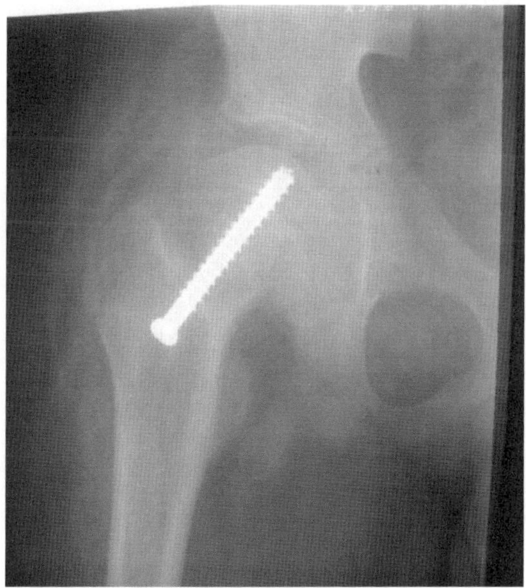

Fig. 6.20 A 13 years old boy with stable SCFE was treated with fixation of the physis using one screw. This will stabilize his physis and prevents further progression

- Ultrasound: to detect fluid in the hip joint.
- MRI: very sensitive to detect joint effusion and nearby bone infection and inflammation (Fig. 21.4 in musculoskeletal infection chapter).

▪ Image guided arthrocentesis:

- The fluid is sent for gram stain, cultures, antibiotic sensitivity, crystals, and **cell counts.**

▪ Laboratory studies:

- Elevated markers of infections (CBC with differential, ESR, and C-reactive protein).

▪ Antibiotics Treatment (see septic arthritis in musculoskeletal infections).

- Urgent orthopedic consultation. (**septic arthritis is a surgical condition**)
  - arthrotomy and debridement of the hip joint.

TRANSIENT SYNOVITIS

Definition:

- Non-specific inflammation of the hip joint.
- It may be related to viral infection or minor trauma.

Clinical picture:

- Transient synovitis has a wide spectrum of presentation.
- It can range from mild limping with moderate pain to inability to walk with severe pain in the hip. The child may have low grade fever.
- Examination of the hip will show painful limitation of the hip range of motion especially flexion internal rotation.

Labs:

- Normal or mild elevation of inflammation markers.

Management:

- NSAID.
- Activity limitation.

How to differentiate between septic arthritis of the hip and transient synovitis.

- **Kocher's criteria** is widely used to differentiate between transient synovitis and septic arthritis. However, some studies showed that it may not be very reliable.

  Kocher criteria

  - History of fever (>38.5).
  - Inability to bear weight on the affected limb.
  - ESR greater than 40 mm per hour.

DIFFERENTIATION BETWEEN SEPTIC ARTHRITIS OF THE HIP AND TRANSIENT SYNOVITIS.

	Septic arthritis of the hip	Transient synovitis
Fever	++	Normal or mild
ESR, CRP, WBCs	+++	Normal or mild elevation
Inability to walk	Common	rare
Aspiration	Positive for gram stain +/- culture Cell count > 50,000/ml	Negative for gram stain and culture Cell count < 50,000/ml
Blood culture	May be positive	negative

- WBC >12,000 cells per mL.
- C-reactive protein level of ≥20 mg/L (not in the original Kocher criteria, but was added later on).

- **The more criteria the child has, the more likely is the diagnosis of septic arthritis.**
- Ultrasound guided aspiration of the hip joint fluid with cell count, gram stain, and culture will confirm or exclude the diagnosis Table 6.1.

IMPINGEMENT OF THE HIP (FEMORO-ACETABULAR IMPINGMENT)

Definition:

- Developmental condition of the hip joint in which the femoral neck impinges against the rim of the acetabulum (Fig. 6.21).

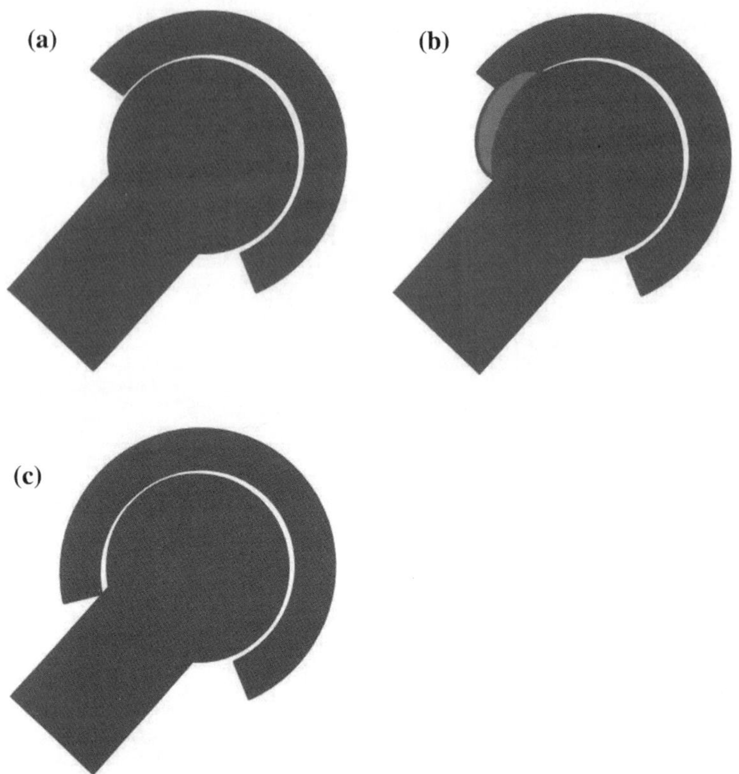

Fig. 6.21 Pathology of femoral acetabular impingement (FAI). (**a**) normal articulation between femoral hip and acetabulum.In Cam impingement (**b**), a bony prominence abuts against the acetabular wall. In Pincer impingement (**c**), a deep or abnormal acetabular orientation causes the edge of the acetabulum to hit the femoral neck

Pathology:

- There are two main pathological types of impingement (Fig. 6.21):
  - Cam impingement:
    - There is a bony prominence (bump) in the neck of the femur that abuts against the edge of acetabulum when the hip is flexed.

- Pincer impingement:
  - Deep acetabulum or abnormal orientation of the acetabulum that results in impingement between the neck femur and the acetabulum during movement of the hip joint.
- Combined type.

Clinical presentation:

- More common in girls.
- Common in activities that require extreme range of motion of the hip as: dancers, cheer leaders, gymnastics, horseback riders, and football players.
- Hip pain:
  - Timing:
    - With activities that require excess hip flexion (see before).
    - After sitting for long period (e.g., traveling in a car).
  - Place:
    - The patient will point to the lateral aspect of his hip joint with the palm of the hand (C-sign) (Fig. 6.22)
- Examination of the hip will show **positive impingement sign** (pain with flexion internal rotation of the hip) (Fig. 6.23).
- Imaging:
  - Plain radiographs will show the abnormal contour of the head of the femur. The deformity is more obvious in the lateral view (Fig. 6.24).
  - MRI: will better delineate the deformity. Also can show associated pathology (labral tear).

Management:

- Avoiding the predisposing activities: this will result in improvement of symptoms in most of the cases of FAI.
- If no improvement with avoiding the predisposing activities, orthopedic referral.
- Orthopedic management will be in the form of either open or arthroscopic surgery to remove the impinging part.

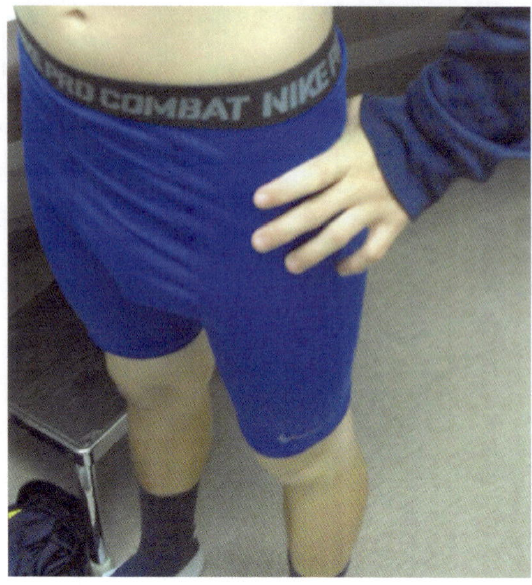

Fig. 6.22 C-sign. When the patient is asked to point his hip pain, he will hold the outer aspect of his hip with the palm of the hand (similar to the letter C)

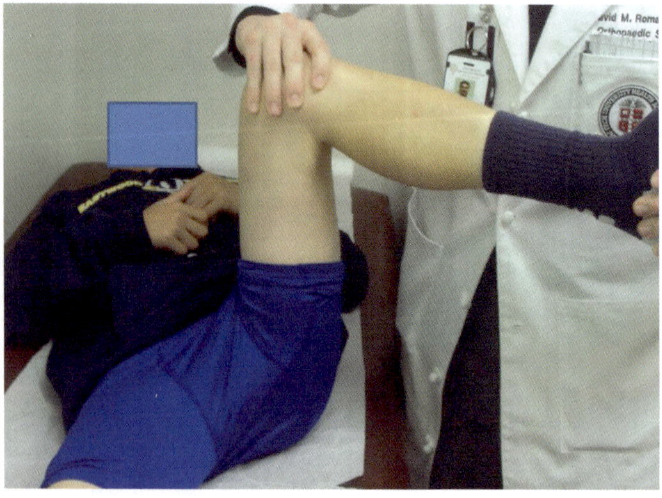

Fig. 6.23 Impingement sign. Flexion internal rotation of the examined hip will cause pain

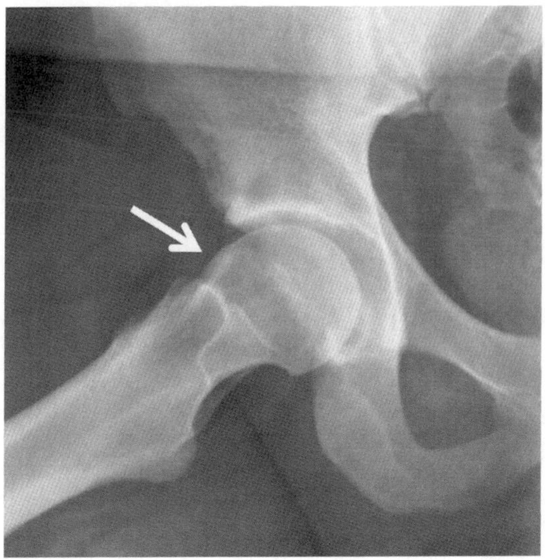

Fig. 6.24 FAI (femoroacetabular impingement). A 16-year-old football player complaining of right hip pain. Lateral radiograph of the hip shows cam impingement (bone exostosis on the anterior neck) (arrow)

Pelvic causes of hip pain:

- Appendicitis
- Psoas abscess
- Mesenteric adenitis

  - These conditions cause **irritation of the psoas muscle** (arises from the lumbar spine, travel through the pelvis, and then inserts in the lesser trochanter of the proximal femur).
  - How to differentiate between septic arthritis of the hip joint and intrapelvic causes of hip pain:

    - Flex of the hip to 90°, this will lead to

      - Relaxation of the psoas muscle and decrease the pain in cases of intrapelvic causes.
      - Increase the pressure inside the hip joint and increase the pain in cases of septic arthritis of the hip joint.

HIGH YIELD FACTS

DEVELOPMENT DYSPLASIA OF THE HIP

- DDH risk increase in first born, female, breech presentation, and positive family history for DDH.
- Physical examination is most important diagnostic tool in diagnosing DDH in neonates.
- No need to order hip ultrasound for newborn positive for Ortolani or Barlow test. Referral to orthopedics is warranted.
- Delay in diagnosis of DDH can lead to significant disability.
- The most reliable physical finding for DDH in older child is limited hip abduction.
- The most important and severe complication of DDH is AVN of the capital femoral epiphysis. This complication occurs only after treatment of DDH. Untreated DDH does not develop AVN.
- Missed DDH is not a painful condition until the development of hip arthritis around the forth or fifth decade.

Legg–Calve Perthes Disease:

- Legg–Calve–Perthes disease commonly occurs between 4–8 years of age.
- Legg–Calve–Perthes disease is more common in boys than girls.

Slipped Capital Femoral Epiphysis (SCFE):

- SCFE is common in obese boys, and usually present between ages 11–14 years of age
- Systemic factors associated with SCFE include hypothyroidism, panhypopituitarism, hypogonadism, and irradiation.
- Half of the children with SCFE will present with knee pain. Any child with knee pain has to have his hip evaluated.
- Diagnosis of SCFE is more obvious in the lateral view.
- SCFE needs urgent orthopedic consult.

Septic arthritis and transient synovitis:

- With significant improvement of joint pain and limping after the use of analgesics or NSAID only, the diagnosis of septic arthritis will be very unlikely.
- Afebrile child with normal CBC, CRP, and ESR does not rule out septic hip.

- Do not give antibiotic treatment before confirming the diagnosis of septic arthritis.
- Septic arthritis is a surgical condition, urgent orthopedic consult is warranted.

Impingement syndrome:

- Most cases of impingement syndrome will respond to cessation of predisposing activities.

CLINICAL SCENARIOS

The presenting patient	The most probable diagnosis and plan of action
6-year-old boy with limping and pain in the left hip for 3 months	**LCPD** Get radiographs of the pelvis (AP and frog lateral) Orthopedic referral
14-year-old male complain of left knee pain and limping for 3 weeks, his BMI > 95 %	**SCFE** Get radiographs of the pelvis (AP and frog lateral) Admit with urgent orthopedic consult
4-year old is having cough and nasal congestion for 7 days, now is complaining of leg pain and not able to walk	**Transient synovitis** NSAID and rest
3-year-old girl, adopted from east Europe, has limping on the left side, limited left hip abduction.	**Missed DDH** Get radiographs of the pelvis (AP and frog lateral) Orthopedic referral
6-year old with high fever, limping, hip ultrasound is positive for large effusion in the left hip, labs are positive for leukocytosis, and shift to the left, ESR and CRP are elevated	**Septic hip** Admit with urgent orthopedic consult

REFERENCES

Clinical practice guideline: early detection of developmental dysplasia of the hip. Committee on quality improvement, subcommittee on developmental dysplasia of the hip. American Academy of Pediatrics. Pediatrics. 2000 Apr;105(4 Pt 1):896-905.

Dezateux C, Rosendahl K. Developmental dysplasia of the hip. Lancet. 2007;369(9572):1541–52.

Sultan J, Hughes PJ. Septic arthritis or transient synovitis of the hip in children: the value of clinical prediction algorithms. J Bone Joint Surg Br. 2010;92(9):1289–93.

Kim HK, Herring JA. Pathophysiology, classifications, and natural history of Perthes disease. Orthop Clin North Am. 2011;42(3):285–95.

Peck D. Slipped capital femoral epiphysis: diagnosis and management. Am Fam Physician. 2010;82(3):258–62.

Wenger DR, Kishan S, Pring ME. Impingement and childhood hip disease. J Pediatr Orthop B. 2006;15(4):233–43.

Maroo S. Diagnosis of hip pain in children. Hosp Med. 1999;60(11):788–93.

Chapter 7
The Knee/Leg

Amr Abdelgawad and Osama Naga

ANATOMY OF THE KNEE JOINT

- The knee joint is a hinge joint
- It is the largest synovial joint in the body.
- The main motion in the knee joint is flexion–extension. Mild internal rotation-external rotation and adduction-abduction can occur.
- The range of motion of the knee is from full extension to about 150° flexion.
- Three bones form of the knee joint (Fig. 7.1):
  - Lower femur.
  - Proximal tibia.
  - Patella:
    - The largest sesamoid bone in the body (bone impeded in a tendon)
- The growth plates (physis) of the distal femur and proximal tibia are:
  - The most active growth plates in the lower extremity
    - The distal femur grows about 9 mm/year.
    - Proximal tibial grows about 6 mm/year.
    - Most of the neoplastic conditions in the lower extremity occur around the knee joint.
  - The growth plates are prone to growth disturbance when they are affected by Salter–Harris injuries.

A. Abdelgawad and O. Naga (eds.), *Pediatric Orthopedics*,
DOI: 10.1007/978-1-4614-7126-4_7,

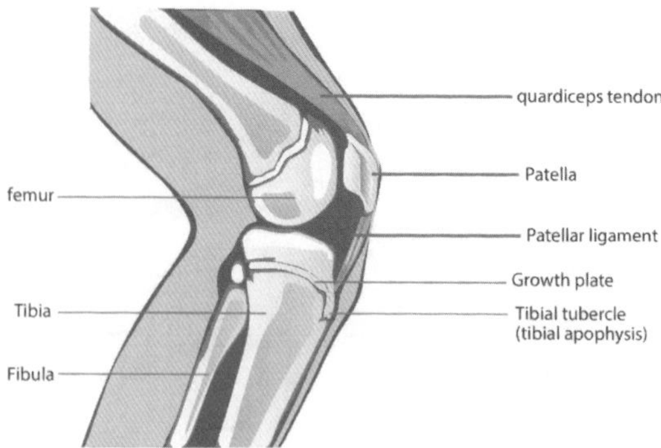

Fig. 7.1 Anatomy of the knee joint

THE MENISCUS

- Two cartilaginous crescent-shaped structures that act like a cushion inside the knee (Fig. 7.2).
- The meniscus lies on the surface of the tibial plateau, one medial and one lateral.
- The medial meniscus is more prone to injury because it is more fixed to the joint capsule, more likely to be caught in between femur and tibia in case of injury.

STABILITY OF THE KNEE JOINT

- The stability of the knee joint depends on strong ligaments connecting the femur with the tibia and the fibula (Fig. 7.3):
  - **Anterior cruciate ligament** (**ACL**):
    - Extends from the **anterior** part of the tibia to posterior femoral notch.
    - It prevents **anterior** displacement of the tibia on the femur.

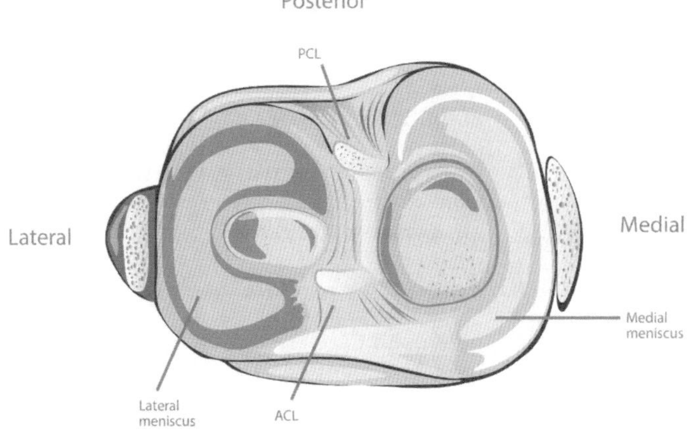

Fig. 7.2 Medial and lateral meniscus

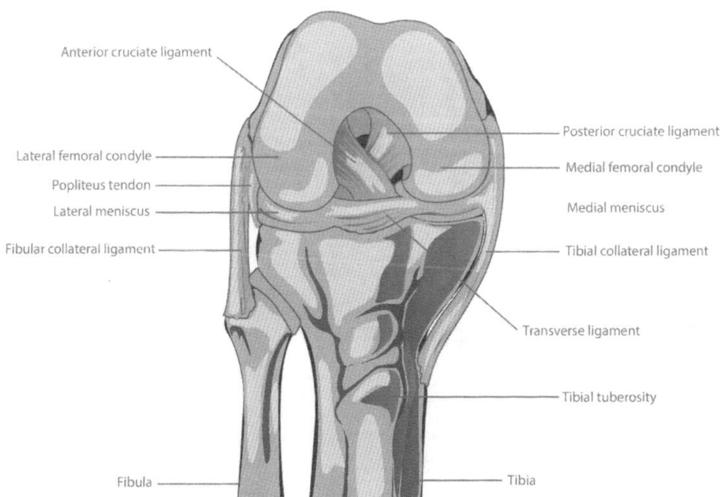

Fig. 7.3 Ligaments of the knee

- ACL is prone to sport injuries especially in adolescent females playing sports with cutting movements (e.g., soccer).

- **Posterior cruciate ligament** (**PCL**):
  - Extends from the **posterior** surface of the tibia to the anterior part of the femoral notch.
  - It prevents **posterior** displacement of the tibia on the femur.
  - PCL is less prone to sports injury than ACL.

- **Medial collateral ligament** (**MCL**):
  - Extends from the medial femoral epicondyle to the medial aspect of the tibia.
  - It consists of two parts: superficial and deep.
  - Primary restrain of the knee joint against drifting into valgus (the tibia point laterally)

- **Lateral collateral ligament** (**LCL**):
  - Extends from lateral femoral epicondyle to the upper end of the fibula.
  - Primary restrain of the knee joint against drifting into varus (the tibia points medially).

HOW TO EXAMINE THE KNEE JOINT

(See the general orthopedic exam in the introduction chapter)

- **Inspection**:
  - Alignment and deformity
  - Swelling and effusion (Fig. 7.4).
  - Scars of previous surgery.
  - Color changes.

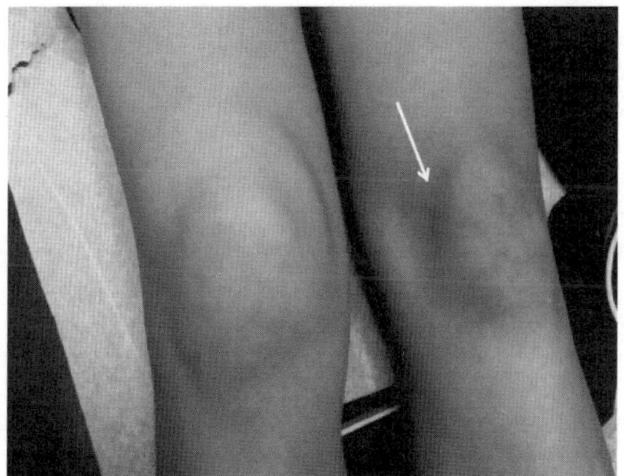

Fig. 7.4 Effusion of the knee. Note the right knee swelling. The medial side of left knee shows the normal groove (*arrow*). The medial groove on the right knee had been obliterated due to knee effusion

- **Palpation**:
  - Bony landmark (patella, tibial tuberosity, medial and lateral femoral epicondyles)
  - Tenderness (joint line, patella, distal femur, proximal tibia, posterior knee)
- **Movement** (**Range Of Motion** (**ROM**)):
  - Active and passive range of motion.
  - Restriction of movement may be due to contracture or pain.
  - **Decreased ROM is a very sensitive indicator of joint inflammation.**
- Special test
  - Assessment of effusion.
    - Disappearance of the groove medial to the patella (Fig. 7.4): this is an early sign of knee effusion.
    - Ballottement test (Fig. 7.5)

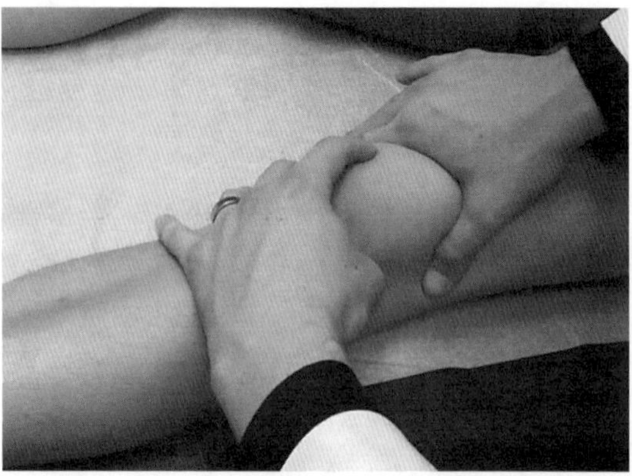

Fig. 7.5 Ballottement test. One hand squeezes the suprapatellar pouch to push the fluid underneath the patella. The index of other hand presses the patella downward. Feeling the patella 'float' in the effusion is a positive sign

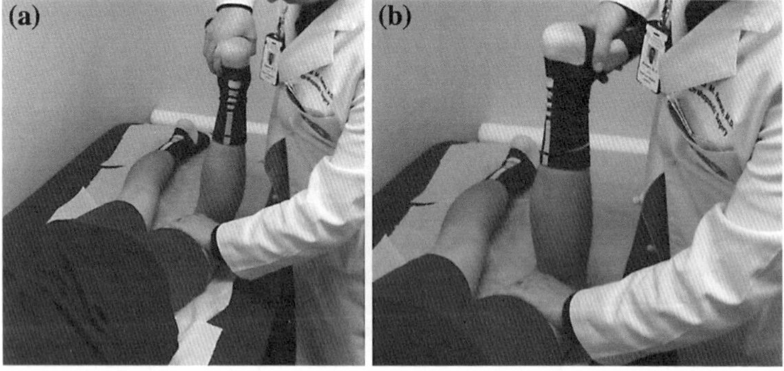

Fig. 7.6 Apley grinding test. The patient is positioned prone with the hip extended and knee flexed. The examiner holds the foot moving the leg internally (**a**) and externally (**b**) while pushing it down against the femur. If there is meniscal tear, the patient will feel pain

- Assessment of meniscal pathology:
  - Apley Grinding test (Fig. 7.6).
  - McMurray test: (Fig. 7.7).
- Other tests for assessment of stability of the knee (see Chap. 10).

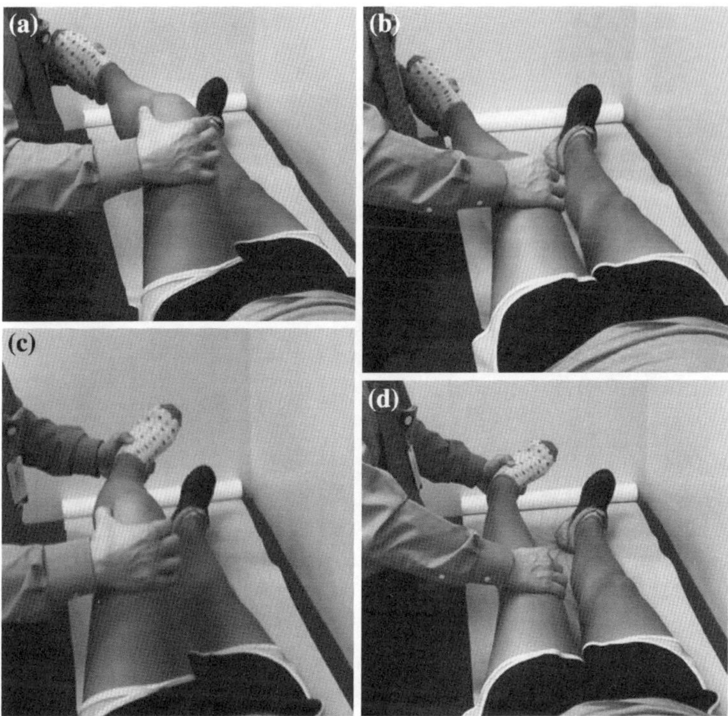

Fig. 7.7 McMurray test: (**a**) The knee is flexed with one hand holding the knee at the joint line and the other hand holding the foot. The knee is put in the position of valgus external rotation. (**b**) The knee is gradually extended with the leg kept in the position of valgus external rotation. Pain or a 'click' constitutes a positive McMurray test for tear in the medial meniscus. (**c** and **d**) The same test is performed with leg in the position of internal rotation and varus. Click or pain is a positive test for lateral meniscus tear

NORMAL KNEE ALIGNMENT

- The knee joint is in varus until **2** years of age (Fig. 7.8).
- The alignment of the knee changes to valgus which reach maximum around the age of **3** years.
- The normal adult alignment (**7 degrees of valgus**) is usually reached by the age **8** years.
- Clinical Method of assessment of knee alignment:

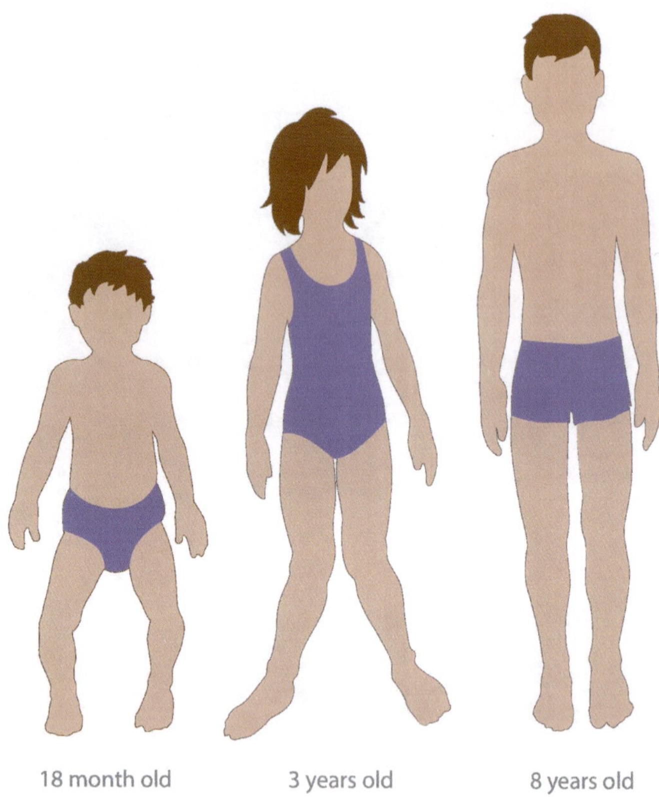

Fig. 7.8 Normal alignment of the knee. The knee joint is in varus at 2 years of age then reaches maximum valgus around the age of 3 years and then normal adult alignment by the age 8 years

- **The intercondylar distance** (Fig. 7.9):
  - Intercondylar distance of more than hand breadth is an indication for genu varum.
- **The intermalleolar distance** (Fig. 7.9):
  - The intermalleolar distance of more than hand breadth is an indication genu valgum.
- **The clinical thigh-leg angle** (Fig. 7.10)

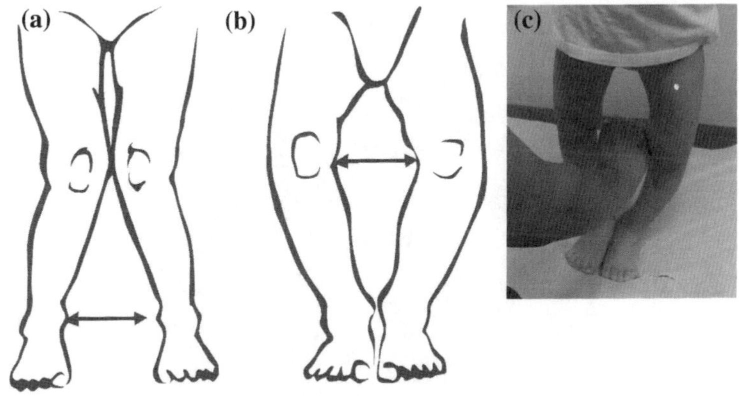

Fig. 7.9 (**a**) Intermalleolar distance. This distance is increased in cases of genu varum (**b**) Intercondylar distance: this increases in cases of genu varum. (**c**) 3-year-old boy with genu varum and intercondylar distance of more than hand breadth

GENU VARUM (BOW LEG)

Definition:

- Deformity of the knee in which the lower leg is pointing medially (see Introduction chapter) (Figs. 7.8, and 7.9).
- The child will have an increase in the intercondylar distance of more than one hand breadth.
- Can be normal development until 2 years of age.

Common cause of genu varum:

Table 7.1: cause of genu varum.

Imaging:

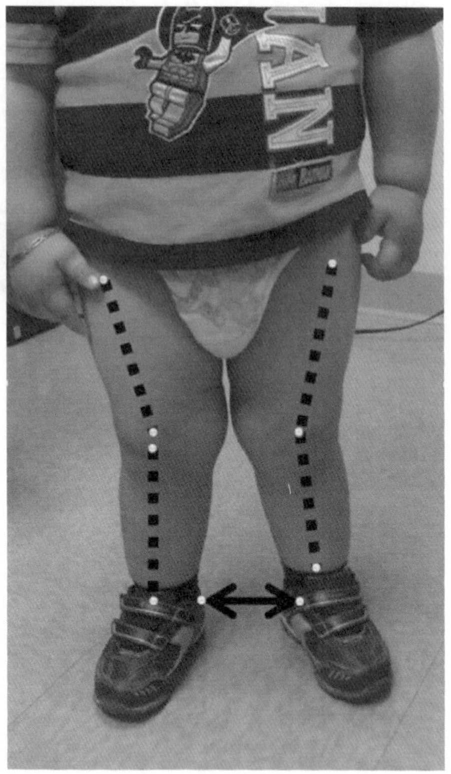

Fig. 7.10 Physiological genu valgum. 30-month-old boy with physiological genu valgum. Notice the increased angle between the leg and the thigh dotted lines and the increased intermalleolar distance (*double headed arrow*)

Indication for plain radiographs in cases of genu varum:

- **Persistence of genu** varum after 24 months.
- **Worsening** genu varum after the age 1 year.
- **Unilateral** genu varum.
- **Severe** genu varum (clinical angle between thigh and leg of more than 20° or intercondylar distance of more than 6 cm).
- Associated deformities of the **other joints**.
- If suspecting **general medical** condition (e.g., rickets).

TABLE 7.1 CAUSES OF GENU VARUM

Physiological	Normal development up to the age of 2 years
Developmental	Blount disease ■ Infantile tibia vara ■ adolescent tibia vara
Metabolic	rickets
Traumatic	Growth plate injury (Salter-Harris injury)
Infective	Growth plate infection
Dysplasia	Achondroplasia
Others	Tibial hemimelia osteogenesis imperfect

GENU VALGUM (KNOCK KNEE)

Definition:

- Deformity of the knee in which the lower leg is pointing laterally (Fig. 7.8 and 7.10).
- Genu valgum is a normal finding in children around 3 years of age (**physiological genu valgum**).
- The condition usually improves gradually to reach the adult alignment by 8 years of age (7° valgus angle between the femur and the tibia).

Causes of genu valgum:

- Physiologic genu valgum (Fig. 7.10).
- Rickets and renal osteodystrophy.
- Posttraumatic physeal arrest.
- Proximal tibial fractures:
    - Proximal tibial fracture can result in genu valgum few months after the injury due to abnormal growth of the proximal tibial physis (**Kozin fracture**).
- Tumor of the proximal tibia.

- Infection of the proximal tibia.
- Dysplasia (e.g., Multiple epiphyseal dysplasia)

Physiological genu valgum:

- Part of the normal development of children (Fig. 7.10).
- Reaches maximum around at the age of 3 years and then improve with time to reach normal alignment by the age of 8 years.
- **Clinical presentation**:
    - Symmetrical deformity of the knee.
    - Increased the intermalleolar distance.
- **Treatment**
    - Reassurance: physiologic valgus can improve up to the age of 8 years.

BLOUNT DISEASE

Definition:

- It is a developmental deformity resulting from abnormal endochondral ossification of the medial aspect of the proximal tibia physis leading to varus deformity and internal rotation of tibia.
- It is also known as **tibia vara**.

Types:

- Infantile type.
- Adolescent type.
    - Infantile type of Blount's disease is more progressive than the adolescent type due to greater growth potential.

Infantile type:

Incidence:

- Occurs in infant and young children (2–4 years).
- More common in **black obese infants**.

Pathology:

- Affection of the proximal medial tibial physis
  - Decrease growth from the medial side with continued growth from the lateral side of the physis results in varus deformity.

Clinical presentation:

- Severe progressive genu varum with internal rotation of the lower leg (Fig. 7.11).
- The condition is usually bilateral.
- In unilateral cases, the condition can be associated with leg-length discrepancy.

Radiographs

- Metaphyseal-diaphyseal angle (Fig. 7.12).
  - More than 16°: is specific for infantile Blount's.
  - Less than 11°: is indicator of physiological genu varum.

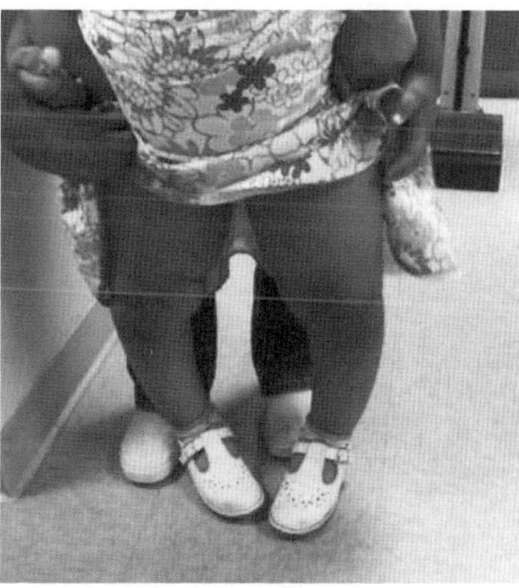

Fig. 7.11 Infantile tibia vara. 3-year-old girl weighing 44 kilograms presenting with bilateral genu varum with internal tibial torsion more on the right side

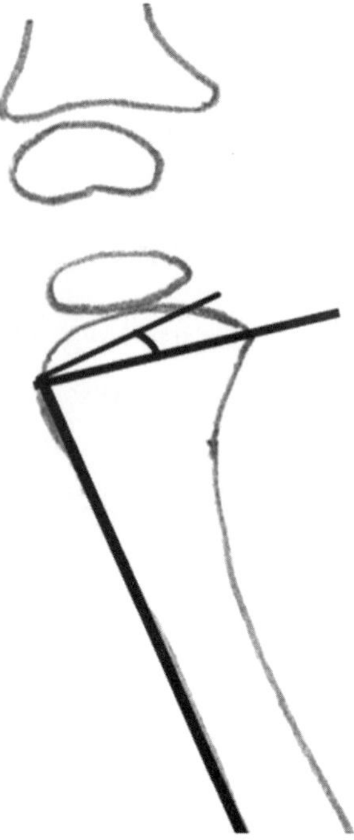

Fig. 7.12 Metaphyseal diaphyseal angle. This is the angle between the line perpendicular to the lateral border of the tibia and the line across the widest area of the metaphysis. Angle >16° indicates Blount's disease and angle <11° indicates physiologic genu varum

- Between 11–16°: can be either physiological genu varum or infantile Blount's.

▪ Growth plate changes in the medial aspect of the proximal tibial (Fig. 7.13).
▪ Medial metaphyseal peaking is often present (Fig. 7.13).

Treatment:

- Knee Brace to correct varus before the age of 3 years.
- If no improvement or if the patient is more than 3 years old: orthopedic referral for surgical treatment.

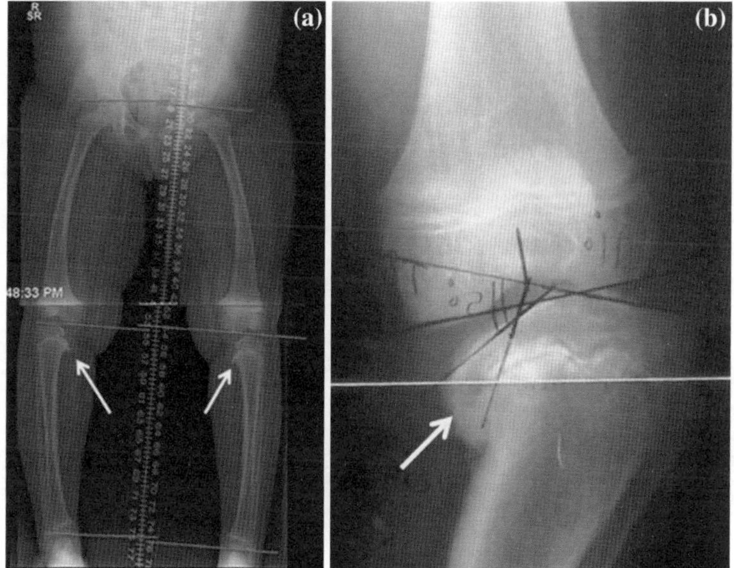

Fig. 7.13 Radiological changes in Blount's disease. (**a**) Long radiographs (*scanogram*) of a 3-year-old girl showing the proximal tibial metaphyseal beaking (*arrow*). (**b**) A 4-year-old boy with depression of the medial tibial plateau and fusion of the growth plate on the medial side (*arrow*). Note the difference between the medial and lateral sides of the tibial growth plate

Adolescent type:

Incidence:

- Less common than the infantile type.
- The disease is common in adolescent obese boys.

Clinical picture:

- Can be unilateral or bilateral.
- Radiograph will show varus deformity of distal femur and proximal tibia with less obvious affection of the growth plate (Fig. 7.14).

Treatment:

- Orthopedic referral of surgical intervention (osteotomy).

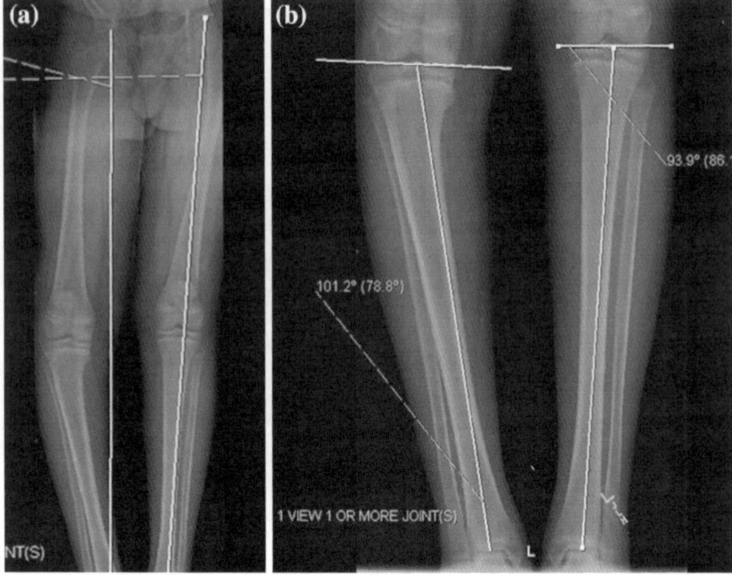

Fig. 7.14 Radiographic changes of adolescent tibia vara. A 15-year-old black male presented with unilateral adolescent tibia vara on the right side. (**a**) Scanogram shows varus alignment on the right side with the mechanical axis medial to the joint. (**b**) Radiographs of the leg shows varus deformity of the proximal tibia

KNEE PAIN IN CHILDREN

Cause:

- Patellofemoral pain:
  - Patellar overload.
  - Chondromalacia patellae.
  - Patellar subluxation.

- Extensor mechanism inflammation:
    - Osgood–Schlatter.
    - Jumper's knee.
    - Sinding–Larsen–Johansson Disorder.
- Tumor:
    - Osteosarcoma.
    - Ewing sarcoma.
    - Osteoid osteoma.
    - Unicameral bone cyst.
- **Vascular**:
    - Osteochondritis dissecans.
- **Traumatic**:
    - Meniscal tear.
    - Ligament injury.
    - Knee plica.
    - Stress fractures:
        - Proximal tibial stress fractures.
- **Infections**.
    - Septic arthritis.
    - Osteomyelitis of the proximal tibia or distal femur.
    - Septic bursitis (Fig. 7.15)
        - Prepatellar bursitis.
        - Infrapatellar bursitis.
- **Rheumatologic condition**:
    - Juvenile rheumatoid arthritis.
- **Referred pain**:
    - Hip pathology, e.g., SCFE.

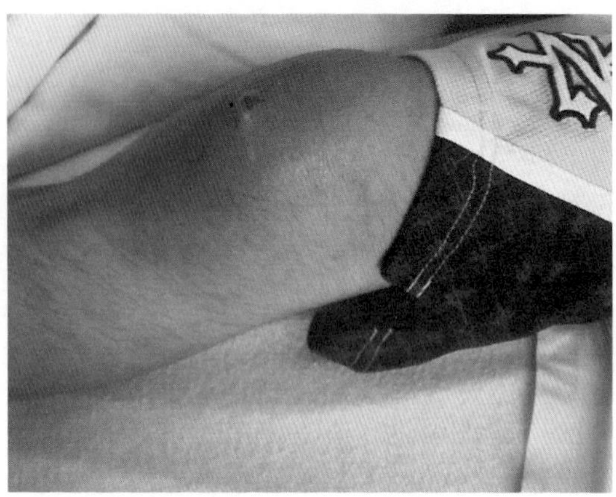

Fig. 7.15 Knee bursitis. A 14-year-old boy with 4 days history of anterior knee pain, swelling, and redness. Examination shows inflammation of the prepatellar bursa (pre patellar buritis). The patient was treated with antibiotic with complete resolution of his symptoms

- **Miscellaneous**:
  - Growing pain.
  - Bipartite patella.

Approach to child with knee pain

- History:
  - Pain:
    - Onset, duration, progression, and exact location.
  - Precipitating factor:
    - The exact mechanism of injury.
  - General manifestation of infection (fever, chills)
  - Ability to bear weight

- **Ability of the child to continue his/her usual activities**.
  - **Children with simple growing pain can continue all their regular activities**.

- Physical exam:
  - **Examination of the ipsilateral hip**.
  - Examination of the contralateral knee (for comparison).
  - Examination of the affected knee.
    - Range of motion, active and passive, is the most sensitive indicator of arthritis.

- Imaging:
  - Radiographs of the affected knee.
  - Radiographs of the ipsilateral hip.
  - If there is persistence of pain with negative plain radiographs, consider obtaining MRI.

OSGOOD–SCHLATTER DISEASE

Definition:

- Inflammation of the insertion of the patellar tendon in the tibial tubercle (tibial tubercle apophysitis).

Incidence:

- More common in
  - Boys.
  - In children active in sports that require repeated of knee movement like soccer.

Clinical presentation:

- Patient will complain of anterior knee pain and swelling.
    - □ The pain is related to physical activity.
- On examination; tender swelling at the tibial tubercle (Fig. 7.16).

Radiographs of the knee (Fig. 7.17)

- Enlargement of the tibial tubercle (tibial apophysis).
- Possible fragmentation of the tibial apophysis.

Treatment:

- First line:
    - □ Decrease activity (the child may have to stop practicing sports for few months).
    - □ NSAIDs.

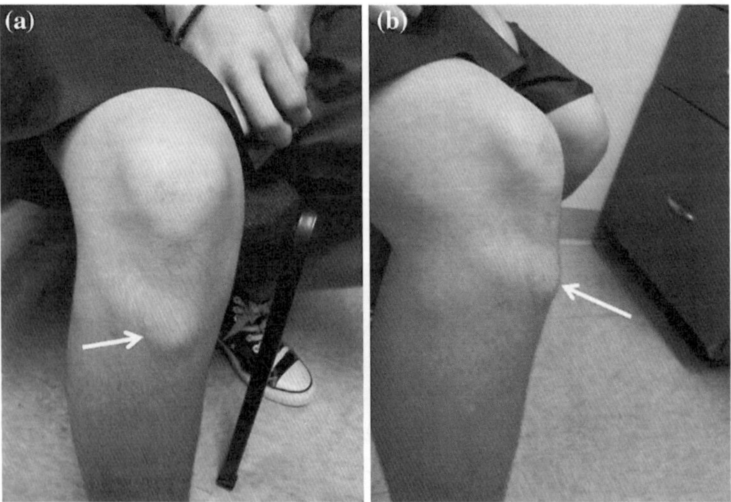

Fig. 7.16 Osgood Schlatter. (A and B) A 14-year-old boy soccer player with right knee pain. Examination shows anterior knee swelling over the tibial tubercle (*arrow*)

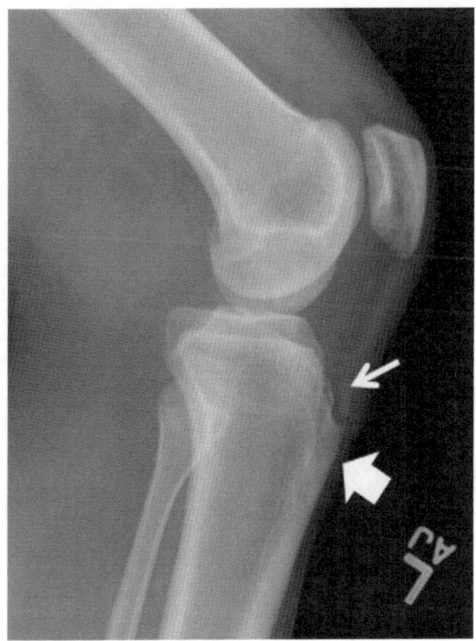

Fig. 7.17 Radiological signs of Osgood Schlatter. Radiographs of a patient with Osgood–Schlatter disease. *Wide arrow* points to the enlarged tibial tubercle. *Small arrow* points to the small fragment of calcification and fragmentation within the patellar ligament

- If no improvement:
  - Physical therapy.
    - Stretching of the hamstring.
    - Quadriceps strengthening.
  - Brace (knee immobilizer).
- Orthopedic referral is rarely needed.

SINDING–LARSEN–JOHANSSON DISORDER

- Inflammation of the distal pole of the patella (traction apophysitis).
- Affected population and clinical presentation is similar to Osgood–Schlatter disease except that pain in related to the lower end of the patella.
- Treatment: as Osgood–Schlatter disease.

Jumper's knee:

- Inflammation of the patellar tendon.
- Affected population and clinical presentation is similar to Osgood–Schlatter disease except that pain in related to the patellar tendon.
- Treatment: as Osgood–Schlatter disease.

OSTEOCHONDRITIS DISSECANS

Definition:

- Osteochondritis dissecans occurs when an area of the bone close to the articular cartilage becomes avascular and ultimately separates from the underlying bone.

Causes:

- The exact cause is unknown. Theories include:
  - Trauma.
  - Repeated stresses.
  - Familial predisposition.

Location:

- Most lesions located on the **lateral portion of the medial femoral condyle** (Fig. 7.18).

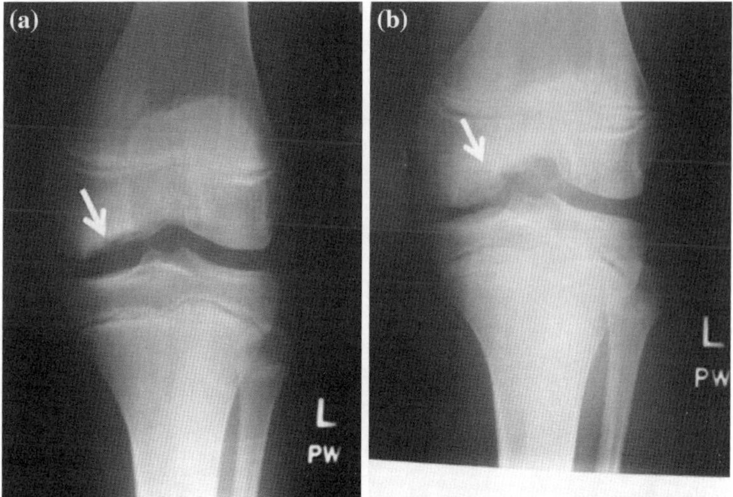

Fig. 7.18 Osteochondritis dissecans. Radiographs of left knee (**a**: anteroposterior; **b**: Notch view) showing osteochondral defect on the medial femoral condyle

Clinical presentation:

- Vague knee pain.
- **Recurrent effusion**.
- If the fragment become loose or separated, there can be crepitation, popping, and occasionally locking of the knee.
- Physical finding:
  - Parapatellar tenderness.
  - Quadriceps atrophy.
  - Pain with range of motion.
  - Knee effusion.

Diagnosis:

- Radiograph will show:
  - Subchondral fragment with a lucent line separating it from the condyle (Fig 7.18).

- MRI is more sensitive and can detect early cases.
- Arthroscopy is the most reliable method in evaluating the status of the lesion.

Treatment

- Most stable lesions will heal spontaneously.
- Orthopedic referral.
  - MRI will guide the treatment plan:
  - If the lesion is stable (non detached) from underlying bone:
    - Activity modification.
    - Physical therapy for strengthening.
  - If the lesion is detached from the underlying bone or no improvement with non operative management:
    - Operative treatment (arthroscopy) for either fixation of the fragment or excising it.

PATELLAR INSTABILITY (RECURRENT PATELLAR SUBLUXATION AND DISLOCATION)

Anatomical considerations:

- The patella lies in the trochlear groove of the distal femur.
- The patella almost always dislocate **laterally**.
- The line of pull of the quadriceps tendon is not in line with patellar tendon. The angle between them is called Q angle (Fig. 7.19).
  - Factors that increase the Q angle will cause more susceptibility to dislocation and subluxation.

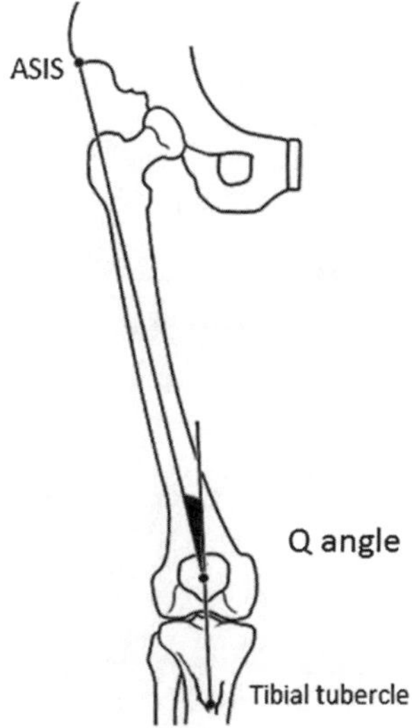

Fig. 7.19 Q angle is the angle between the axis of the femur (from the ASIS to the patella) and the axis of the patellar ligament (from patella to tibial tubercle)

- The main restrain against lateral patellar dislocation is **the medial patello-femoral ligament** which extends from the medial femoral condyle to the medial patella.

Predisposing factors for recurrent dislocation and subluxation:

- Dysplastic trochlear groove.
- Patella alta (high riding patella).
  - The patella will not be seating in the trochlear groove as it will lie above it.
- Increase Q angle:
  - Genu valgum.
  - Increased femoral anteversion.
  - External tibial torsion.
  - Laterally positioned tibial tuberosity.

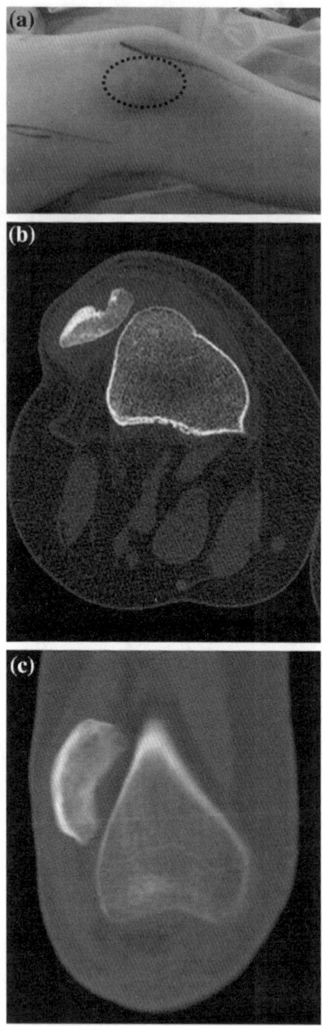

Fig. 7.20 Chronically dislocated patella. A 17-year-old patient with right chronically dislocated patella since early childhood. (**a**) The patella lies on the outer aspect of the knee (*dotted circle*). Axial CT (**b**) and coronal reformat (**c**) shows the abnormal shape of the patella which is lying outside the groove

- VMO (vastus medialis obliqus) insufficiency:
  - The muscle fibers of the quadriceps responsible for pulling the patella medically.
- Syndromes associated increased laxity.
  - **Down syndrome**.
  - Ehlers–Danlos syndrome.
  - Marfan's syndrome.
  - Turner's syndrome.

CLINICAL PRESENTATION

Classification of patellar dislocation by history

- Recurrent patellar dislocation.
  - History of repeated dislocation.
  - With the dislocation event the patella will lie on the lateral side of the knee and has to be reduced back by the patient himself or someone else.
- Recurrent patellar subluxation.
  - History of repeated subluxation. The patient feels that the patella is unstable, but no full dislocation.
  - **Usually associated with knee pain**.
- Habitual dislocation of the patella.
  - Dislocation of the patella each time the patient bends his knee.
- Chronically dislocated patella.
  - The patella had been always in a dislocated position (Fig. 7.20).

- Examination of the lower extremity for the predisposing factors.
- General examination for signs of increased laxity (e.g., elbow hyperextension).
- The condition may be bilateral.
- Parapatellar tenderness.
- Mild effusion.
- **Specific test for patellar stability**:
  - **Tracking of the patella (J sign)**
    - Assess patellar tracking by flexing and extending the knee.
    - Positive J sign with patella deviating laterally at the end of extension.
  - **Apprehension sign**
    - Positive result (quadriceps contraction or apprehension look on the face) indicates instability (Fig. 7.21):.

Imaging:

- **Radiographs**:
  - Sunrise view (Fig. 7.22) will show the lateral tilt of the patella.
- **CT and MRI**
  - Can better delineate the tilt of the patella.
  - May show trochlear hypoplasia.

Treatment

- After first dislocation:
  - Knee immobilizer for 1–2 weeks followed by physical therapy.
- Recurrent dislocation:

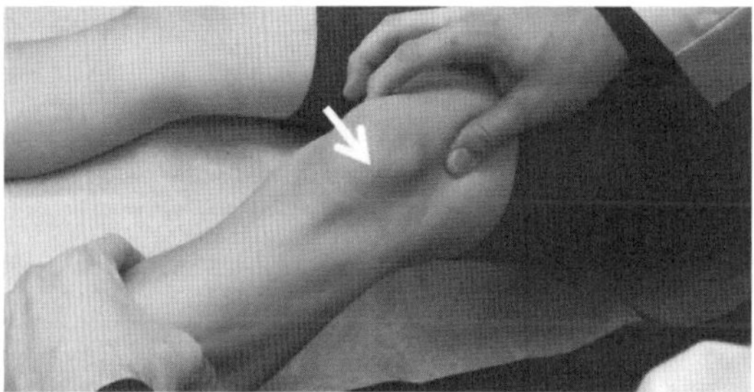

Fig. 7.21 Apprehension sign. The patient lies supine on the table with the knee in 20–30° of flexion and the quadriceps relaxed. The examiner carefully glides the patella laterally observing for the apprehension sign. A positive test is the presence of this reaction by the patient

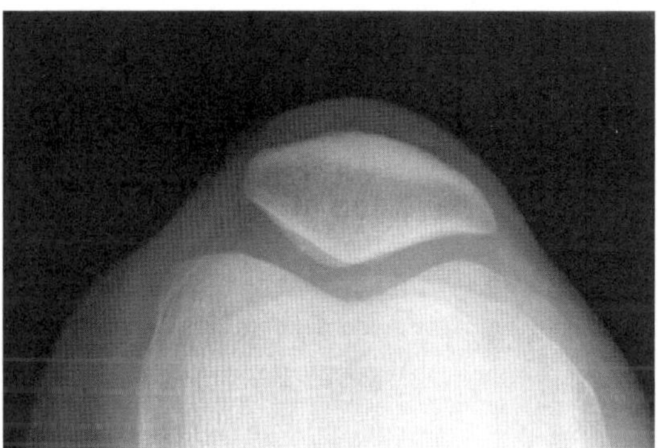

Fig. 7.22 Sunrise view. This view shows the position of the patella in the trochlear groove

- Therapy: isometric quadriceps-strengthening exercise
- Orthopedic referral: Surgery is indicated if conservative treatment fails.
  - □ Correction of underlying deformity (e.g., genu valgum)
  - □ Reconstruction of the medial patellofemoral ligament.

POPLITEAL CYST (BAKER CYST)

Definition:

- Baker cyst is common in children.
- It is a cystic mass filled with gelatinous material that develops in the popliteal fossa.

Clinical presentation:

- It is more common in boys.
- Usually found on the medial side of the popliteal fossa (Fig. 7.23).
- Painless.
- It can disappear spontaneously within 6–24 months.

Treatment

- **A prolonged period of observation is recommended before considering surgical excision**.
- Indication of further diagnostic evaluation (Atypical finding):
    - □ Tenderness.
    - □ Firmness (solid mass).
    - □ History of rapid enlargement.
    - □ Pain.
- If swelling persists for more than 12 months or atypical findings, orthopedic referral for excision.

PATELLOFEMORAL PAIN SYNDROME

Other names

- Chondromalacia patella (misnomer as the patellar cartilage is intact).
- Patellar overload syndrome.

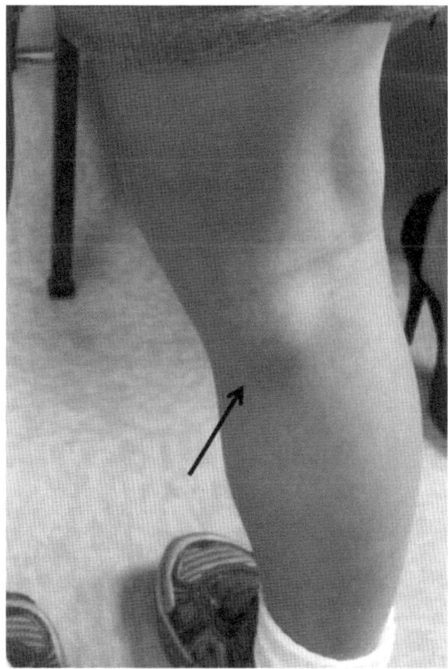

Fig. 7.23 Popliteal Cyst (Baker Cyst). A 6-year-old boy brought with his family because of non painful swelling on the back of the right the knee. The *arrow* shows the baker's cyst on medial side of the back of the knee

Definition:

- Knee pain due to increased loads of the patellofemoral joint.

Clinical presentation:

- A common cause of knee pain in **adolescent girls**.
- Anterior knee pain that increases with activity.

Predisposing factor:

- Certain mechanical factors lead to increased stress on the patellar cartilage by causing uneven distribution of stresses through the articulation between patella and trochlea.

- Miserable malalignment syndrome:
  - Common rotational malalignment in adolescent females.
  - It consists of the following three elements (Fig. 7.24):
    - Increased femoral anteversion.
    - External tibial torsion.
    - Pes planus (flat foot).
- Increased Q angle.

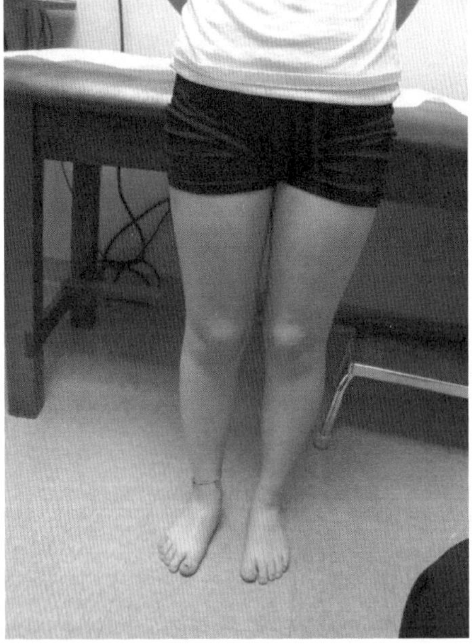

Fig. 7.24 Miserable malalignment syndrome. A 15-year-old girl with 2 years history of knee pain. Patient had excess femoral anteversion as manifested by her patellas pointing inward. Despite the inward position of the patella, her foot is still pointing forward due to her external tibial torsion

Treatment

- Ice, rest, NSAID.
- Physical therapy:
  - Quadriceps strengthening and hamstring stretching.
- Patellar stabilizing braces may be needed.
- If no improvement: orthopedic referral (surgery is rarely indicated, results are not always very promising).

CONGENITAL CONDITION AFFECTING THE LEG

Fibular hemimelia:

Definition:

- Congenital condition with abnormal development of the fibula.
- Considered type of longitudinal deficiency of the limb.

Incidence:

- One in every 100,000 live birth.

Clinical presentation:

- **Limb length discrepancy** (**LLD**). The affected side will be shorter than the other side (Fig. 7.25).
  - Positive Galeazzi sign.
  - Limping.
- Foot:
  - Deficiency of the lateral rays of the foot (Fig. 7.25).
  - Abnormal development of the carpal bone.
  - Valgus deformity of the foot.

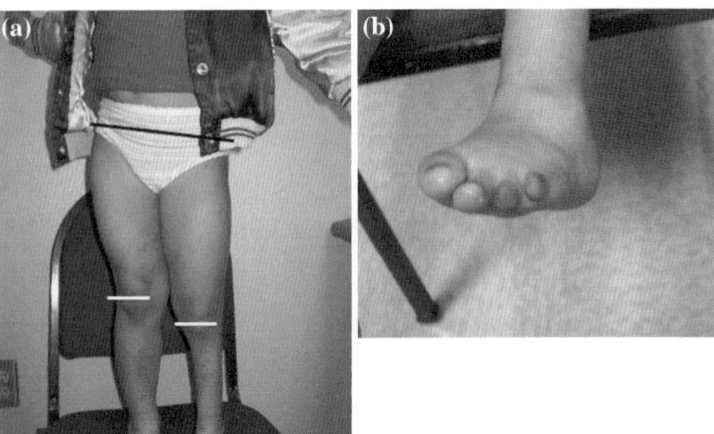

Fig. 7.25 Fibular hemimelia. A 4-year-old girl with left side fibular hemimelia. (**a**) The patient has 5 cm limb length discrepancy (*white line* indicating the knee level bilaterally), with pelvic obliquity (*black line*). (**b**) The left foot shows the absence of the most lateral ray

- Knee:
  - Deficiency of the anterior cruciate ligament.
  - Valgus deformity of the knee due to abnormal shape of the lateral femoral condyle.

Radiographs:

- Scanogram (radiographs of the whole lower extremity (Fig. 7.26):
  - LLD.
  - Valgus deformity to the extremity.

Management:

- Orthopedic referral (see Chap. 2).

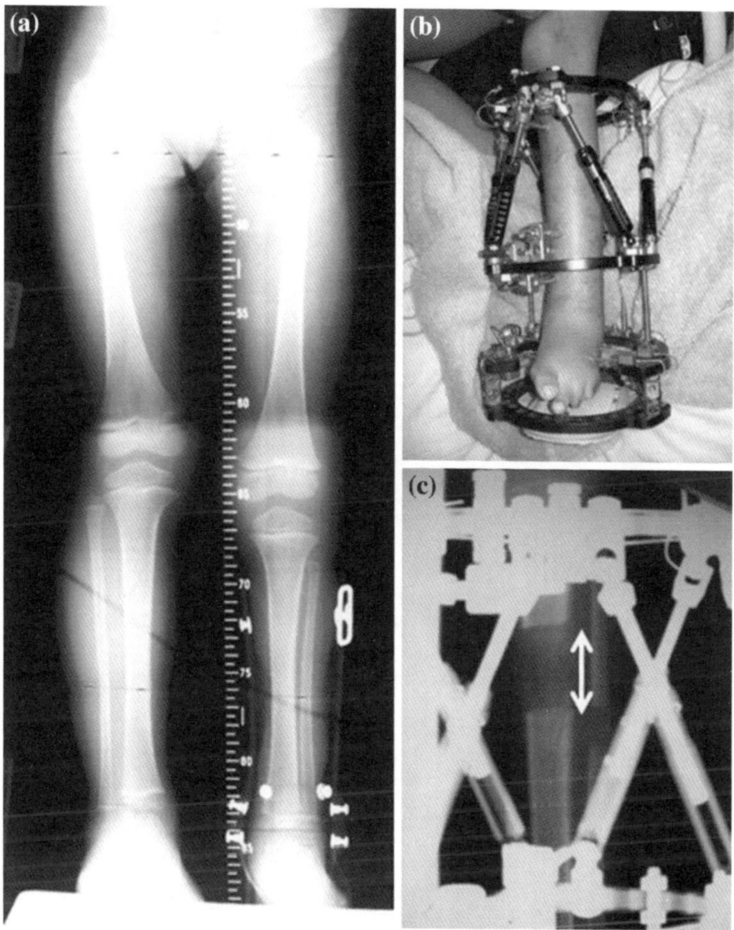

Fig. 7.26 Long radiographs of both lower extremity (*scanogram*) of the patient in Fig. 7.25. (**a**) The radiograph shows the 5 cm difference between both sides. (**b**) External fixator was applied and distraction osteogenesis was done to lengthen the affected bone. (**c**) 5 cm of new bone regenerate was formed (*arrow*)

CONGENTIAL PSEUDOARTHROSIS OF THE TIBIA

Definition:

- Developmental condition of persistent non union of distal part of tibia.
- Pseudoarthrosis: means non union with excess motion between the two ends of the bone (false joint).

Clinical presentation:

- The child will have anterolateral bowing of his tibia (Fig. 7.27).
- The condition usually occurs spontaneously in the second or third years of life.
    - Spontaneous fracture of the leg will occur (with minimal or no history of trauma).
- About 50 % of these children will have **neurofibromatosis**.
- Persistence of non union (or recurrence of fracture) despite multiple surgical interventions.
- Pain is minimal.

Radiograph:

- Anterolateral Bowing of the tibia (Fig. 7.27).
- Atrophic non union of the distal tibia and fibula (atrophy and sclerosis of the bone ends).

Management:

- Orthopedic referral.
    - **The non union is very resistant to healing** (one of the most tough conditions to treat in pediatric orthopedic).
    - Sometimes amputation of the extremity is the only possible method of treatment especially after multiple failures to achieve union or multiple re-fractures.

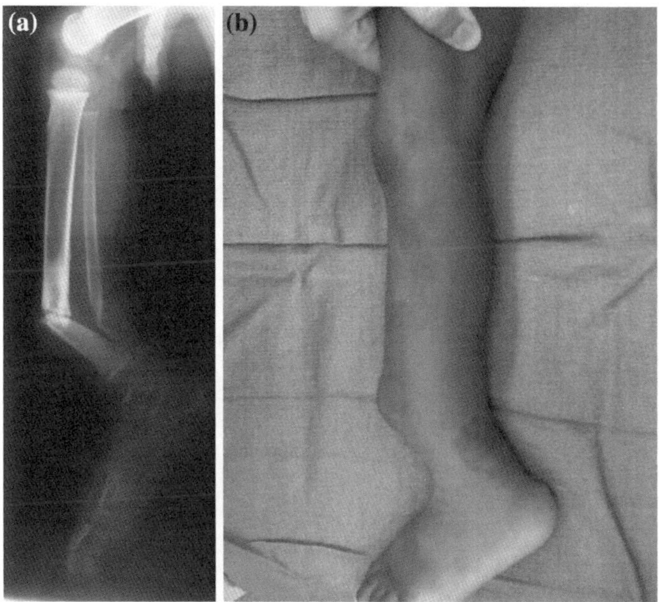

Fig. 7.27 Congenital pseudoarthrosis of the tibia. A 3-year-old boy with spontaneous fracture of the left leg. (**a**) Radiograph shows fracture with non union (pseudoarthrosis) of the tibia and fibula. (**b**) Clinical picture of the leg shows the anterior bowing of the leg

Bowing of the leg:

- There are different types of bowing of the leg.
- The direction of the bow is the direction of the apex of the bow.

Anterolateral bowing:

- Usually associated with congenital pseudoarthrosis of the tibia (Fig. 7.27).
- Most dangerous type of tibial bowing.
- Treatment:
  - Orthopedic referral for bracing.

Posteromedial bowing of the tibia

- Usually resolve spontaneously with growth.
- Takes about 7–10 years to remodel.
- Associated with:
  - Calcaneovalgus deformity of the foot.
  - LLD (the affected leg is usually shorted by about 3–5 cm at the end of growth).
- **Treatment**:
  - Orthopedic referral for management of LLD.
  - No need for bracing (no increased risk of fractures).

Anteromedial bowing of the tibia:

- Associated with fibular hemimelia.

HIGH YIELD FACTS

- Genu varum is normal finding until the age of 2 years old, and then the knee alignment changes to valgus that reaches maximum by the age of 3 years old.
- At about the age of 8 years, most children will reach adult alignment of 7 degrees of valgus.
- Presence of bowlegged after 24 months, unilateral, and > 20 degree clinically should be evaluated.
- Children with infantile Blount's disease who are older than 3 years or failed brace treatment should be referred to orthopedics for surgical correction.
- Patellofemoral pain is common in adolescent girls. Treatment is mainly non operative.
- Genu valgum, patella alta, and hypoplastic trochlear groove are among the predisposing factors for patellar instability.
- Patellar instability can present with recurrent attacks of patellar dislocation or patellar subluxation and pain.
- Popliteal cyst is a common condition in children. Observation for up to 12 months is the appropriate first treatment.

- **Rest**, **NSAIDs**, quadriceps stretching and strengthening, and cross training is the most appropriate initial management of Osgood–Schlatter disease.
- Anterolateral bowing of the tibia is associated with congenital pseudoarthrosis of the tibia (a condition which is very resistant to treatment).
- Posteromedial bowing of the tibia is associated with limb length discrepancy.

CLINICAL SCENARIOS

The presenting patient	The most probable diagnosis and plan of action
13-year-old girl soccer player complaining that she had three dislocation of her "knee cap" in the last year during her practice. On exam, the patient has obvious bilateral genu valgum	Patellar instability with genu valgum ▪ Orthopedic referral for correction of the deformity
15-year-old boy basketball player complaining of right knee pain and swelling during and after practice, he said his knee is locking. Physical examination showed atrophy and weakness of the quadriceps muscle, tenderness on the media condyle of the femur, and mild joint effusion, radiograph on the right knee revealed lucency in the medial femoral condyle. What is the most likely diagnosis?	Osteochondritis dissecans Orthopedic referral ▪ MRI ▪ If the lesion is stable (not separated from the underlying bone), conservative treatment for 3 months

(continued)

(CONTINUED)

The presenting patient	The most probable diagnosis and plan of action
12-year-old football player complained of leg pain for the last 1 month which is more after the games, physical examination showed swelling, tenderness to palpation of tibial tuberosity.	Osgood-Schlatter disease Treatment ■ NSAID ■ Avoid excessive sport activities for few weeks
18-month-old boy brought to the clinic by his mother for deformity of the left leg. On exam, patient has multiple cafe au lait patches on the trunk and back. The left leg is bowed with abnormal movement in the lower third. Radiographs show a fracture of the tibia and fibula with sclerotic edges	Neurofibromatosis with congenital pseudoarthrosis of the tibia ■ Orthopedic referral ■ Warn the family that the condition will need multiple surgeries and may end in amputation

REFERENCES

Staheli LT. Knee and tibia. In: Staheli LT, editor. Practice of pediatric orthopedics. 2nd ed. Philadelphia: Lippincott Williams and Wilkins; 2006. p. 143–58.

Sponseller PD. Bone, joint, and muscle problems. In McMillanJA, Feigin RD, DeAngelis C, Jones MD, editors. Oski's Pediatrics: Principles and practice. 4th ed. Philadelphia: Lippincott Williams and Wilkins; 2006. p. 2470–2504.

Kocher MS, Tucker R, Ganley TJ, Flynn JM. Management of osteochondritis dissecans of the knee: Current concepts review. American Journal of Sports Medicine. 2006;34(7):1181–91.

Davids JR. Pediatric knee. Clinical assessment and common disorders. Pediatric Clinics of North America. 1996;43(5):1067–90.

Lehman WB, Abdelgawad AA, Sala DA. Congenital tibial dysplasia (congenital pseudoarthrosis of the tibia): an atypical variation. Journal of Pediatric Orthopaedics B. 2009;18(5):211–3.

Herzenberg JE, Paley D. Leg lengthening in children. Current Opinion in Pediatrics. 1998;10(1):95–7.

Chapter 8
Foot

Amr Abdelgawad and Osama Naga

INTRODUCTION

Normal anatomy of the foot:

- The foot bones are:
  - 7 carpal bones:
    - Talus, Calcaneus, Navicular, Cuboid, and three Cuneiforms. (Fig. 8.1)
  - 5 metacarpals
  - 14 phalanges (two phalanges in the big toe and three in the lateral four toes)
- Subtalar joint is the joint between the talus and calcaneus

Nomenclature (see also\introduction):

- Supination: inward rotation of the subtalar joint (Fig. 8.2).
- Pronation: outward rotation of the subtalar joint (Fig. 8.2).
- Forefoot: the anterior part of the foot (metatarsus and phalanges).
- Hindfoot: the posterior part of the foot (talus and calcaneus).
- Taleps: foot
- **Positions and deformities of the foot** (Fig. 8.3):
  - Equines: plantar flexion of the ankle and the foot.
  - Calcaneus: dorsiflexion of the ankle and the foot.
  - Varus: inward position of the foot and ankle.
  - Valgus: outward position of the foot and ankle.
  - Cavus: high arch deformity.

A. Abdelgawad and O. Naga (eds.), *Pediatric Orthopedics*,
DOI: 10.1007/978-1-4614-7126-4_8,

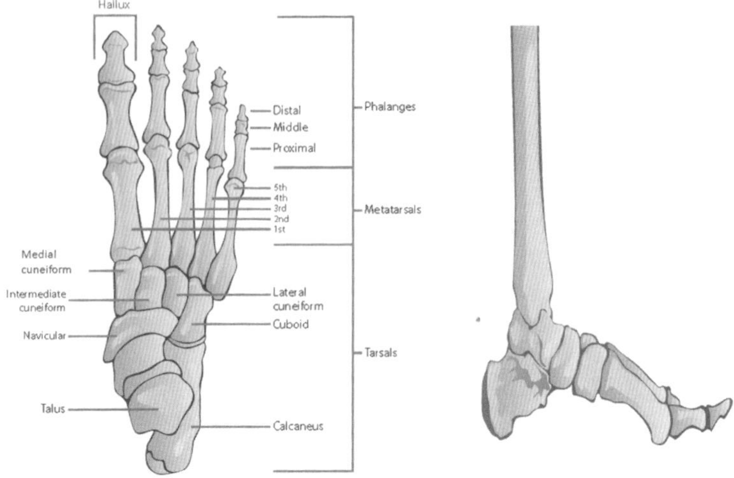

Fig. 8.1 Anatomy of the foot

INTOEING

- **One of the most common pediatric complaints related to musculoskeletal system.**
- **The vast majority of cases of intoeing represents a normal development and does not need orthopedic referral.**

Causes of intoeing:

- **Foot causes:**
  - **Metatarsus adductus**.
- **Leg causes:**
  - **Internal tibial torsion (ITT).**
- **Hip causes:**
  - **Excess femoral anteversion**.

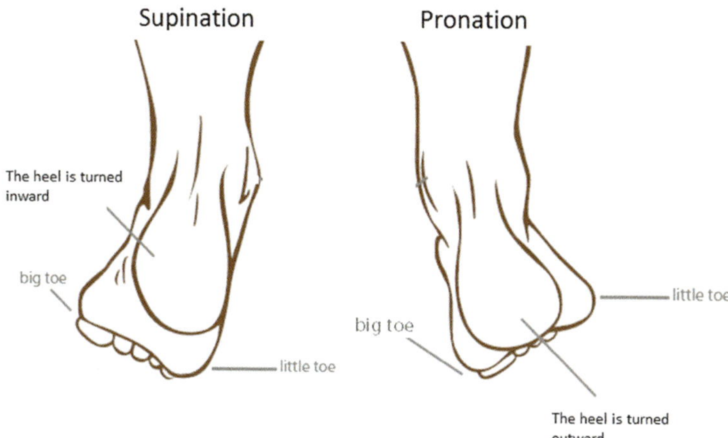

Fig. 8.2 Movement of the subtalar joint. Right foot (seen from the *back*) in supination (*inward rotation*) and pronation (*outward rotation*). These movements occur at the level subtalar joint

Approach to a child with intoeing:

Four steps are used to assess the child with intoeing:

- **First: Foot progression angle**
  - To assess the direction of the foot when the child walks.
  - The child should walk about 30 feet.
    - It has to be a relatively long distance (in the hallway not in the exam room). (Fig. 8.4)
    - Most children will walk in front of the physician different than they would do in their real life.
    - When the child walks back and forth many times, he/she will be distracted enough to start walking in his/her "normal pattern".
- **Second: Assessment of the hip range of motion (assessment of version of the hip)**
  - Normally, external rotation is similar to or slightly more than internal rotation. If internal rotation is more than external rotation, this indicates excess femoral anteversion. (Fig. 8.5):

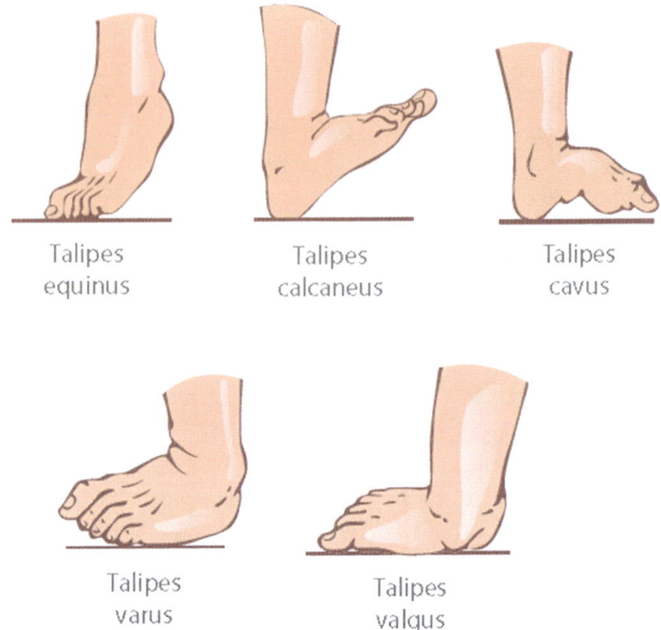

Fig. 8.3 Different position of the foot

- **Third: Assessment of the thigh foot angle (assessment of the tibial torsion)**
  - The thigh foot angle assesses the torsion of the tibia.
  - By the age of 8 years, the torsion of the tibia reaches its adult value which is about 15° externally. (Fig. 8.6)
- **Fourth: Assessment of the relation between the forefoot and the hindfoot (assessment of metatarsus adductus).**
  - Draw an imaginary line bisecting the ankle, this line should pass by the second toe (Fig. 8.7).
  - If it passes lateral to the third toe, this indicates metatarsus adductus.

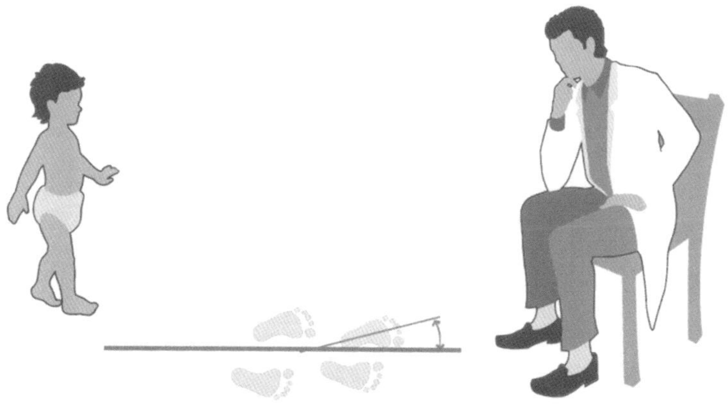

Fig. 8.4 Foot progression angle. The pediatrician should examine the child's gait and assess the relationship between the direction of the gait and the axis of the foot

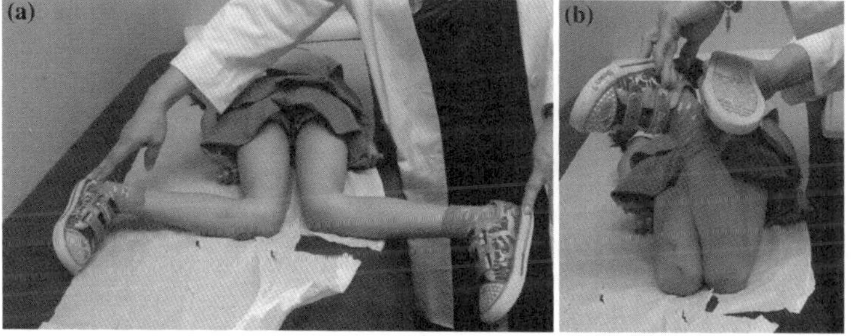

Fig. 8.5 Assessment of the hip range of motion. The patient is positioned prone with the knee flexed. Both hips are turned inward and then outward. Picture for 7-year-old girl with intoeing. Internal rotation in both hips is approximately 85° and external rotation is approximately 15°. This indicates excess femoral anteversion. **a** Assessment of hip internal rotation with the patient lying prone. **b** Assessment of hip external rotation with the patient lying prone

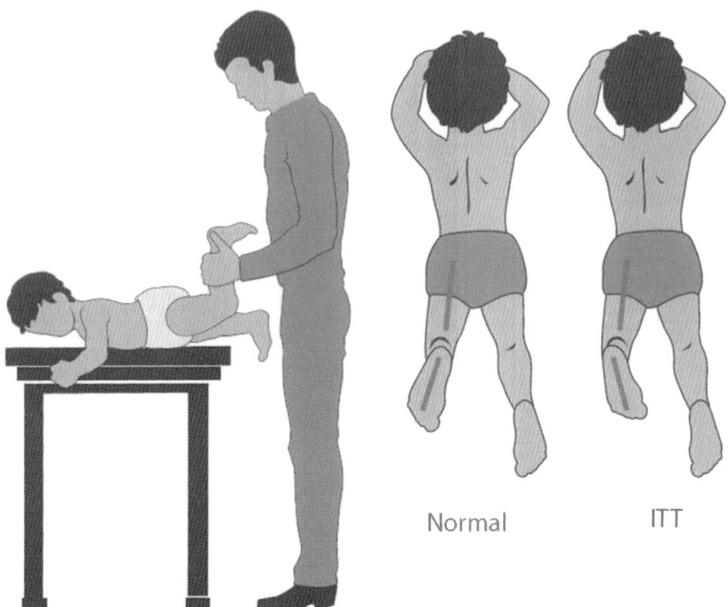

Fig. 8.6 Assessment of the tibial torsion (*thigh foot angle*). The child lies prone on the table and the physician assesses the angle between the thigh and foot with the knee flexed

EXCESS FEMORAL ANTEVERSION

Definition:

- Femoral anteversion is the angle between the neck of the femur and the shaft in the sagittal plane (Fig. 8.8).
- This angle is about 40° at birth and decreases when the child starts walking.
- Reaches the normal value (about 17°) by the age of 8 years.
- In diseases which affect the child's ability to walk (e.g., cerebral palsy), the child continues to have increased angle of femoral anteversion.
- Commonest cause of intoeing **between the ages of 3 and 8 years.**

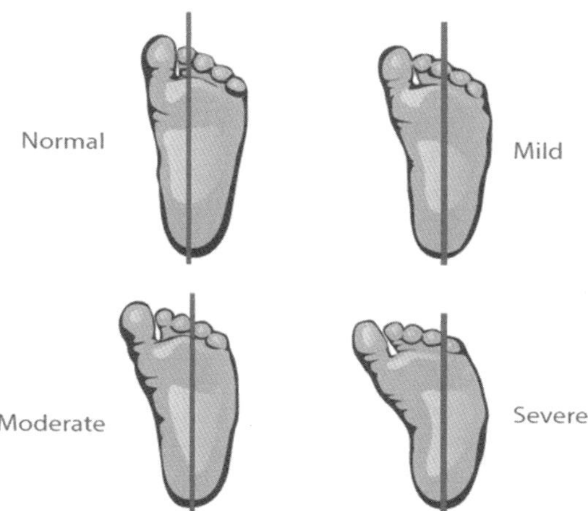

Fig. 8.7 Assessment of the relation between forefoot and hindfoot. An imaginary line is drawn bisecting the hindfoot. This line normally should pass by second toe. If the line passes lateral to second toe, it indicates metatarsus adductus

- Examination will show that hip internal rotation exceeds hip external rotation (Figs. 8.5, 8.9)
- Treatment:
  - No treatment is required.
    - Usually resolves spontaneously around the age of 8 years.
    - Bracing and orthotics do not change natural history of the condition.
    - If the condition does not improve by 9 years of age, orthopedic referral (Fig. 8.9):
      - Surgery (osteotomy to externally rotate the femur) is rarely indicated (Fig. 8.10).

INTERNAL TIBIAL TORSION

- Definition:
  - Inward rotation of the shaft of the tibia (Figs. 8.6, 8.11).

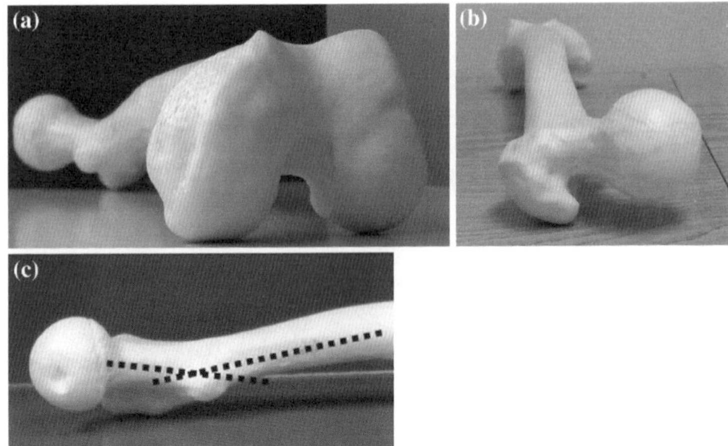

Fig. 8.8 Femoral anteversion. **a** and **b** Notice when the femur rests on the flat surface, the femoral head is elevated on that surface by the anteversion of the neck. **c** femoral anteversion is the angle between the femoral neck and the shaft in the sagittal plane (dotted lines)

- It is considered normal finding in newborn due to intrauterine position.
- **ITT is the most common cause of intoeing**.
    - Usually seen in infants around the age of 2–3 years.
- The thigh foot angle will show the ITT (Fig. 8.11)
- Treatment:
    - No treatment is required.
        - Usually resolves spontaneously over the first few years of life.
        - Bracing and orthotics do not change natural history of the condition.
        - If the condition does not improve by 4 years of age, orthopedic referral (Fig. 8.12):
            - Surgery (osteotomy to externally rotate the leg) is rarely indicated.

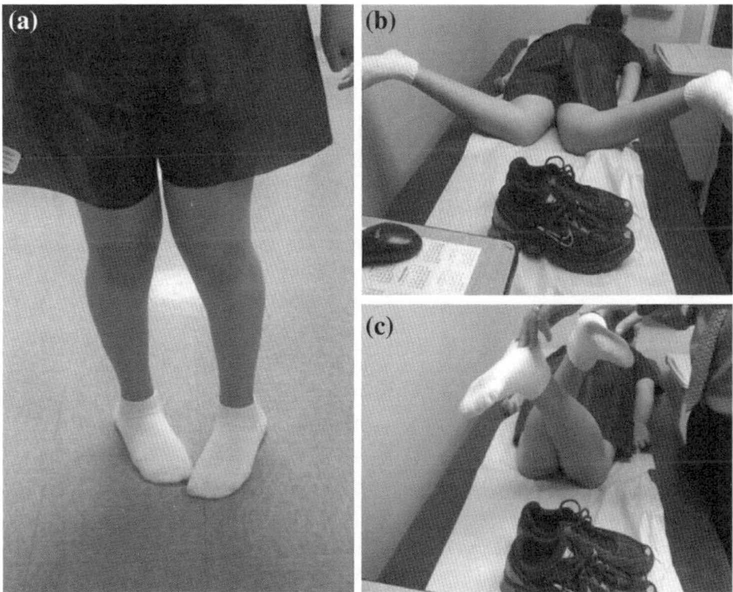

Fig. 8.9 A 12-year-old girl with severe intoeing (notice the inward position of both patellae) (**a**). Examination shows increase hip internal rotation (**b**) compared to external rotation (**c**)

METATARSUS ADDUCTUS (METATARSUS VARUS)

Definition:

- Adduction and inward position of the forefoot (Figs. 8.7, 8.13).

Etiology:

- Unknown.
- It may be related to intra-uterine position.

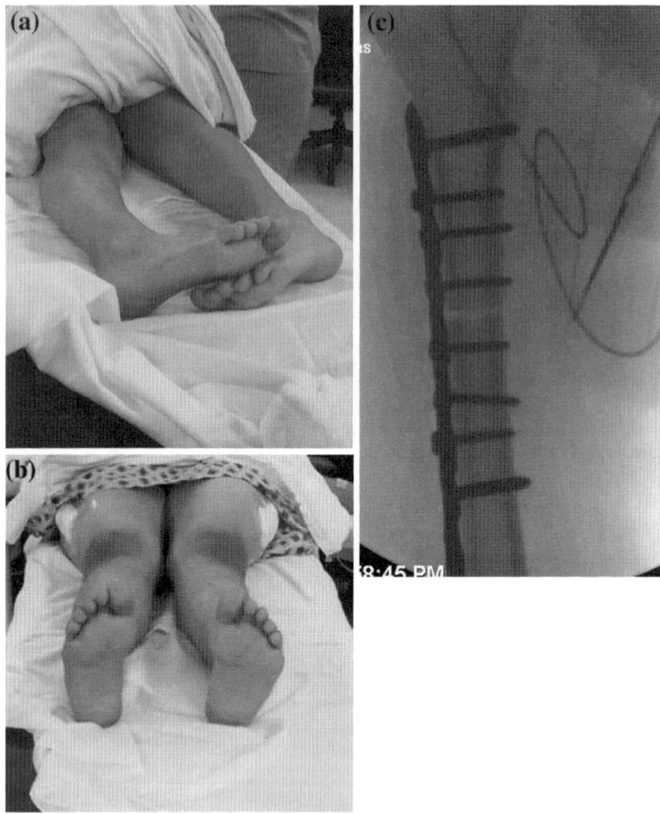

Fig. 8.10 The girl in Fig. 8.9 had been referred to orthopedic management. To the *left* (**a**), the patient is lying on the operating room bed before surgery with knees, legs, and feet internally rotated. Surgery (external rotation osteotomy) of both femurs was done. **b** Shows the patient immediately after surgery, **c** shows right intra-operative radiographs of the osteotomy with fixation using plate and screws

Clinical presentation:

- **The foot has a curved lateral border rather than being straight.** The forefoot will be adducted in relation of the hindfoot.
- Intoeing.

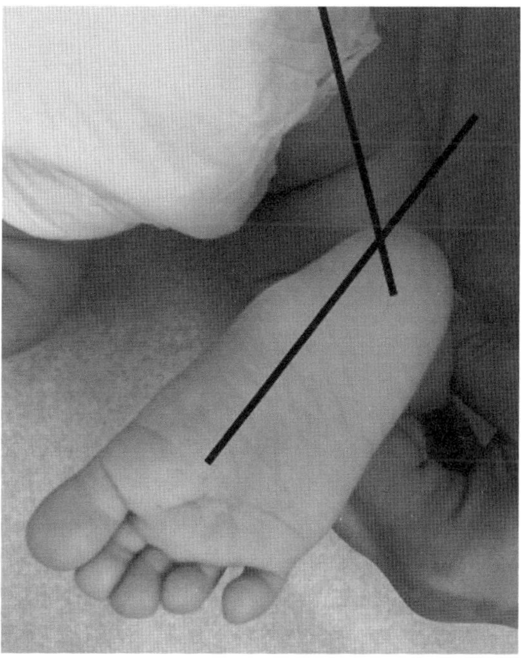

Fig. 8.11 Internal tibial torsion. A 16-month-old girl brought by her mother to the physician because of intoeing. Examination shows internal tibial torsion (notice the thigh foot angle)

- May be associated with other conditions related to uterine malposition (e.g. Hip dysplasia).
- Differentiated from clubfoot by the:
    - Absence of ankle equines (plantar flexion).
    - Absence of hindfoot varus (inward position of the heel).

Classification of severity:

- By drawing an imaginary line bisecting the ankle **with the foot in the maximum corrected position** (Figs. 8.7, 8.13).
    - Normally this line should be along the second toe.

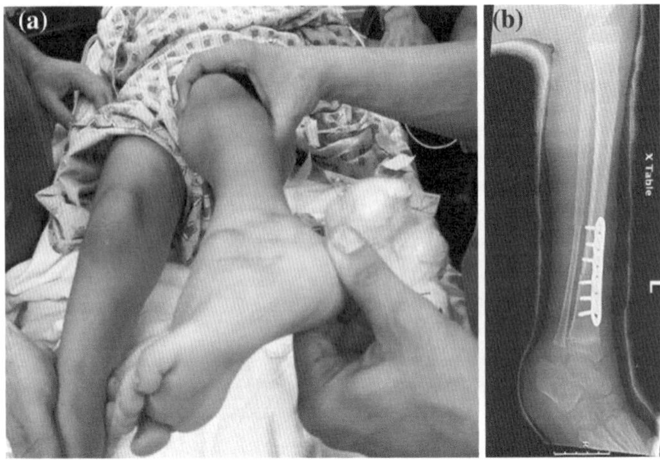

Fig. 8.12 A 10-year old with severe internal tibia torsion of the *left leg*. The foot is turned 90° in relation to the knee (**a**). Osteotomy was done to externally rotate the leg (**b**)

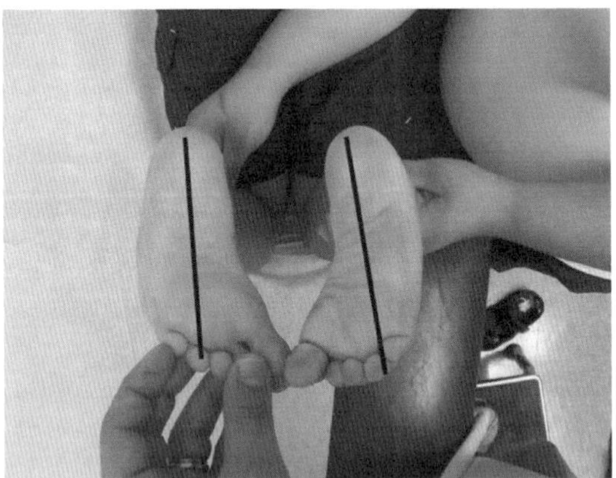

Fig. 8.13 Metatarsus adductus. Four years old with moderate metatarsus adductus on the *left side* and severe on the *right side* (patient is prone with flexed knee). Notice the curved lateral border of the foot

TABLE 8.1 THE CHANGES OF LOWER EXTREMITY ROTATION BY AGE

The structure	At birth	Adult value/age at which it is achieved
Tibial Tosion	About 0°	About 15° externally by the age 3 years old.
Femoral Aneversion	About 40° anteversion	About 17° by the age of 8 years old

- If it passes lateral to the third toe, it is considered moderate deformity.
- If it passes lateral to the fourth toe, it is considered a severe deformity.

Treatment:

- Most of the infants with metatarsus adductus will improve without interference.
- Observation in the first 6 months of life.
- **If the condition persists beyond 6 months of age and the deformity is rigid**, orthopedic referral for either serial casting or bracing. Surgery is rarely indicated.

Table 1 shows the changes in lower extremity rotation by age.

CLUBFOOT (TALIPES EQUINOVARUS)

Definition:

- Complex rigid deformity of the ankle and the foot.
- The foot will be in equines, varus, and forefoot adduction (Fig. 8.14).

Etiology:

- Unknown.
- Muscular, neurogenic, genetic, and connective tissue theories have been proposed.

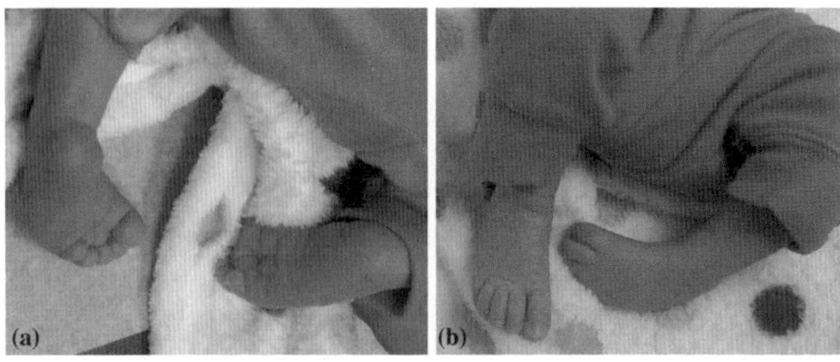

Fig. 8.14 Clubfoot. A 2-week-old girl with left clubfoot. Notice the deformity of the *left foot* (equinus, varus, forefoot supination, and cavus).(**a**), notice the hindfoot varus and equinus.(**b**), notice the forefoot adduction and equinus

Incidence:

- Affects about one in 1,000 live births.
- The condition runs in families and the incidence increases if there is positive family history:
  - **10 %** incidence of clubfoot if one sibling has clubfoot.
  - **25 %** incidence of clubfoot if one sibling and one parent have clubfoot.
- More common in boys (2:1)
- 50 % of the cases are bilateral.

Types:

- **Idiopathic:**
  - No other congenital condition can be found.
  - Most common type.
- **Postural:**
  - The deformity can be corrected easily by the examiner. **Not considered as a "real clubfoot"** (Fig. 8.15)
  - Will improve with time even without treatment.

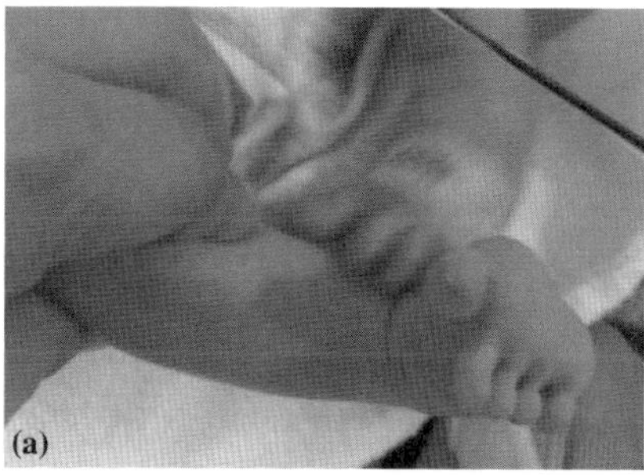

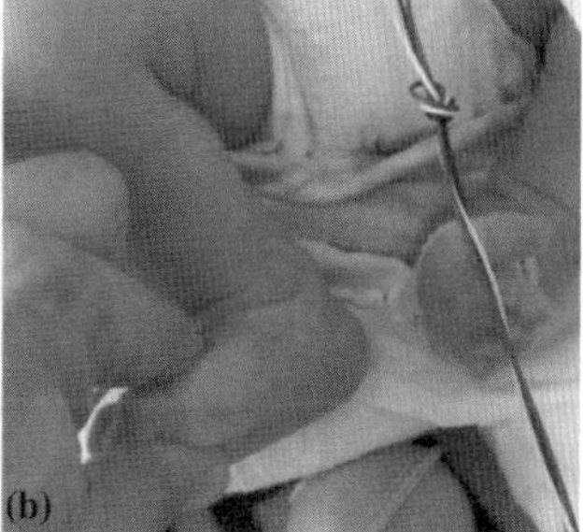

Fig. 8.15 Postural clubfoot.**(a)** A 2-day-old girl with orthopedic consult for 'right clubfoot.' **(b)**The deformity can be corrected fully by passive stretch. This is postural clubfoot with no treatment needed

- **Syndromic**:
  - Some congenital conditions are associated with clubfoot deformity e.g.:
    - **Arthrogryposis.**
    - Diastrophic dwarfism.
    - Freeman-Sheldon ("whistling face") syndrome.
- **Neuromuscular conditions**:
  - Myelomeningocele:
    - May have clubfoot deformity either at birth or shortly after (from the muscular imbalance).
  - Cerebral palsy:
    - Equinovarus deformity due to spasticity of gastrocnemius muscle and tibialis posterior muscle.

Clinical presentation:

- The disease can be diagnosed intra-uterine by ultrasound.
- The sensitivity of prenatal diagnosis improved after the 3D ultrasound.
- The deformity must be **rigid** (cannot be corrected by the examiner).
- Clubfoot has **three main deformities** (Fig. 8.14):

- Ankle and foot **equines** (plantar flexion of the ankle and the foot)
- Hindfoot **varus** (inward deviation of the heel)
- Forefoot **adduction** (inward position of the forefoot in relation to the hindfoot)

- Other components of the deformity:
  - Cavus of the foot (high arch foot).
  - ITT of the leg.
  - The size of the foot and the calf are smaller than the contra lateral side.

Management:

- NO radiographs are needed.
- Orthopedic referral:
  - **Two treatment options are currently utilized:**
    - Serial casting by Ponseti method.
    - Physical therapy and stretching (French method).
- The early referral is preferred (first weeks in life) as the foot is more flexible, however:
  - No need for urgent orthopedic consultation in the neonatology unit.
  - The treatment is still effective in older infants (results continue to be good up to the age of 6 months)

Ponseti Casting method

- New casting technique that became the standard of treatment for this condition. (Fig. 8.16):
- The success rate in correcting the foot is more than 90 %.
- It consists of serial casting with cast change every week.
- Correction usually requires 4–7 cast changes.
- After correction of the foot by serial casting, **brace (corrective shoes with a bar in-between the shoes to turn the feet outward) is then worn for about 2 years** (Fig. 8.17).
- Family compliance with using the brace was found to be associated with lower recurrence rate.

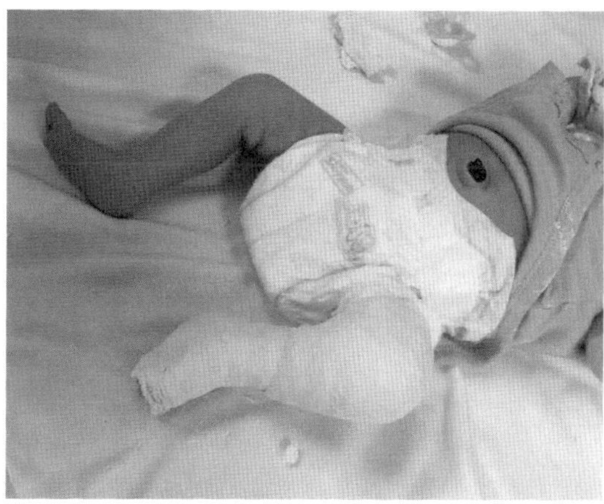

Fig. 8.16 Ponseti casting. Serial casting is done for the clubfoot to obtain correction

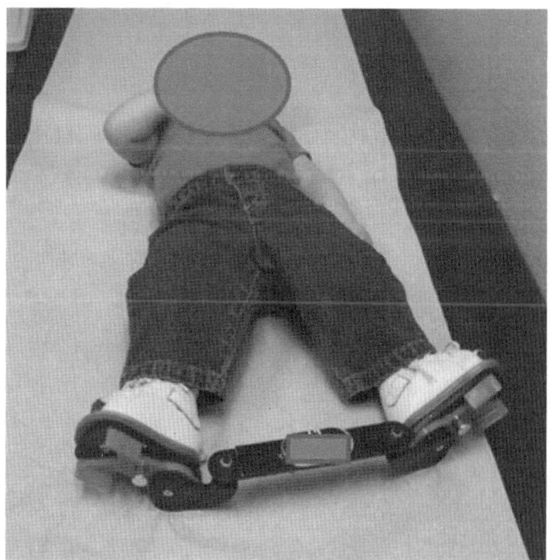

Fig. 8.17 Foot orthosis after Ponseti casting. The child has to wear special braces to keep the foot in external rotation (foot abduction orthosis)

Physical therapy and stretching method (French method):

- This treatment option is used more commonly in Europe than in United States.
- Requires intensive therapy sessions, more involvement and commitment from the parents' side.

CALCANEOVALGUS FOOT

Definition:

- The foot is in excessive dorsiflexion and valgus (Fig. 8.18).

Etiology:

- It is related to intrauterine position

Clinical Picture:

- The foot is in excess dorsiflxion and valgus to the degree that the dorsum of the foot is touching the front of the tibia.

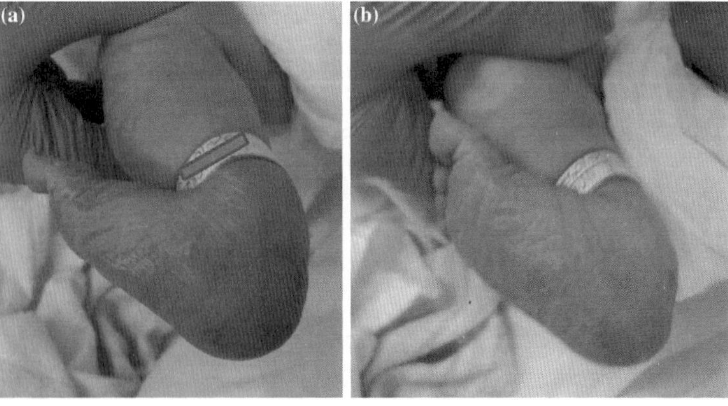

Fig. 8.18 Calcaneo-valgus foot. (**a**–**b**) Newborn baby with right foot deformity. The foot is in valgus and dorsiflexion (calcaneus position). No treatment required as the condition is self-limiting

- Calcaneovalgus may be associated with posteromedial bowing of the leg. In these cases it may lead to limb length discrepancy (see Chap. 7 The Knee/Leg).

Treatment:

- Most cases do not require treatment as they will improve with growth.
- If associated with posteromedial bowing of the leg, orthopedic referral for assessment of limb length discrepancy.

CAVUS FOOT

Definition:

- High Arched foot (Fig. 8.19)

Etiology:

- Cavus foot is an indication of **neurological affection**.
- In some cases, the neurological affection is very subtle and the cavus foot is the first and the only manifestation of the disease.
- **Causes:**
  - Charcot-Marrie-Tooth disease (most common cause of cavus foot in developed world)
  - Spina bifida (sacral level affection)
  - Intra thecal pathology (e.g. diastiatomelia, cord lipoma, tethered cord)

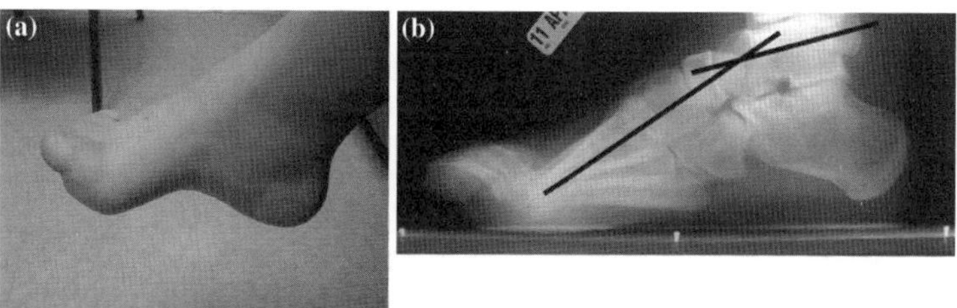

Fig. 8.19 Cavus foot. 15-year-old boy with Charcot-Marrie Tooth. Patient has right foot high arch deformity (cavus). Lateral radiograph of the foot (Standing) shows increased lateral talar—1st metatarsal (Meary's) angle

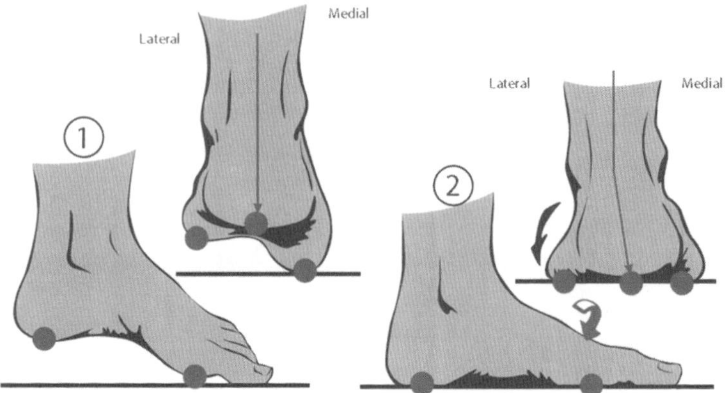

Fig. 8.20 Tripod theory: the foot rests on three pillars (heel, first ray, and fifith ray). With plantar flexion of the first ray (increased arch), the fifth metatarsal can only contact the ground through varus of the hindfoot

Pathophysiology:

- The foot normally rest on the floor on three pillars (the first ray, the fifth ray, and the heel) (the tri-pod theory) (Fig. 8.20).
- Tibialis anterior muscle becomes weaker than peroneus longus muscle, this will cause plantar flexion of the first ray. The foot will be resting on two pillar only (the heel and first ray).
- In order to keep the 5th toe on flat surface, the heel will turn into varus (cavo-varus foot) (Fig. 8.20).

Diagnosis:

- The foot will have high arch appearance (Fig. 8.19).
- It can be either unilateral or bilateral.
- Thorough neurological exam has to be done to identify the underlying cause.
- Assessment of the varus component of the deformity in order to identify if it is reversible or rigid by **Coleman block test** (Fig. 8.21).
- **Radiographs:**
  - Normally in the lateral view of the foot: a line across the talus should form a zero degree (in line) with a line drawn across

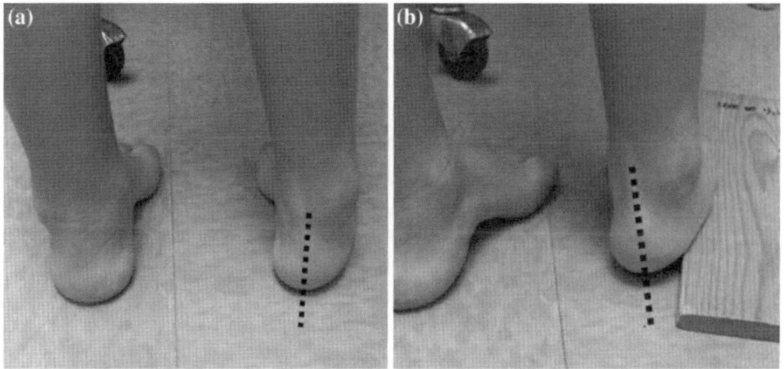

Fig. 8.21 Coleman block test. An 8-year-old boy with spina bifida and cavus foot. **a** Patient has varus deformity (heel pointing inwards, dotted line). **(b)** The heel varus was revered with applying ½″ block on the lateral aspect of the foot

the first metatarsal (lateral talar—1st metatarsal (Meary's) angle).

- In cavus foot: this angle is more than 5° convex dorsally (Fig. 8.19).

Treatment:

- Identification and treatment of the underlying cause. The patient may need MRI of the lumbar spine or Neurology/neurosurgery referral.
- Orthopedic referral:
  - Early: bracing by ankle foot orthosis (AFO)
  - If the condition becomes fixed, surgical intervention is indicated.
    - Plantar fascia release.
    - Osteotomy of the first ray to correct the deformity.

CLEFT FOOT

Definition and Clinical presentation:

- Congenital malformation of the foot with deep cleft in the foot (Fig. 8.22).

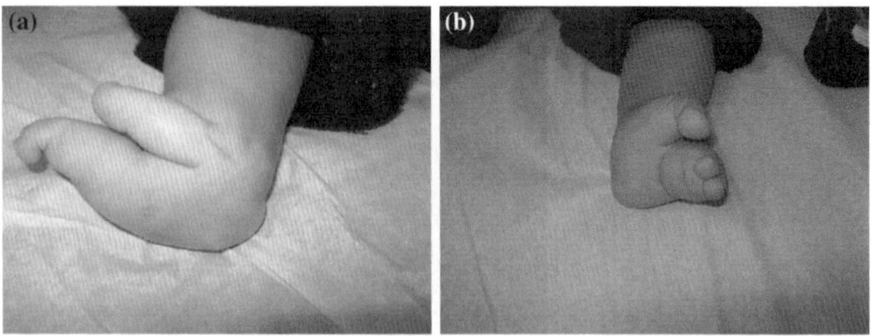

Fig. 8.22 A 1-year-old boy with bilateral cleft foot (**a**, **b**). Patient was able to walk with minimal affection of the gait

Treatment:

- Most cases function relatively good and no treatment is indicated.
- Orthopedic referral for possible reconstruction (rarely needed).

FLAT FOOT (PES PLANOVALGUS)

Development of the medial arch of the foot:

- The flatness of the infant's foot is due to a combination of abundant subcutaneous fat and joint laxity common in infants.
- **The medial arch of the foot does not develop until the age of 4 years and reaches close to the adult value by the age of 8 years.**

Types:

- Flexible flat foot
- Rigid (tarsal coalition, vertical talus)

Flexible flat foot:

Definition and incidence:

- Loss of the medial arch support when the child stands.
- This is normal finding in about 10 % of the population.

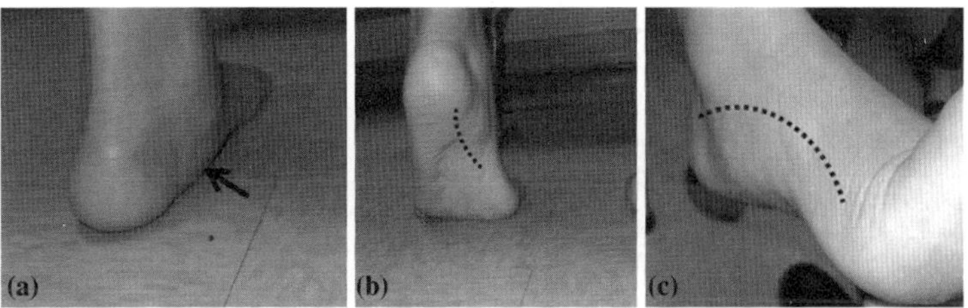

Fig. 8.23 Flexible flat feet. A 9-year-old girl with bilateral flexible flat feet. When patient stands there is loss of arch (*arrow*) (**a**). When she tip toes (**b**) or with dorsiflexion of the big toe (**c**), there is restoration of the arch (*dotted arch*)

- It is universal finding in neonates and toddlers and is associated with physiological ligamentous laxity and excess fat at the sole of the foot.
- Improvement will be seen in the majority of cases when longitudinal medial arch develops between 5 and 10 years of age

Clinical picture:

- Loss of the arch of the foot (the heel will be in valgus) when the patient stands.
- With tip toeing or with dorsiflexion of the big toe (tightening of the plantar fascia), restoration of the arch (Fig. 8.23).
- "too many toes" sign (Fig. 8.24).
- Normal subtalar joint movement.
- The condition in the vast majority of cases is asymptomatic for the children and parents are seeking medical treatment because of the deformity.
- Some cases are associated with tight Achilles tendon (heel cord).
- Some cases may be associated with generalized laxity of the joints.
- Rarely, the condition can cause pain at the medial aspect of the foot over the tarsal head.

Treatment:

- Re-assurance (the condition is a normal variation).
- Achilles tendon stretching for the children with tight Achilles tendon.

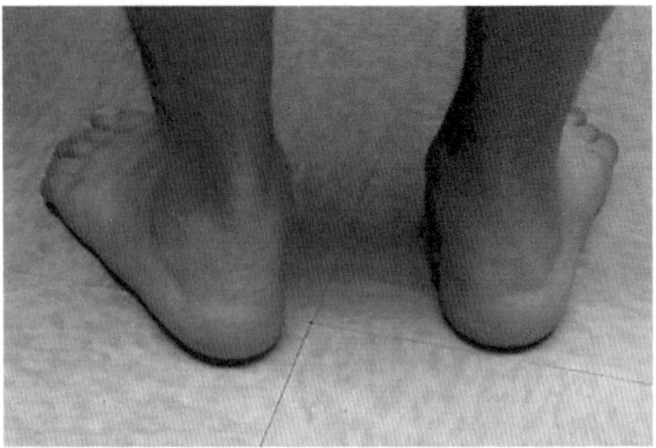

Fig. 8.24 A 14-year-old boy with bilateral flat feet more on the *left side*. Viewing the feet from the *back* shows more toes on the left side than the *right side* 'too many toes' sign

- **Soft** medial longitudinal arch support can be prescribed.
- Orthopedic referral in cases of persistence of pain (for possible calcaneal osteotomy, very rarely indicated).
- **Arthroereisis:** insertion of implant at the subtalar joint laterally to correct the flat foot.
  - This surgery had become more popular recently.
  - **It can cause synovitis of the subtalar joint and convert an asymptomatic condition to a symptomatic one.**

Tarsal coalition (peroneal spastic flat foot)

- **Definition:**
  - Abnormal connection (bridging) between two of the tarsal bone.
- The condition usually starts as fibrous or cartilaginous connection and then matures to bony bridge between two bones by the age of adolescence.

Incidence:

- About 5 % of the population has tarsal coalition.
- The condition is usually asymptomatic and bilateral.

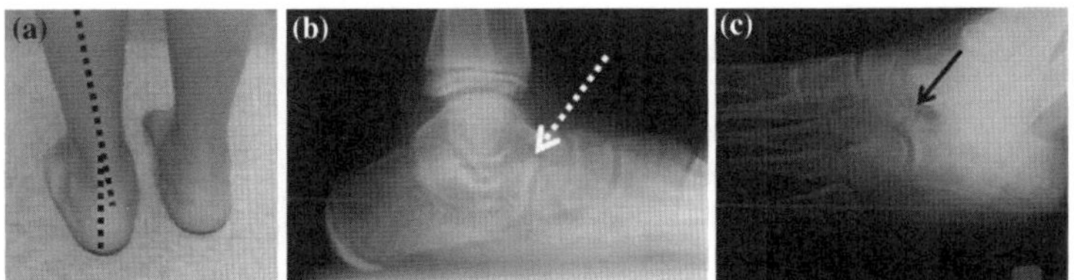

Fig. 8.25 Calcaneonavicular coalition. An 11-year-old boy with left flat foot and valgus heel (**a**) (*dotted line*) and foot pain for 6 months. Lateral standing radiograph (**b**) shows flat foot with no arch and bony prominence of the calcaneus (*white arrow*) (ant eater sign). Oblique radiograph (**c**) shows the calcaneonavicular coalition (*black arrow*)

- Some cases are transmitted by autosomal dominant transmission.
- Most common coalition is calcaneonavicular and subtalar (talo-calcaneal) fusion.

Clinical presentation

- Usually presents in the second decade (around 10 years for calcaneonavicular coalition and 14 years in the talocalcaneal coalition).
  - Patients present at this age as this is the time where bony coalition starts to develop.
- **Stiff flat foot with foot pain (**Fig. 8.25**).**
- Recurrent ankle sprains with persistence of the pain after the injury.
- Decreased subtalar movement (supination and pronation of the hindfoot).
- The peroneal tendons are spastic and tender (hence the old name) trying to stabilize the foot.

Imaging:

- Radiographs can show the bony fusion especially calcaneonavicular type (ant eater sign) (Fig. 8.25).
- Subtalar (talo-calcaneal) coalition is harder to detect in plain radiographs. C-sign (Fig. 8.26) is usually seen in cases of subtalar fusion.

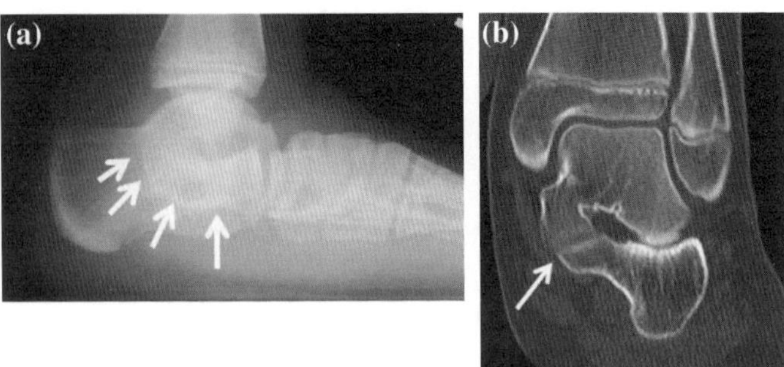

Fig. 8.26 Subtalar (tibio-calcaneal) colation. A 14-year-old boy with left flat foot and 1-year history of left foot pain. **a** Lateral radiograph of the foot shows C-sign (*arrows*). **b** CT scan shows bony coalition at talo-calcaneal joint (*arrow*)

- If radiograph is normal and the condition is suspected clinically, CT of the foot is indicated.
- CT will show the extent of coalition in a more precise way (Fig. 8.26).

Treatment:

- If discovered accidentally during foot radiographs taken for other reasons: no treatment is needed.
- Orthopedic referral for symptomatic cases only.
    - Treatment is first symptomatic (NSAIDs, bracing, casting).
    - If pain persists: surgery.

CONGENITAL VERTICAL TALUS

Definition:

- It is a rigid rocker-bottom foot deformity in which the talus does not articulate normally with the navicular bone.

Causes:

- Idiopathic
- Syndromic (e.g. Larsen Syndrome)

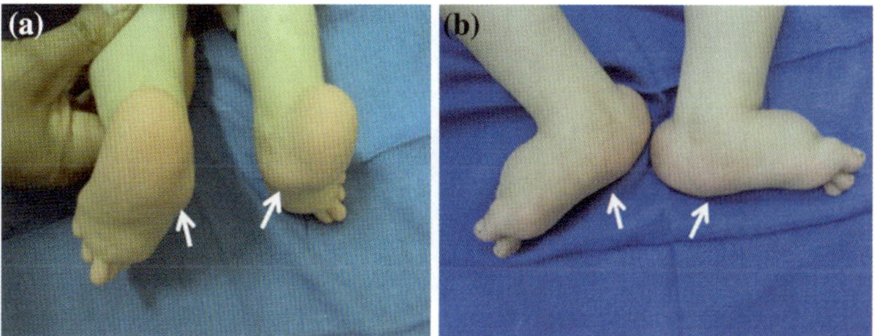

Fig. 8.27 Rocker button deformity. A 7-month-old boy with bilateral rocker button deformity. (**a** and **b**) Notice the loss and arch and the bony prominence at the medial sole representing head of talus (*arrows*) (Courtesy of Dr Thabet)

- Neuromuscular

Clinical presentation:

- Rigid rocker-bottom foot deformity (Fig. 8.27).
  - The foot is convex plantarly
  - Reversal of the normal arch
- If left untreated, it results in painful callus over the talar head with weak push off power.

Radiographs:

- The talus is vertical in position (almost in line with the tibia) (Fig. 8.28).
- Radiograph with maximum planter flexion of the foot: the talus does not line up with first metatarsus.

Treatment:

- Orthopedic referral.
  - The deformity is sometimes resistant to casting and surgical intervention may be needed.

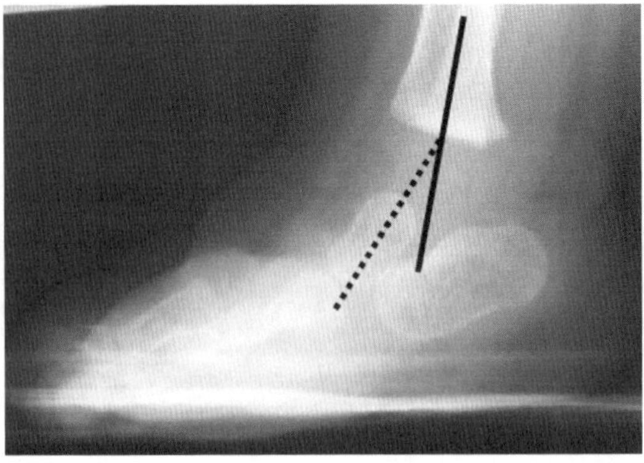

Fig. 8.28 Lateral foot radiograph for a 1-year-old boy with congenital vertical talus. Note the talus alignment (*dotted line*), which is in line with the tibial alignment (*continuous line*) (normal position is nearly perpendicular)

TIP TOE WALKING

Definition:

- Pattern of walking in which the child walks on his toes with ankle plantar flexion.
- If no underlying neurological cause is identified, it is referred to as "Habitual toe walking" or "idiopathic toe walking".
  - It is a diagnosis of exclusion.

Clinical presentation:

- The child walks on his/her toes with no pain.
- Common in toddlers and young children when they are starting to learn to walk.
- Tight Achilles tendon especially with the knee extended.
- Sometimes, the toe walking is associated with autism or speech delay.

Management:

- Full neurological exam to exclude underlying neurological disease.

- If the child had just learned how to walk, less than 24-months old or the toe walking is occasional, observation and reassessment is after 6 months.
- If the child is older than 24 months and the toe walking is constant:
  - Physical therapy for Achilles tendon stretching.
  - If no improvement after 6 months of therapy:
    - Orthopedic referral:
      - Botox injection of the calf muscle.
      - Achilles tendon lengthening (rarely indicated).

Differential diagnosis of idiopathic toe walking:

- Cerebral palsy:
  - Sometimes, it is very hard to differentiate between idiopathic toe walker and mild cerebral palsy.
  - Upper extremities movement during gait is normal in idiopathic toe walking and restricted in mild cerebral palsy.
- Duchene Muscular dystrophy:
  - positive Gower sign
  - pseudo hypertrophy of the calf
- Tether cord syndrome
- Limb length discrepancy:
  - will cause unilateral toe walking (on the short side)

ADOLESCENT HALLUX VALGUS

Definition:
Bunion deformity of the foot that develops in adolescence.

Pathology:
Adolescent hallux valgus has the following characteristics:

- Ligamentous laxity.

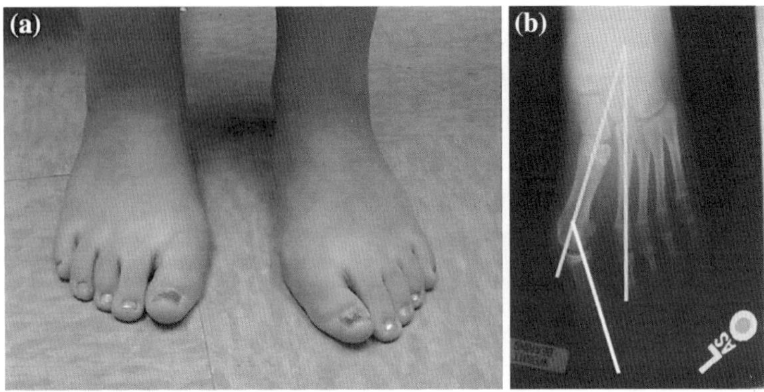

Fig. 8.29 Adolescent hallux valgus. An 8-year-old girl with bilateral hallux valgus more in the left side (**a**). Weight bearing radiographs (**b**) show 28° of the 1st metatarso-phalangeal angle and 18° of 1st metatarsal-2nd metatarsal angle

- Positive family history.
- Metatarsus pimus varus: the first metatarsal bone is pointing medially.

Clinical presentation:

- Deformity (Bunion) (Fig. 8.29).
- The condition is usually bilateral.
  - Most cases are asymptomatic. However, sometimes, pain develops over the medial prominence.

Radiographs:

Standing AP foot radiographs will show the following (Fig. 8.29):

- 1st metatarso-phalangeal angle more than 15
- metatarsus pimus varus
- 1st metatarsal-2nd metatarsal angle of more than 10°

Treatment:

- For asymptomatic cases, no treatment required.
- If symptomatic:

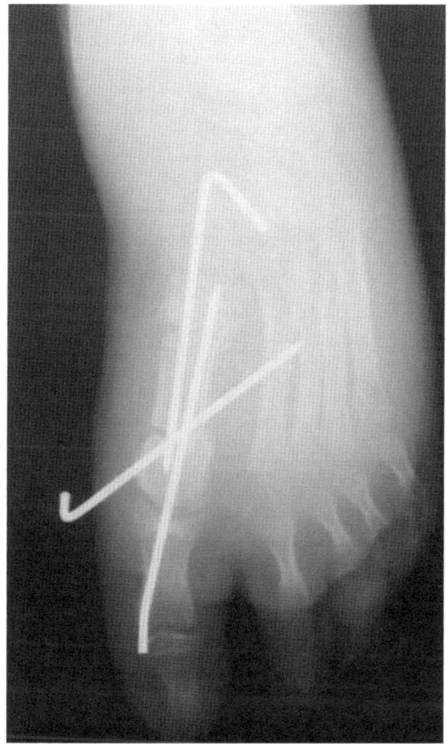

Fig. 8.30 The patient in Fig. 8.29 had persistent foot pain despite conservative measures. Double osteotomy of the left foot to correct the deformity was done

- Conservative treatment: wide shoe box.
- If conservative treatment fails: orthopedic referral for possible surgical intervention (Fig. 8.30).

EXTRA DIGIT (POLYDACTYLY)

Definition:

- Presence of extra digit (Fig. 8.31).

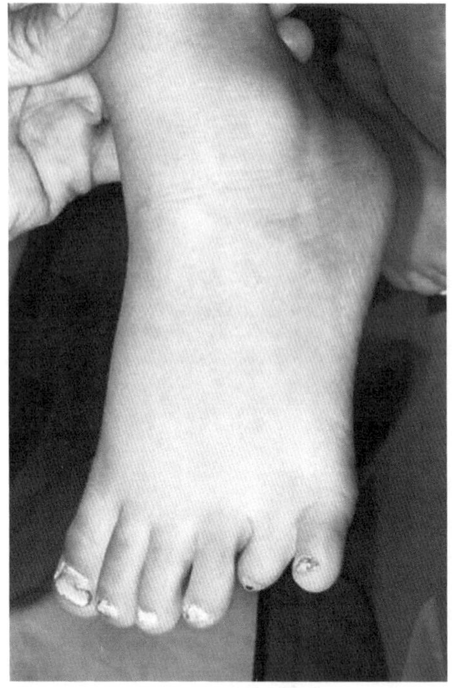

Fig. 8.31 A 3-year-old girl with foot polydactyly

- It ranges from fully formed digit (bones, tendons) to a small knob

Treatment:

- Orthopedic referral if the family is interested in excision of the extra digit.

Foot infections:

- **See musculoskeletal infections**

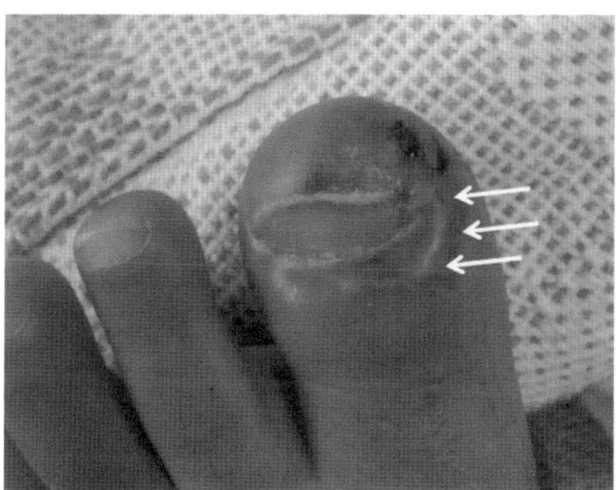

Fig. 8.32 A 6-year-old with ingrowing toe nail. Notice the pocket of pus (*arrows*)

INGROWING TOENAIL

Definition:

- The penetration of the border of the nail plate into the nail fold causing pain and inflammation in the surrounding tissue (Fig. 8.32)

Etiology:

- Unknown.
  - Theories include: tight-fitting shoes, trauma to the toe, incorrect trimming of toenails and genetic susceptibility.

Clinical Presentation

- The condition is common in the pediatric age group.
- Ingrown toenails will cause significant pain and discomfort.
- Upon examination, the following may be present:
  - Inflammation of tissue surrounding the nail bed (edema, redness, tenderness)

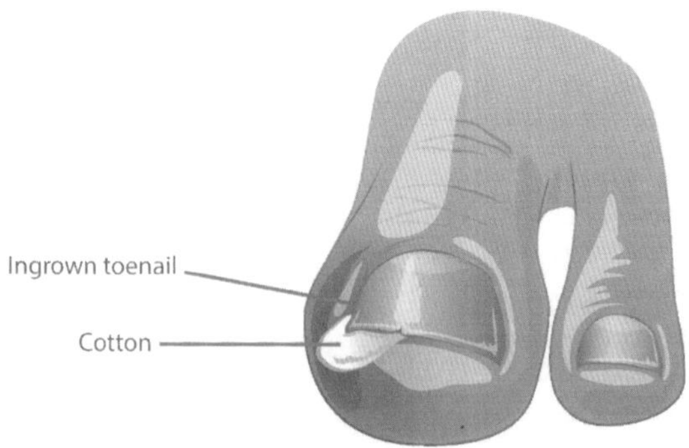

Fig. 8.33 Placing a small piece of gauze between the nail and the nail fold

- Drainage
- Crusting
- Hypertrophy of the nail folds

Treatment

- Proper care of the nail:
  - A comfortable wide toe box or open-toed shoes
  - The nail should be cut straight across and avoid cutting back the lateral margins
  - The nail edge should extend past the tissue
- Frequent soaking of the foot in warm water
- Local antibiotic application (Oral antibiotic can be prescribed if the infection is advanced)
- Elevating the offending edge of the nail from the soft tissue, and placing a small piece of gauze between the nail and the skin (Fig. 8.33).

Surgical Treatment

- If no improvement with the above measures: Orthopedic or Podiatry referral:
  - Wedge excision of the nail edge with possible chemical treatment of the nail bed with phenol.

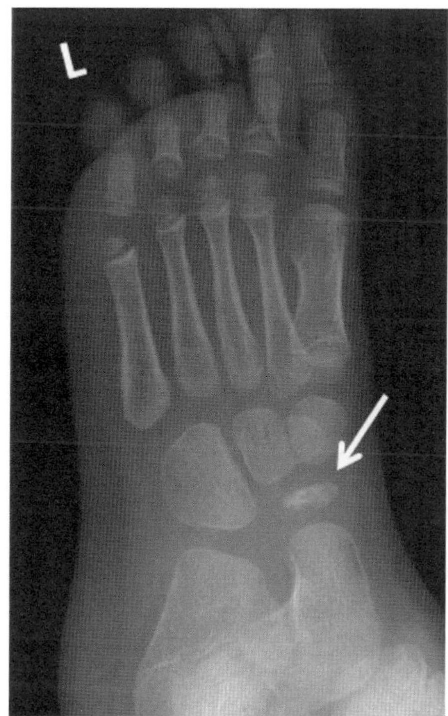

Fig. 8.34 Kohler disease. A 6-year-old boy with 3-month history of left foot pain. Radiograph showed Kohler disease. The navicular bone is collapsed and sclerotic (*arrow*)

Osteochondritis of foot bone:

- **Kohler disease**.
- **Freiberg disease**.

KOHLER DISEASE

Definition:

- Avascular necrosis of the navicular bone.

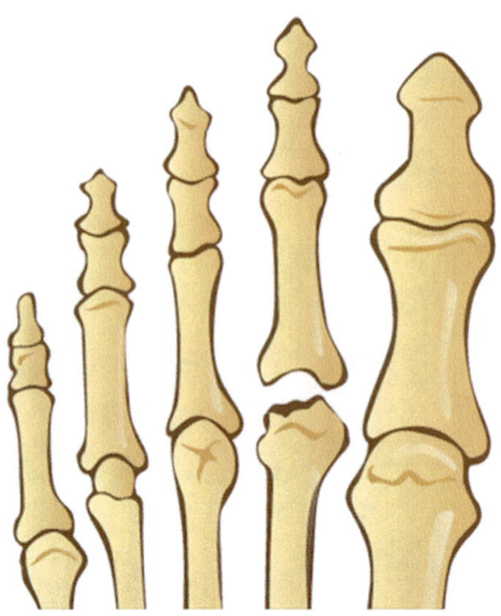

Fig. 8.35 Freiberg disease. Avascular necrosis of the metatarsal head leading to collapse and loss of contour of the metatarsal head

- The condition is self-limiting.

Clinical presentation:

- Common in boys between 4 and 10.
- Pain over the medial aspect of the foot.
- Radiographs will show collapse and sclerosis of the navicular bone (Fig. 8.34).

Treatment:

- Symptomatic treatment.
- If the pain is not controlled by NSAIDs, orthopedic referral for possible casting for few weeks.

FREIBERG DISEASE

Definition:

- Avascular necrosis of the metatarsal head (most commonly in the 2nd metatarsal head) (Fig. 8.35)

Clinical presentation:

- Common in adolescent girls.
- Pain over the middle of the forefoot.

Treatment:

- Symptomatic treatment (decrease activity, NSAIDs, shoe inserts (toeplate) to relief stress over the metatarsal heads).
- If the pain is not controlled, orthopedic referral of possible intervention.

SEVER DISEASE

Definition:

- Traction apophysitis of the calcaneal tubrosity.

Clinical presentation:

- Pain over the heel.
- Sclerosis and fragmentation of the calcaneal tuberosity is a normal finding in children and does not signify a specific disease.

Treatment:

- Symptomatic treatment.
    - Rest, NSAID, stretching exercise.

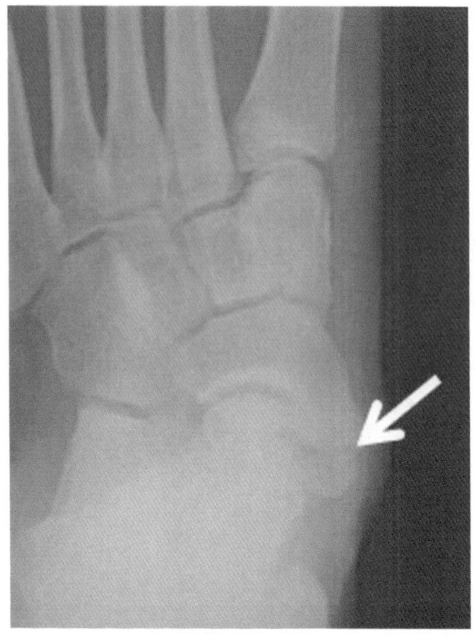

Fig. 8.36 A 9-year-old girl with medial foot pain. Radiograph showed accessory navicular bone (arrow).

ACCESSORY NAVICULAR

Definition:

- Accessory ossicle on the medial aspect of the foot just medial to the talar head (Fig. 8.36).
- Present in 10 % of the population.
- Rarely can cause pain at the medial aspect of the foot.

Treatment:

- If asymptomatic: no treatment required.
- If painful: rest, NSAIDs, shoe inserts to relief pressure from the accessory navicular.
- Orthopedic referral for excision is rarely indicated.

Table 2: Common Causes of Foot Pain:

TABLE 8.2 COMMON CAUSES OF FOOT PAIN

Trauma	• Fractures • Sprains • Laceration
Infections	• Osteomyelitis • Septic arthritis • Puncture wound • Ingrowing toenail.
Osteochondritis	• Freidberg disease • Kohler disease
Deformity	• Tarsal coalition • Hallux valgus
Miscellaneous	• Sever's disease • Accessory navicular • Plantar warts

What is the best shoe to wear?

A common question asked by parents:

- Soft comfortable shoe.
- No high heels.
- Cushioned sole.
- Built-in arch will not result in long-lasting effect regarding the foot shape.
- Shoes are mainly protective for the child foot and not corrective for deformities.

HIGH YIELD FACTS

- Most cases of intoeing represent normal development and do not need orthopedic referral.
- Tibial torsion usually improves by the age of 3 years and femoral anteversion usually improves by the age of 8 years.
- If the foot deformity in cases of metatarsus adductus is flexible (the forefoot can be abducted), stretching exercises are sufficient.

- The most important component of clubfoot is equinovarus deformity which has to be rigid.
- The best treatment method of clubfoot is serial casting at early age.
- Calcaneovalgus, if not associated with posteromedial bowing, will improve spontaneously without intervention.
- Cavus foot is an indication of neurological affection.
- Flexible flat foot is normal finding, does not require treatment or referral.
- The longitudinal foot arch does not develop until the age of 4 years.
- Tarsal coalition can be found as incidental finding in foot radiographs.
- Idiopathic toe walker is treated with Achilles tendon stretching exercises. If no improvement, Botox injection or surgery may be indicated.
- Adolescent hallux valgus is better treated by shoe modification.
- Ingrowing toenail is a common cause of foot pain, conservative treatment is usually effective in most cases.
- Kohler disease is necrosis of the navicular bone.
- Sever disease is a common cause of heel pain; it is traction apophysitis of the calcaneal tuberosity.

CLINICAL SCENARIOS

The presenting patient	The most probable diagnosis and plan of action
10-year-old runner came to your clinic complain in intermittent heel pain, the pain is worse when running or jumping, on physical examination there is pain with deep palpation at the Achilles insertion and pain when performing active toe raises, radiograph on the foot showed fragmentation of the calcaneal apophysis	Sever disease or calcaneal apophysitis ■ The best recommendation is heel stretching exercise and decrease activity

(continued)

(CONTINUED)

The presenting patient	The most probable diagnosis and plan of action
13-year-old had three ankle sprains in the last 6 months. He comes to the clinic complaining of persistence of the ankle pain after the last ankle sprain which was 2 months ago. Examination shows mild valgus deformity of the foot, tenderness over the hindfoot, and limited subtalar motion	Tarsal coalition XR and CT of the foot Rest, brace, and activity modification, if no improvement, orthopedic referral for possible surgical intervention
6-year-old boy brought to the clinic by his mother complaining the child has flat feel. On examination, patient has valgus feet when he stands. Patient regains his arch when he stands on his tip toe. The child has good ROM of the subtalar joint	Flexible flat foot No treatment is required

REFERENCES

Abdelgawad AA, Lehman WB, van Bosse HJ, Scher DM, Sala DA. Treatment of idiopathic clubfoot using the Ponseti method: minimum 2-year follow-up. J Pediatr Orthop B. 2007;16(2):98–105.

Sass P. Hassan G Lower extremity abnormalities in children. Am Fam Physician. 2003;68(3):461–8.

Karol LA. Rotational deformities in the lower extremities. Curr Opin Pediatr. 1997;9(1):77–80.

Dietz FR Intoeing-fact, fiction and opinion. Am Fam Physician. 1994;50 Suppl 6:1249–59, 1262–4.

Schwend RM, Drennan JC. Cavus foot deformity in children. J Am Acad Orthop Surg. 2003;11 Suppl 3:201–11.

Choudry Q, Kumar R, Turner PG. Congenital cleft foot deformity. Foot Ankle Surg 2010;16(4):e85–7.

Chiodo WA, Cook KD. Pediatric heel pain. Clin Podiatr Med Surg. 2010;27(3):355–67.

Zaw H, Calder JD. Tarsal coalitions. Foot Ankle Clin. 2010;15(2):349–64.

Lemley F, Berlet G, Hill K, Philbin T, Isaac B, Lee T. Current concepts review: tarsal coalition. Foot Ankle Int. 2006;27(12):1163–9.

Yang G, Yanchar NL, Lo AY, Jones SA. Treatment of ingrown toenails in the pediatric population. J Pediatr Surg. 2008;43:931–5.

Kean JR. Foot problems in the adolescent. Adolesc Med State Art Rev. 2007;18 Suppl 1:182–91, xi.

Hendrix CL. Calcaneal apophysitis (sever disease). Clin Podiatr Med Surg. 2005;22 Suppl 1:55–62, vi.

Staheli LT. Shoes for children. In: Staheli LT, Song KM, editors. Secrets of pediatric orthopedic. 3rd ed. Philadelphia: Mosby Elsevier; 2007. p. 84–7.

Chapter 9
Hand and Upper Extremity

Miguel Pirela-Cruz

HAND EMBRYOGENESIS

- First visualization of the limb bud is noted **26–33 days** after fertilization when the hand becomes a recognizable paddle.
- **8 weeks after fertilization**, all limbs are present.
- Digital separation occurs between days 47 and 54.
- Hand development is essentially complete by the end of the first trimester.
- Myelination of the peripheral nerves takes place over the next 2 years.

Signaling Centers

- There are three signaling centers which control the development and guide the growth of the upper extremity.
- Signaling from all three centers is required to have proper development of the limb
  - Apical Ectodermal Ridge (AER)
    - Responsible for the **proximal to distal** development of the limb.
    - Disruption of this signal can lead to transverse deficiencies with a shortened limb (Fig. 9.1).
    - These developmental deficiencies are usually spontaneous and not inherited.
  - Zone of Polarizing Activity (ZPA)
    - Responsible for development of the limb in a radial to ulnar direction (sometimes referred to as pre-and post-axial development).

A. Abdelgawad and O. Naga (eds.), *Pediatric Orthopedics*,
DOI: 10.1007/978-1-4614-7126-4_9,

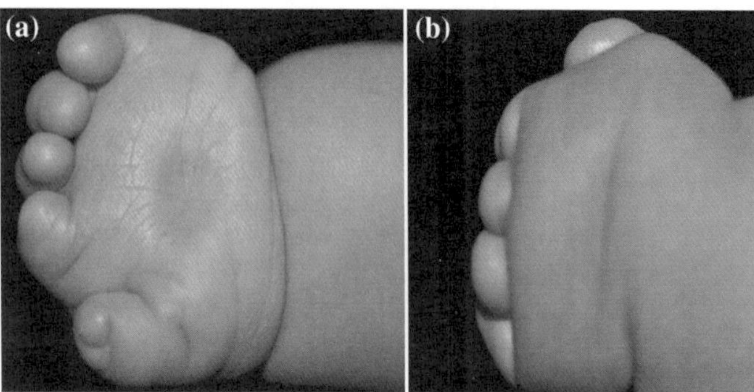

Fig. 9.1 (**a** and **b**) Transverse deficiency of the hand at the level of the metacarpophalangeal joint

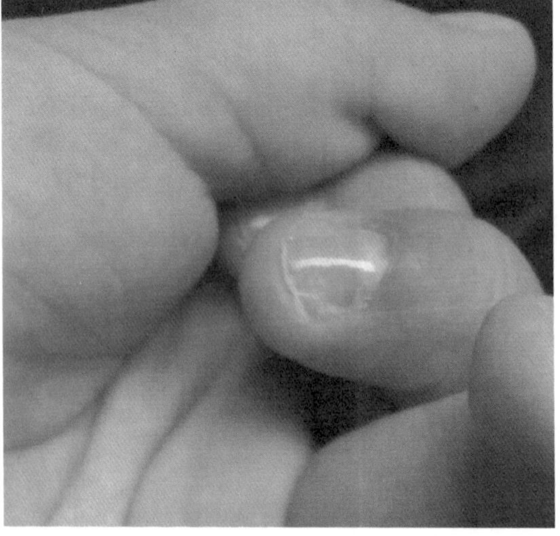

Fig. 9.2 Nail–patella syndrome. A 9-year-old girl with nail–patella syndrome. Notice the poorly developed ridged nail of the middle finger

- Disturbance of this signal can lead to the duplication or absence of digits.
- The so-called "Mirror hand" is the classic example of deformities arising from disturbances involving the ZPA

- Wingless Signaling Center (Wnt)
  - Responsible for the dorsal-palmar limb development.
  - It arises from the dorsal ectodermal ridge.
  - The nail–patella syndrome is an example of a deformity that occurs when this signal is altered (Fig. 9.2).

Congenital hand deformities:

- Congenital hand anomalies are relatively common. It is estimated to occur in 2-3 per 1,000 live births.
- The majority of these anomalies are of minor consequence and do not interfere with hand function.
- Parents seek treatment for their children to obtain a normal appearing hand that will hopefully allow the child to have acceptance by peers.

International classification for congenital limb malformation

- It includes seven categories.
- Table 9.1 summarize these categories

Systemic evaluation of patients with hand anomalies:

- It is important to distinguish clinical deformities that occur in isolation versus the deformities that are associated with other congenital anomalies.
- Some clinical problems can be life-threatening; therefore, it is important that a thorough evaluation be performed by the appropriate consultants.
  - The classic example is radial hypoplasia that may be associated with cardiac, renal, gastrointestinal, or hemopoietic anomalies.

COMMON CONGENITAL ANOMALIES

Phocomelia (Figs. 9.3):

TABLE 9.1 CLASSIFICATION FOR CONGENITAL LIMB MALFORMATION

Type	Categories	Examples
I	**Failure of formation**	Transverse arrest - Can be at any level from shoulder to phalanx Longitudinal arrest Preaxial - Varying degrees of hypoplasia of the thumb or radius Central - Divided into typical and atypical types of cleft hand Postaxial - Varying degrees of ulnar hypoplasia to hypothenar hypoplasia Intercalated longitudinal arrest - Various types of phocomelia
II	**Failure of differentiation**	• Soft tissue - Syndactyly, trigger thumb, Poland syndrome, camptodactyly • Skeletal - Various synostoses and carpal coalitions • Tumorous conditions - Include all vascular and neurologic malformations
III	**Duplication**	• May apply to whole limb, mirror hand, polydactyly
IV	**Overgrowth**	• Includes conditions such as hemihypertrophy and macrodactyly
V	**Undergrowth**	• Most commonly, radial hypoplasia, brachysyndactyly, or brachydactyly
VI	**Constriction band syndromes**	• Occurs with or without distal lymphedema; may involve amputation at any level
VII	**Generalized anomalies and syndromes**	

- A form of longitudinal deficiency due to transverse arrest of the developing limb bud.
- Thalidomide, a drug that was taken by many females during the first trimester for morning sickness in the 1950s and 1960s, has been associated with this anomaly.

Polydactyly (Supernumerary digit)

- **Definition**: the presence of an extra digit (or duplication),

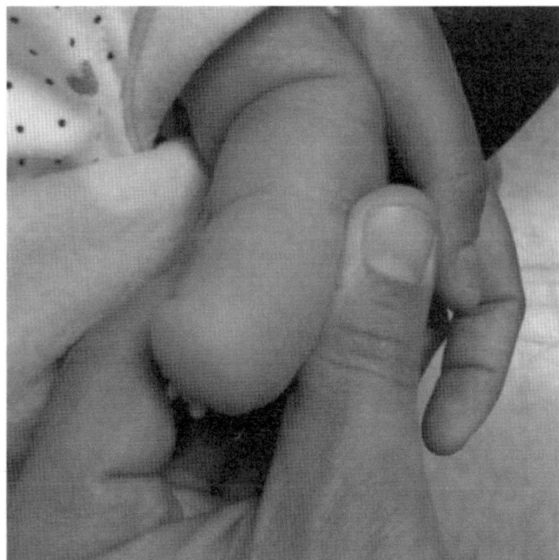

Fig. 9.3 Phocomelia with absent hand. Only small 'knobs' are attached to the forearm

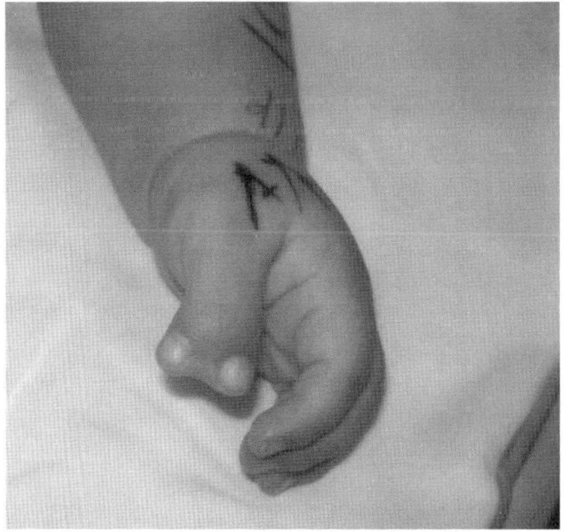

Fig. 9.4 Thumb polydactyly. A 1-year-old boy with radial polydactyly

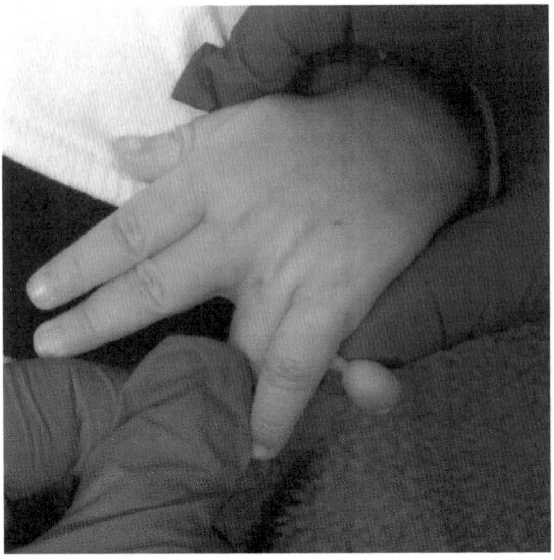

Fig. 9.5 Ulnar polydactyly. A small extra digit on the ulnar side of the hand attached with to the hand with a stalk

- **Polydactyly is the most common congenital digital anomaly of the hand and foot.**
- A common form of polydactyly is an extra thumb (radial polydactyly or pre-axial polydactyly) (Fig. 9.4). More common among Caucasians
- Ulnar (post axial) polydactyly is usually a small poorly formed extra digit attached by a thin stalk of soft tissue (Fig. 9.5). More common among African Americans.
- Central polydactyly (rare) involves duplication of the second, third, or fourth digit or ray.
- It may appear in isolation or in association with other birth defects.
    - Isolated polydactyly is often autosomal dominant or occasionally random, while syndromic polydactyly is commonly autosomal recessive

Assessment of a child with polydactyly:

- About 15–20 % of children born with polydactyly have other congenital anomalies, usually as part of a defined syndrome (more common among preaxial polydactyly).
- **Unless there is a clear family history of isolated polydactyly, any newborn with polydactyly should be investigated for the presence of associated anomalies**.
- Hand postaxial polydactyly is less often associated with other congenital anomalies.

Management

- Genetic workup and thorough medical examination in these patients is recommended especially for radial (preaxial) polydactyly in Caucasian patients
- In cases of preaxial polydactyly, a thorough ultrasound evaluation should be performed, especially of the heart, nervous system, limbs, and kidneys, to identify any associated anomalies or syndromes.
- **Radiographs**
  - Radiographs of the affected limb are recommended to show whether the rudimentary digit contains skeletal elements or not.
- **Surgical Removal**:
  - For small rudimentary ulnar polydactyly attached by a thin stalk:
    - **The base can be tied with a suture in the newborn period**, and it will fall off spontaneously.
  - For More developed extra digits, radial polydactyly, or polydactyly in older children: Orthopedic referral for surgical excision. Radial polydactyly usually requires more extensive planning and surgery to reconstruct the thumb.

RADIAL HYPOPLASIA (RADIAL LONGITUDINAL DEFICIENCY SYNDROME, RADIAL CLUB HAND)

- **Definition**: Longitudinal deficiency of the radial side of the forearm
- Classification is dependent on the degree of deficiency.
- Type I (Short distal radius):
  - The distal radial epiphysis is present but delayed in development
  - The radius has some mild shortening, but the carpus is well supported with minor radial deviation of the hand.
  - The thumb is hypoplastic
- Type II (Hypoplastic radius)
  - The radius is severely shortened; however, both proximal and distal ends are present.
  - The carpus is poorly supported, and the ulna is bowed. Moderate radial deviation of the hand is noted
- Type III (Partial absence of the radius)
  - Absence may occur in the proximal, middle, or distal segments of the radius.
  - The elbow is stable and the ulna has a bow.
  - The carpus is unsupported by radius. Severe radial deviation of the wrist is noted (Fig. 9.6)
- Type IV (Complete absence of the radius)
  - The most common type.
  - The ulna has a severe bow. It is short and thickened.
  - There is no support of the carpus. Radial deviation of the wrist is severe.

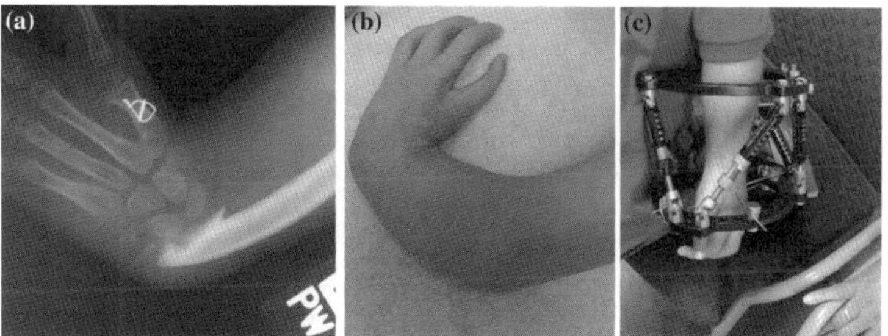

Fig. 9.6 Radial club hand. A 6-year-old boy with VACTERL syndrome and radial club hand. **a** Radiograph shows small bowed ulna, wrist deviation, and presence of small part of the proximal radius. **b** Clinical picture showing the severe radial deviation of the wrist. **c** Ring external fixator was applied to correct the deformity and lengthen the extremity

SYNDROMES ASSOCIATED WITH RADIAL HYPOPLASIA

Thrombocytopenia-Absent Radius syndrome (**TAR syndrome**):

- Bilateral radial aplasia
- Exhibits a low platelet count that is usually present at birth and often continues to improve after the first 2 years.

Fanconi's anemia:

- **Definition**: an aplastic crisis that is not present at birth but usually develops in early childhood.
- Blood count may reveal trilineage pancytopenia or may only show RBCs that are macrocytic for age.
- This condition can be fatal but can be treated successfully with a bone marrow transplant.

VACTERL syndrome:

- This syndrome is characterized by **V**ertebral anomalies, **A**nal atresia, **C**ardiac abnormalities, **T**racheoesophageal fistula,

Esophageal atresia, **R**enal disorders, and/or **L**imb (including lower) anomalies.

Holt-Oram syndrome

- **Definition**: is a cardiac anomaly that is associated with radial hypoplasia.
- The most common anomaly is a cardiac septal defect.
- This syndrome is usually transmitted as an autosomal dominant disorder with variable expression.

General management of radial hypoplasia:

- **Children with radial hypoplasia require medical workup of their cardiac, renal, and hematologic systems**.
  - Evaluation by a pediatric genetist may be helpful in identifying associated anomalies and syndromes.
  - Cardiology consultation, Hematology consultation, EKG, and an echocardiogram should be obtained.
  - **CBC and platelet count** are essential laboratory studies that should be included in the evaluation.
  - Renal studies including ultrasound and urine analysis (UA) are important in this workup.
- Management of the hand deformity:
  - The initial treatment for the radial club hand should be **passive stretching** and **splinting** to prevent radial deviation of the hand.
  - Orthopedic referral
    - Alignment of the carpus (centralization) in relation to the forearm and distraction lengthening of the ulna (Fig. 9.6).

Ulna Hypoplasia

- Less common than radial hypoplasia.
- Unlike radial hypoplasia, systemic or visceral associated anomalies are usually not present, however it may be associated with other musculoskeletal conditions:

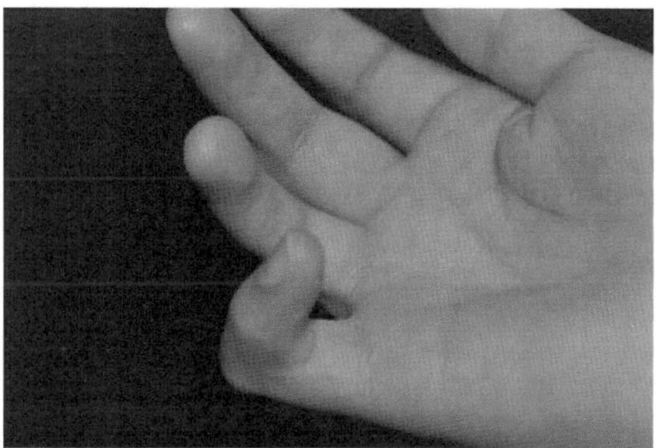

Fig. 9.7 Camptodactyly. A 13-year-old girl with Camptodactyly involving the middle and small fingers

  - Transverse absence of the forearm, cleft hand with bifid thumb, absence of ring and small fingers, and hemimelia of the fibula.

- Treatment of ulnar hypoplasia
  - Mild cases: no treatment needed.
  - Orthopedic referral for surgical reconstruction.

CAMPTODACTYLY

Definition:

- A flexion deformity of the fingers most commonly seen in the small digit (Fig. 9.7).

Etiology:

- The etiology is unknown but it is generally accepted to be an imbalance between the flexor digitorum superficialis (FDS) and the intrinsics of the finger (interossei and lumbricals).

Clinical presentation:

- It is typically progressive, the deformity increases during the adolescent period.
- Most patients experience little functional deficits.
- **Cosmesis is main reason for seeking medical treatment**.

  - There are 3 types

    - Type I (congenital):

      - Isolated finding, may be unilateral or bilateral, normal child otherwise

    - Type II (Adolescent):

      - Presents later in age, child is normal otherwise.

    - Type III (syndromic):

      - May involve multiple digits, identified shortly after birth, the camptodactyly is more severe

CLINODACTYLY

- **Definition and clinical presentation**:

  - This is an angulatory deformity involving the fingers, most commonly the small finger. The angulation is in the radio-ulnar plane.

- **Etiology**:

  - An abnormal middle phalanx is the most common cause. The morphology of the middle phalanx can vary from an abnormal appearing tubular phalanx to a triangular (delta shaped) or trapezoidal phalanx.

- **Management**:

  - For the most part, this is more of a cosmetic problem and rarely do the children have a functional problem.

SYNDACTYLY (CONGENITAL WEBBING)

- **Definition and clinical presentation**:
  - It is the joining of adjacent fingers.
  - One of the common congenital anomalies.
  - Syndactyly most commonly involves the long and ring fingers (Fig. 9.8).
- **Etiology**:
  - This anomaly is presumed to be a derangement in the signaling pathway that occurs during weeks 6–8 of gestation that allows for complete differentiation of the fingers.
  - This anomaly is usually transmitted as a autosomal dominant trait and can have variable degrees of penetrance.
- **Types**:
  - **Simple Versus Complex**
    - Simple syndactyly
      - Only the skin and soft tissue are involved.

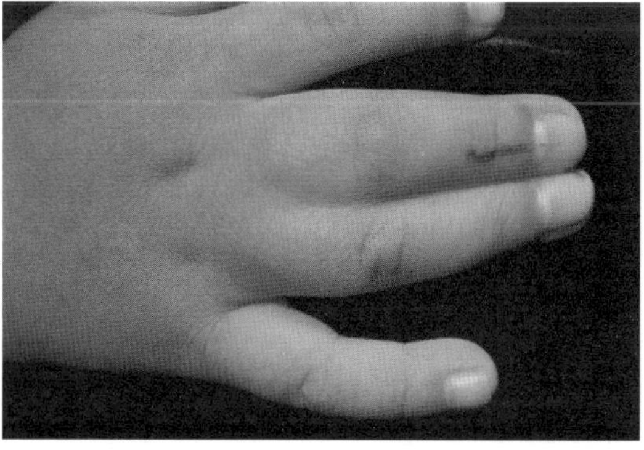

Fig. 9.8 Syndactyly affecting the middle and ring finger

- Complex syndactyly
    - The union involves bone fusion and skin tissue.

- **Complete Versus Incomplete**
    - Incomplete:
        - The two fingers are joined **partially** along the length of the fingers.
    - Complete:
        - The two fingers are joined **entirely** along the length of the fingers (up to the finger tip).

- **Treatment of syndactyly**
    - Orthopedic referral for surgical release and creation of web space.
    - The separation of the digit is not a 'simple division of the joint fingers.' The procedure can be associated with various possible complications.
    - Timing of surgical release:
        - For syndactyly between the index and middle or middle and ring fingers: surgery can be performed around the age of 12–18 months.
        - For border digits (syndactyly between the thumb and index or ring and small fingers): there is different rate of growth between the fused digit, so surgery has to be done at earlier age to avoid angular deformity of the digits.
        - If a syndactyly involves both the radial and ulnar sides of a digit, one side should be released at a time to have adequate skin flap for coverage.

Some congenital syndromes that have hand affection:

1. Apert's syndrome.
2. Poland's syndrome.

Apert's syndrome.

- **Definition and clinical presentation**:
  - Apert's syndrome (Acrocephalosyndactyly) is a congenital condition that includes malformations of the face, skull, hands, and feet.
  - Fusion of the cranial and facial sutures occurs resulting in cranial and facial deformities.
- **Hand deformities associated with Apert's syndrome**
  - Hypoplasia of the hand.
  - Complex syndactyly involving the middle three rays.
  - Thumb: shortened and radially deviated.
  - Symphalangism (congenital ankylosis of the joints of the fingers) affecting the middle and ring fingers.
  - Synostosis (bony fusion) of the ring and small metacarpals.
  - Contracture of the first web space.

Poland's syndrome

- **Definition and clinical presentation**:
  - Poland's syndrome is a rare congenital anomaly that involves absence of the sternal portion of the pectoralis major muscle and ipsilateral hand manifestations.
  - It is estimated to occur between one in 10,000 and 100,000 births per year.
- **Etiology**:
  - The etiology is unknown but one of the more common theories is an interruption in the blood flow to the upper extremity shortly after gestation causing developmental compromise to the upper limb structures.
- **Hand findings in Poland's syndrome**
  - Hypoplasia of the hand (especially the thenar part) with brachydactyly (short fingers).
  - Syndactyly.

- Oligodactyly (missing fingers).
- Humerus is absent or abnormal.

CONGENITAL TRIGGER THUMB

- **Clinical presentation**:
  - **Relatively common condition that affect the thumbs**.
  - Characteristic posture of the **flexed** interphalangeal (IP) of the thumb (Fig. 9.9)
  - The parents will have difficulty extending the joint or the child will have pain when passive extension is performed.
  - Large nodule (Notta's node) is often present along the tendon and can be felt at the level of the metacarpophalangeal joint of the thumb.
- **Pathology**:
  - The underlying anatomical problem is a mismatch between the large size of the flexor pollicis longus tendon and the relatively small fibro-osseous tunnel for the tendon to slide.
  - The condition occurs at the level of A1 pulley (fibrous bands across the tendon sheath at the level of metacarpophalangeal joint).

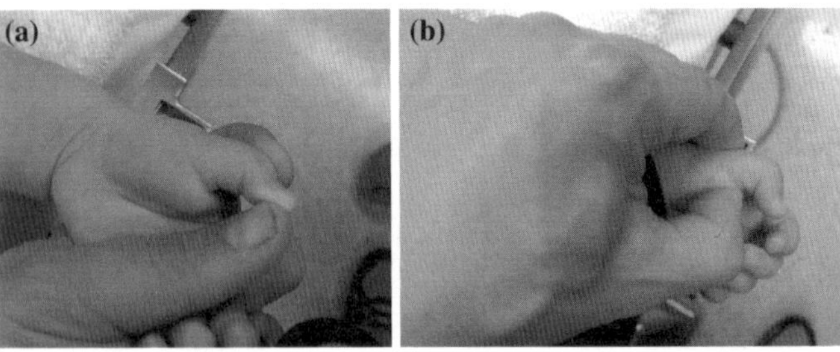

Fig. 9.9 Congenital trigger thumb. **a** An 18-month-old girl with inability to extend the terminal phalanx of the thumb. **b** A nodule can be felt at the base of the thumb

- **Management**:
  - Initial treatment involves referral to a hand therapist that can perform passive range of motion extension exercises, splinting, and other modalities.
  - **If no improvement by 12 months of age after an adequate period of non-operative treatment, the child is a candidate for surgery**.
    - Orthopedic referral for surgical intervention which involves decompression of the A1 pulley (the fibrous constriction band over the base of the thumb).

MADELUNG'S DEFORMITY

- **Definition**:
  - Madelung's deformity (MD) is a physeal growth arrest involving the ulnar-volar portion of the distal radius growth plate. This arrest results in a characteristic appearance of the distal radius and ulna.
- **Etiology**:
  - Madelung deformity can be an isolated finding or a manifestation of a systemic process.
  - It may be associated with: dyschondrosteosis, achondroplasia, multiple exostoses, Ollier's disease (multiple enchondromas), and **Turner's syndrome**.
- **Clinical presentation**:
  - Patients present with a shorten forearm, loss of supination of the forearm, loss of ulna deviation, and lack of extension of the wrist.
  - Additionally, patients complain of the unsightly appearance of the wrist due to dorsal dislocation of the distal radioulnar joint (DRUJ).
  - **Despite the deformity, many individuals function quite well**.

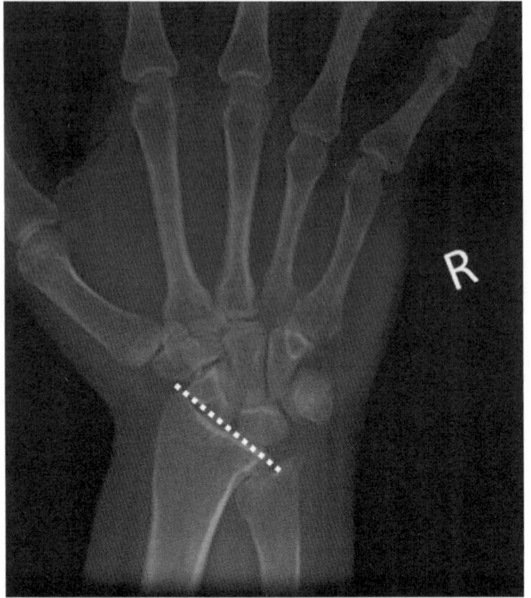

Fig. 9.10 A 19-year-old girl with Turner syndrome and wrist deformity. Radiograph of the *right hand* showed Madelung deformity with increased radial inclinational (*dotted line*)

- Wrist pain (mild, uncommon).
- **Radiology** (Fig. 9.10):
  - □ increase radial tilt
  - □ increase palmer tilt
  - □ carpus subluxation

▪ **Management**:

- Most cases of Madelung deformity need no intervention.
- If there is marked deformity or pain: orthopedic referral.

CONGENITAL DISLOCATION OF THE RADIAL HEAD

- **Clinical presentation**:
  - Most cases are bilateral
  - Most patients are asymptomatic early in life.
  - During adolescence the child may become symptomatic due to arthritic changes in the proximal radioulnar and radio-capitellar joints.
- **Management**:
  - Most cases need no intervention.
  - If symptomatic: Orthopedic referral.

CONGENITAL PROXIMAL RADIO-ULNAR SYNOSTOSIS

- **Definition**:
  - Congenital bony fusion between the proximal parts of the radius and ulna.
- **Clinical presentation**:
  - Relatively common condition.
  - Fixed position of the forearm rotation: inability to supinate or pronate the forearm (Fig. 9.11)
  - Normal elbow flexion and extension.
  - Despite having inability to rotate the forearms, patients are quite functional.
  - Parents often discover the inability of the child to rotate their forearms when the child participates in sporting activities such as holding a bat to play baseball and find him/her self not able to perform these activities.
  - **Radiographs of the elbow**: show the bony fusion (Fig. 9.11).

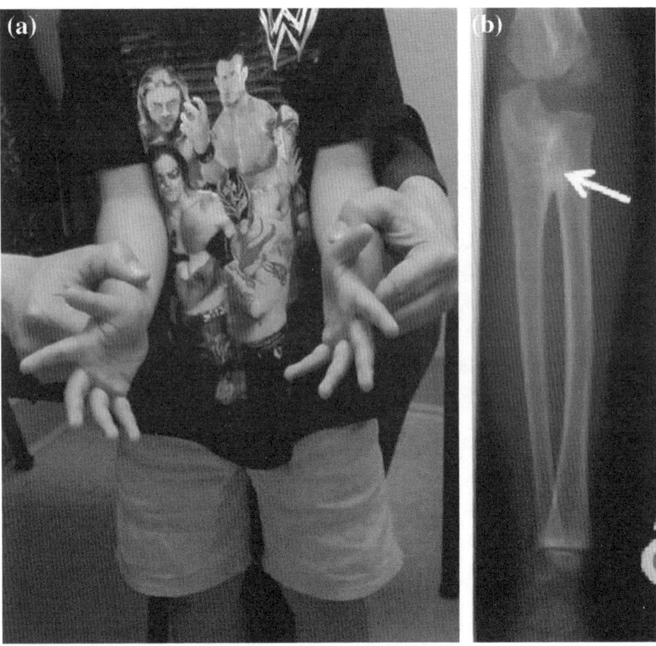

Fig. 9.11 Bilateral radio-ulnar synostosis. **a** A 7-year-old boy, brought by his parents because they noticed that he cannot rotate both forearms. No supination/pronation could be obtained at the level of the forearm. **b** Radiograph reveals fusion between proximal part of radius and ulna (*arrow*)

- **Management**:
  - Orthopedic referral if the position of the hand is interfering with the patient function.
  - Surgery is rarely indicated for this condition.
    - Surgery aims to reposition the forearm in a better functional position (dominant hand in pronation for writing and typing and non dominant hand supinated for hygiene).
    - An attempt to excise the fusion is usually non successful due to high recurrence rate.

HAND INFECTIONS

PARONYCHIA

Definition

- A paronychia is a superficial infection of nail fold adjacent to the nail plate (see nail anatomy later).

Etiology

- Acute paronychia is most commonly caused by *Staphylococcus aureus* or *Streptococcus* species.
- A mixed bacterial infection is common, particularly in patients with diabetes.
- Recurrent or Chronic infection can be caused by *Candida albicans*.

Predisposing factors:

- Nail biting
- Finger sucking
- Trivial finger trauma
- Finger exposure to chemical irritants
- Acrylic nails
- Nail glue, sculpted nails
- Frequent hand immersion in water

Clinical Presentation:

- Acute onset of pain and swelling around the nail.
- Hypertrophy of the nail plate indicates fungal infection.
- Abscess (collection of pus material) can be found in advanced cases. The collection will be superficial to the nail plate.
- With advanced cases, the infection will spread deep to the nail plate (subungal abscess).

Investigation:

- **Laboratory studies are not routinely performed in simple cases**
- Gram stain and cultures after incision and drainage if there is extensive infection with surrounding cellulitis

- Potassium hydroxide (KOH) and fungal cultures if Candidal infection is suspected
- Tzanck smear or viral culture may be helpful when herpetic whitlow is suspected
- Skin biopsy may be indicated in chronic cases where malignancy is suspected

Management

- If there is no abscess formation:
    - Local treatment is usually sufficient:
        - Rinsing in warm water for few minutes several times a day.
        - Local antibiotic treatment.
- If there is a superficial abscess:
    - Drainage of the abscess followed by local treatment as before.
- If there is an abscess formation with surrounding cellulitis:
    - Drainage followed by oral antibiotic (anti staph antibiotic followed by antibiotic according to culture).
- If there is a subungual abscess (the abscess extends underneath the nail plate):
    - Drainage of the abscess with removal of the part of the nail plate followed by oral antibiotics.
- Oral antibiotics
    - Oral antibiotics are not necessary if the incision successfully achieves adequate drainage and no cellulitis is present. Most paronychia infections can be managed without oral antibiotics.
    - If cellulitis is present, antibiotics are indicated.
    - Trimethoprim and sulfamethoxazole (TMP/SMX), doxycycline, or clindamycin may be considered to cover community-acquired MRSA and anaerobic organisms.

- Chronic fungal paronychial infections are usually managed with oral antifungals such as ketoconazole, itraconazole, or fluconazole

TENOSYNOVITIS

Definition

- Tenosynovitis involves inflammation of the tendon and tendon sheath.

Etiology

- Gonococcal tenosynovitis: caused by *Neisseria gonorrhoeae*.
- Nongonococcal infectious tenosynovitis
  - *Staphylococcus aureus* and *Streptococcus* species are the most common etiologic agents, but infection is frequently mixed (aerobic and anaerobic).
  - *Pasteurella multocida* is common with cat bites (about 50 %) and dog bites (about 30 %); *Eikenella corrodens* occurs with human bites. However, human and animal bites may have a mixture of aerobic and anaerobic flora.

Clinical Presentation

The 4 cardinal signs (**Kanavel signs**):

- Pain on passive extension (**the earliest and most consistent sign**)
- Tenderness along the course of the flexor tendon
- Symmetric edema of the involved finger (fusiform swelling)
- Flexed resting posture of finger

Gonococcal tenosynovitis (**see also gonococcal arthritis**)

- part of **Arthritis-dermatitis syndrome**: the classic triad:
  - Tenosynovitis.
    - □ Most common sites affected are the dorsum of the wrist, hand, and ankle.
    - □ Erythema, tenderness to palpation, and painful range of motion of the involved tendon(s) are present

- Dermatitis: small vesicles or pustules
- Migratory polyarthralgia: multiple joint are affected. Tend to involve the upper extremities more than the lower extremities. The wrist, elbows, ankles, and knees are most commonly affected.

Laboratories

- Gonococcal cultures of the urethra or cervix, rectum, and pharynx are appropriate, if gonococcal tenosynovitis is suspected.
- Markers of infection will be elevated in infectious tenosynovitis.
  - CBC count with differential
  - Erythrocyte sedimentation rate (ESR)
  - CRP

MRI and ultrasound:

- Can help establish the diagnosis of tenosynovitis, **however, most cases are diagnosed on clinical basis with a good clinical history.**

Management

- **Gonococcal tenosynovitis**
  - Admit to hospital with intravenous (IV) or intramuscular (IM) antibiotics (e.g., ceftriaxone, spectinomycin)
- **Nongonococcal infectious tenosynovitis**
  - Orthopedic referral:
    - The condition needs **urgent surgical debridement** as delay in treatment may lead to necrosis of the tendons.
  - Antibiotic treatment.
    - Antibiotics should cover both staph and anaerobes.

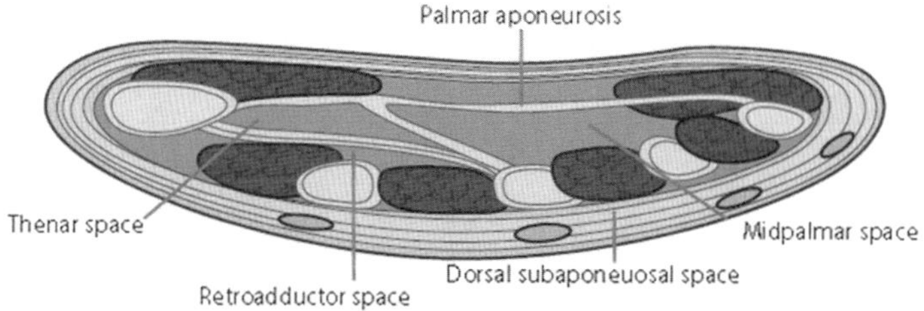

Fig. 9.12 Deep fascial spaces of the hand

DEEP HAND INFECTION

Definition

- The deep fascial spaces of the hand are potential spaces for infection and deep abscess formation in the hand (Fig. 9.12)
  - Dorsal subaponeurotic space.
  - Web space infection.
  - Midpalmar space.
  - Thenar space.

Etiology

- *S aureus* and *Streptococcus* species are the most commonly isolated organisms.
- After animal bite: see tenosynovitis.

Clinical presentation

- Deep fascial space infections present with pain in the hand, swelling, and tenderness over the affected area:
  - **Dorsal subaponeurotic abscesses**:
    - Result in swelling and pain on the dorsum of the hand and pain with passive movement of the extensor tendons (Fig. 9.13).

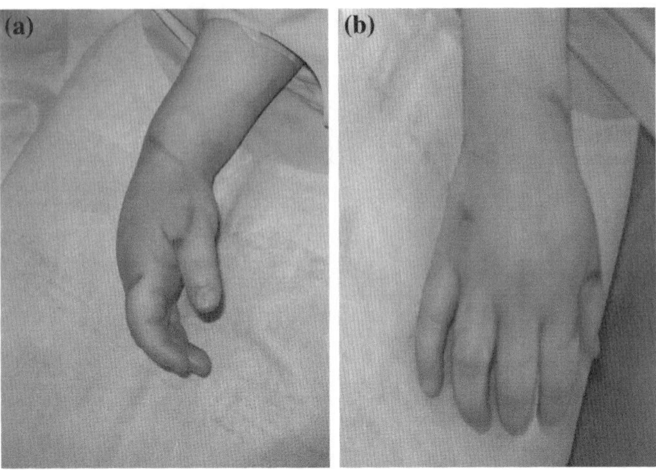

Fig. 9.13 (**a** and **b**) Dorsal hand subaponeurotic abscesses. 2-year-old boy who had a dog bite 3 days earlier presenting with pain, swelling, and redness over the dorsum of the hand

- **Web space infection**:
  - Presents with marked swelling on the dorsum of the hand and the web space in-between two digits.
- **Midpalmar space infections**
  - Present with pain, swelling, loss of palmar concavity, pain with movement of the third and fourth digits, and dorsal swelling secondary to the tracking of infection dorsally along the lymphatics.
- **Thenar space infections**
  - Result in marked swelling of the thumb-index web space.

Management:

- **Orthopedic referral for surgical debridement**.
- Antibiotic coverage:
  - Similar to flexor tenosynovitis.

FELON (PULP SPACE INFECTION)

Definition:

- Felons are closed-space infections of the fingertip pulp (the palmar aspect of the finger tip)

Pathophysiology

- Fingertip pulp has numerous vertical septa that divide the pulp into small compartments.
- Infection occurring within these compartments can lead to abscess formation, edema, and increased pressure in a closed space. This may lead to affection of the blood supply and necrosis of the skin and pulp.

Clinical Presentation

- Predisposing factors include splinters, cuts, or extension of paronychia.
- Fingertip blood glucose measurements have been implicated as an etiology
- Patient will present with pain (usually severe) at the tip of the finger with edema, swelling, and tightness of the pulp.
- Early infection may resolve with antibiotics.
- If resolution does not occur, abscess formation will occur which will present by throbbing pain

Etiology

- *Staphylococcus aureus*: most common organism

Management

- Early (before abscess formation):
    - Antibiotic (Adequate early treatment of a felon can prevent abscess formation)
    - Empirical coverage for *Staph aureus* and streptococcal organisms should be provided.
- After abscess formation:
    - Incision and debridement.

- The felon should be incised in the area of maximum tenderness.
- All the septa should be released to avoid increasing pressure in certain compartment.
- Antibiotic treatment (start with anti staph antibiotic followed by antibiotic according to culture and sensitivity).

HERPETIC WHITLOW

Definition

- Herpetic whitlow is an infection of the hand that typically affects the terminal phalanx caused by viral Herpex simplex infection

Etiology

- Herpes simplex virus (60 % of cases by HSV-1 and 40 % by HSV-2)

Clinical Presentation

- Intense pain and swelling of a finger, typically with characteristic vesicular lesions.
  - Grouped vesicular lesions or ulcers with surrounding erythema.
  - Fluid within the vesicles is usually clear, although it may appear cloudy or hemorrhagic.
- The most commonly involved digits are the thumb and index fingers.
- Presence of gingivostomatitis is very characteristic finding in pediatric patients.

Laboratory studies:

- The diagnosis is mainly clinical.
- Identification of the organism can be done by Tzanck smear or viral culture.

Treatment

- Herpetic whitlow is a self-limited disease. Treatment most often is directed toward symptomatic relief.
- Acyclovir may be beneficial.
  - In primary infections (topical acyclovir, 5 %) has been demonstrated to shorten the duration of symptoms and viral shedding.
  - Oral acyclovir may prevent recurrence
- Use antibiotic treatment only in cases complicated by bacterial superinfection
- Tense vesicles may be unroofed to help ameliorate symptoms, and wedge resection of the fingernail may be used for the same purpose in cases involving the subungual space.
- **Deep surgical incision is contraindicated** because it can lead to:
  - Delayed resolution,
  - Bacterial superinfection
  - Systemic spread

SNAKE BITE

Background

- Most snakebites are non poisonous and are delivered by non-poisonous species. Worldwide, only about 15 % of the more than 3,000 species of snakes are considered dangerous to humans.
- North America has about 25 species of poisonous snakes.

Clinical Presentation

- **Local manifestation**
  - Local swelling, pain, and paresthesias may be present (Fig. 9.14).

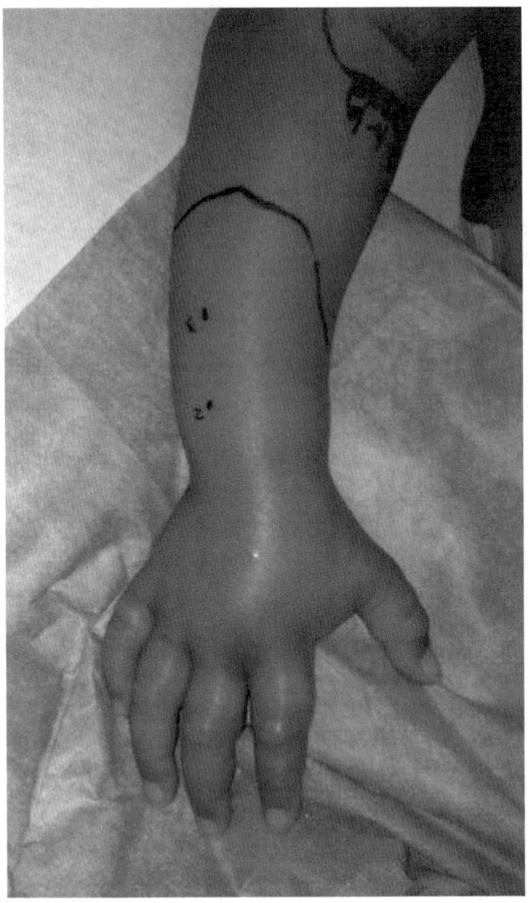

Fig. 9.14 Snake bite to the right hand. 1-year-old boy with bite to the right hand. Notice severe swelling of the hand and finger (Courtesy of Dr S Machen)

- Soft pitting edema that generally develops over 6-12 h, but may start within 5 min
- Bullae
- Streaking
- Erythema or discoloration

Systemic toxicity

- **Assessment of vital signs, airway, breathing, circulation**.
- The time elapsed since the bite is a necessary component of the history.
- Determine history of prior exposure to antivenin or snakebite. (this increases risk and severity of anaphylaxis).
  - Hypotension
  - Petechiae, epistaxis, and hemoptysis
  - Paresthesias and dysesthesias
  - Respiratory distress (more common with coral snakes)

Investigation

- **Laboratory**
  - CBC with differential and peripheral blood smear
  - Coagulations profile
  - Fibrinogen and split products
  - Blood chemistries, including electrolytes, BUN, creatinine
  - Urinalysis for myoglobinuria
  - Arterial blood gas determinations and/or lactate level for patients with systemic symptoms
- Baseline chest radiograph (for assessment of pulmonary edema)
- Plain radiograph on bitten body part to rule out retained fang
- Measurement of forearm or leg compartment pressure to rule out a "compartment syndrome."

MANAGEMENT

- **Pre-hospital care**
  - Monitor vital signs and airway.
  - Restrict activity and immobilize the affected area.
  - Immediately transfer to definitive care with possible need to intensive care admission.
  - Do not give antivenin in the field.

- **Grades of envenomation are defined as mild, moderate, or severe**.
  - **Mild envenomation** is characterized by:
    - **Local signs** are present: local pain, edema.
    - **No signs of systemic toxicity** or abnormal laboratory values.
  - **Moderate envenomation** is characterized by:
    - **Severe local pain**; edema larger than 25 cm surrounding the wound (Fig. 9.14)
    - **Systemic toxicity** starts to occur including nausea, vomiting, and alterations in laboratory values
  - **Severe envenomation** is characterized by:
    - Generalized petechiae and ecchymosis
    - Blood-tinged sputum
    - Hypotension and hypoperfusion leading to renal dysfunction
    - Changes in PT and PTT and other coagulation studies

Indication for antivenom

- Hemodynamic or respiratory instability
- Abnormal coagulation studies
- Neurotoxicity, e.g., paralysis of diaphragm
- Evidence of local toxicity with progressive soft tissue swelling

Anti-venom is relatively specific for snake species against which they designed to protect. Often the anti-venom is administered empirically based of the snake species in a geographic region. The risk of anaphylaxis may occur due to the large protein load be administered.

Orthopedic referral:

- Surgical assessment focuses on the injury site and concern for the development of compartment syndrome.
- Fasciotomy is indicated only for those patients with objective evidence of elevated compartment pressure.

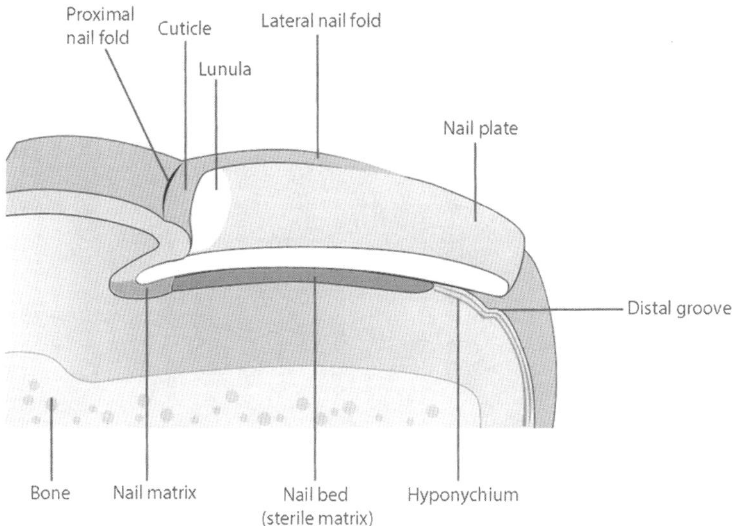

Fig. 9.15 Nail anatomy

- Bitten extremities should be marked proximal and distal to the bite and the circumference at this location should be monitored every 15 min to follow the progression of the condition.

Anatomy of the nail (Fig. 9.15)

- **Nail (nail plate)**: Hard keratinized structure composed of desiccated squamous cells
- **Nail bed**: Soft tissue below the nail connecting it to underlying periosteum of the distal phalanx and consists of the germinal and sterile matrix
- **Paronychium**: Lateral nail folds
- **Hyponychium**: Junction between the nail bed and fingertip
- **Eponychium (cuticle)**: the distal portion of the proximal nail fold where it attaches to the dorsum of the nail
- **Lunula**: White opacity distal to the eponychium

Nail bed and finger tip injuries

- Nail bed and finger tip injuries are common hand injuries in children. It represents about two thirds of hand injuries in children

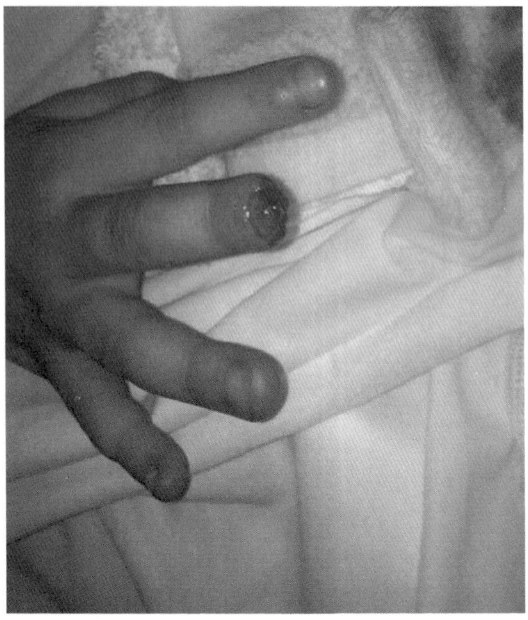

Fig. 9.16 An 8-year-old boy with finger tip amputation by the door closing on the middle finger

Etiology

- Most injuries of the nail bed are due to crushing injuries.
  - The door closing on the fingers (either by self or by other children) is common among children(Fig. 9.16).
- Laceration (by glass or knife) is another cause of nail bed and finger tip injuries.

Clinical presentation

- Most injuries of the nail bed will also involve the fingertip.
- Nail bed and finger tip injuries are usually associated with:
  - Subungual hematomas.
  - Lacerations to the surrounding skin.

- Finger tip amputation.
- Fractures of the distal phalanx.
- The nail may be partially or completely avulsed from the nail fold.
  - Nail plate avulsion is usually accompanied by significant nail bed laceration that requires repair.

Radiology

- Indication for X-ray is depending on the extent of injury
- Radiologic evaluation with anteroposterior, lateral, and oblique views of the injured fingers are useful to rule out:
  - Foreign bodies
  - Fractures or dislocations of the distal finger

Management
Subungual hematoma:

- **Future deformity of the nail can result from nail injuries, so must warn the family in advance**.
- **A subungual hematoma is a common presentation, and the possibility of an underlying nail bed laceration or injury should always be considered**.
- The blood will be incorporated into the surrounding tissues and eventually can cause separation of the nail plate from the nail bed.
- Small non expanding subungual hematomas: ice and NSAIDs.
- If the subungual hematoma covers more than 25 % of the nail bed or is causing pain, it should be evacuated via trephination.
  - local anesthesia (without epinephren) at the base of the finger (both volarly and dorsally).
  - Trephination can be done using an electric cautery, which melts a hole through the nail, another method is to use 16 guage needle tip.

Repair of nail bed laceration:

- Principles of treatment include:
  - Copious irrigation

- Minimal debridement
- Splinting of the repair with the nail plate or an alternative material

- The repair can be done by suture techniques or use of tissue adhesive material as the 2-octylcyanoacrylate (Dermanbond®).
- If immunization is not update, tetanus immunization is indicated
- **Antibiotic**
  - The prophylactic use of antibiotics is indicated depending on the mechanism and extent of injury, such as for crush injuries and human or animal bites

Consultation

- A hand surgeon should be consulted for significantly avulsed nail matrix or for severe crush injuries

REFERENCES

Brook I. Aerobic and anaerobic microbiology of paronychia. Ann Emerg Med. 1990;19:994–6.

Rockwell PG. Acute and chronic paronychia. Am Fam Physician. 2001;63:1113–6.

Goldenberg DL. Gonococcal arthritis. In: McCarty DJ, editor. Arthritis and allied conditions: a textbook of rheumatology. 11th ed. Philadelphia: Lea and Febiger; 1989.

Watson FM Jr. Nonarthritic inflammatory problems of the hand and wrist. Emerg Med Clin North Am. 1985;3:275–82.

Antosia RE, Hand LE. In: Rosen editor, Emergency medicine concepts and clinical practice. 5th ed. Philadelphia: Mosby; 2002. p. 493–535.

Gold BS, Dart RC, Barish RA. Bites of venomous snakes. N Engl J Med. 2002;347:347–56.

Al-Qattan MM, Al-Thunayan A, De Cordier M, Nandagopal N, Pitkanen J. Classification of the mirror hand: multiple hand spectrum. J Hand Surg (Br). 1998;23(4):534–6.

Bamshad M, Van Heest AE, Pleasure D. Arthrogryposis: a review and update. J Bone Joint Surg Am. 2009;91(Suppl 4):40–6.

Bayne LG. Ulnar club hand-ulnar deficiency. In: Green DP, editor. Operative hand surgery. New York: Churchill Livingstone 2009; 198. p. 245–257.

Bayne LG, Klug MS. Long-term review of the surgical treatment of radial deficiencies. J Hand Surg. 1987;12A:169–70.

Carter PR, Ezaki M. Madelung's deformity. Surgical correction through the anterior approach. Hand Clin. 2000 Nov;16(4):713–721, x-xi.

Cleary JE, Omer GE Jr. Congenital proximal radio-ulnar synostosis. Natural history and functional assessment. J Bone Joint Surg Am. 1985;67:539–45.

Ezaki M. Treatment of the upper limb in the child with arthrogryposis. Hand Clin. 2000;16:703–11.

Goldfarb CA. Congenital hand differences. J Hand Surg. 2009;34A(1351–56):2009.

Ito T, Handa H. Deciphering the mystery of thalidomide teratogenicity. Congenit Anom (Kyoto). 2012;52(1):1–7. doi:10.1111/j.1741-4520.2011.00351.

Kelikian H. Reconstructive surgery of congenital hands. Proc Inst Med Chic. 1968;27:52.

Kerby C, Oberg MD, Jennifer M, Feenstra BS, Paul R, Manske MD, Michael A, Tonkin MD. Developmental biology and classification of congenital anomalies of the hand and upper extremity. J Hand Surg. 2010;35A:2066–2076.

Kozin Lamb DW, Wynne-Davies R. Incidence and genetics. In: Buck-Gramcko D, editor. Congenital malformations of the hand and forearm. London: Churchill Livingstone; 1998. p. 21–27.
Madelung O. Die Spontane Subluxation de Hand Nach Vorne. Verh Dtsch Ges Chir. 1878;7:259–76.
McCarroll HR, James MA, Newmeyer WL 3rd, Molitor F, Manske PR. Madelung's deformity: quantitative assessment of x-ray deformity. J Hand Surg Am. 2005;30:1211–20.
Devilliers Minnaar AB. Congenital fusion of the lunate and triquetral bones in the South African Bantu. J Bone Joint Surg Br. 1953; 34-B:45–48.
Nielsen JB. Madelung's deformity. A follow-up study of 26 cases and a review of the literature. Acta Orthop Scand. 1977;48:379–84.
Oberg KC, Feenstra JM, Manske PR, Tonkin MA. Developmental biology and classification of congenital anomalies of the hand and upper extremity. J Hand Surg. 2010;35A:2066–76.
Poland A. Deficiency of the pectoral muscles. Guy's Hosp Rep. 1841;6:191–3.
Ritt MJPF, Maas M, Bos KE. Minnaar type 1 symptomatic lunotriquetral coalition: a report of nine patients. J Hand Surg. 2001;26A:261–70.
Sachar K, Mih AD. Congenital radial head dislocations. Hand Clin. 1998;14(1):39–47.
Swanson AB, Swanson GD, Tada K. A classification for congenital limb malformation. J Hand Surg Am. 1983;8(5 Pt 2):693–702.
Tonkin MA. Thumb duplication: concepts and techniques. Clin Orthop Surg. 2012 Mar;4(1):1–17. Epub 2012 Feb 20.
Wilkie AO, Patey SJ, Kan SH, van den Ouweland AM, Hamel BC. FGFs, their receptors, and human limb malformations: clinical and molecular correlations. Am J Med Genet. 2002;112:266–78.
Zook EG. Anatomy and physiology of the perionychium. Hand Clin. 1990;6:1–7.
Seaberg DC, Angelos WJ, Paris PM. Treatment of subungual hematomas with nail trephination: a prospective study. Am J Emerg Med. 1991;9:209–10.
Kilgore ES Jr, Brown LG, Newmeyer WL. Treatment of felons. Am J Surg. 1975;130:194–8.
Fetter-Zarzeka A, Joseph MM. Hand and fingertip injuries in children. Pediatr Emerg Care. 2002;18(5):341–5.
Langlois J, Thevenin-Lemoine C, Rogier A, Elkaim M, Abelin-Genevois K, Vialle R. The use of 2octylcyanoacrylate (Dermabond(®)) for the treatment of nail bed injuries in children: results of a prospective series of 30 patients. J Child Orthop. 2010 Feb;4(1):61–65. Epub 2009 Nov 13.
Connolly B, Johnstone F, Gerlinger T, Puttler E. Methicillin-resistant staphylococcus aureus in a finger felon. J Hand Surg Am. 2000;25(1):173–5.
Wu IB, Schwartz RA. Herpetic whitlow. Cutis. Mar 2007;79:193–196.
Nikkels AF, Pierard GE. Treatment of mucocutaneous presentations of herpes simplex virus infections. Am J Clin Dermatol. 2002;3:475–87.
Castilla EE, Lugarihno R, da Dutra MG, Salgado LJ. Associated anomalies in individuals with polydactyly. Am J Med Genet. 1998;80:459–65.
Graham TJ, Ress AM. Finger polydactyly. Hand Clin. 1998;14(1):49–64.

Chapter 10
Sport Injury: Lower Extremity

Amr Abdelgawad and Courtney Holland

INTRODUCTION

- Dramatic increase in adolescent sports participation over the past two decades.
- Estimated 30 million children participate in organized athletics per year.
- Primary care physicians are often the first to assess these children and start medical treatment for them.
- Keen understanding of the common pediatric lower extremity (hip, knee, and ankle) injuries is paramount in proper initial evaluation and referral management.
- Unlike in adults, reconstruction procedures are complicated by a growing axial skeleton and potential extended recovery period.

Hip joint:

Avulsion injuries of the pelvic apophyses:

Definition:

- The pelvis has multiple apophyses (see Chap. 1) that act as an origin for pelvic muscle.
- These apophyses can be pulled by excessive muscle contraction during sport activity.

Clinical presentation:

- Pain at affected side:
  - Anterior superior iliac spine (ASIS) (Sartorius) (Fig. 10.1).
  - Anterior inferior iliac spine (AIIS) (rectus femoris).
  - iliac crest (abductor).
  - ischial tuberosity (hamstrings).

A. Abdelgawad and O. Naga (eds.), *Pediatric Orthopedics*,
DOI: 10.1007/978-1-4614-7126-4_10,

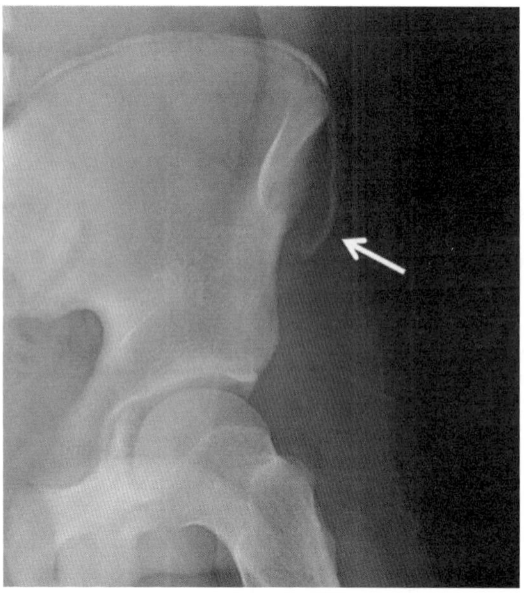

Fig. 10.1 1 ASIS avulsion. A 13-year-old boy was playing basketball and had left hip and pelvis pain. Radiograph showed avulsion of ASIS (*arrow*)

Radiographs:

- Will show the pulled apophysis (Fig. 10.1).

Management:

- The lesion will heal spontaneously, only symptomatic treatment is needed.
  - Rest and decrease activity.
  - NSAIDs
  - Return to sports when patient has no pain (indicating healing of the avulsion fracture).

OTHER HIP SPORT INJURIES

Hip dislocation:

- See Chap. 16.

Acute slipped capital femoral epiphysis:

- See Chap. 6.

KNEE SPORTS INJURY

Special Considerations

- **Knee is the most commonly affected joint in sports lesions**.
- Knee pain can be due to pathology in hip joint, secondary to irritation along the obturator nerve.
- Injury to the knee in skeletally immature children can lead to potential physeal injury of the proximal tibia or distal femur physis.
  - Injury to the physis can lead to increased risk for progressive limb deformity or growth arrest (see Chap. 16).
- Consider infectious, neoplastic, or inflammatory processes with atypical clinical presentation.
  - Knee is common site for benign and malignant processes due to the highly active physis growth, so do not assume that all pain is related to injury **(radiographs should be obtained for any unilateral knee pain)**.
  - **History of trauma does not exclude other non trauma etiologies** as patients and/or their families have the tendency to relate most knee pain to trauma.

Evaluation of the knee after sport injury:

Initial Assessment:

- Thorough history of present illness.
- Attempt to establish exact mechanism of injury if possible:
    - direction of the hit (if it happened by contact with other person)
    - hearing of a 'pop' sound of the knee (indicate a possible ACL injury)
    - timing between injury and swelling:
        - Immediate swelling: possible ACL injury.
        - Swelling of the knee after few hours: possible meniscal injury.
    - Ability to continue playing and/or weight bearing after injury.

Physical Examination:

- Inspection of the injured knee.
    - Note effusion, soft tissue swelling (Chap. 7, Fig. 7.4).
    - Limb alignment (genu varum or valgum).
- Observation of gait and determine ability to weight bear; if possible.
- Palpation of parapatellar tissues and joint line.
    - Note joint line tenderness.
    - Note tenderness about femoral/tibial physis.
- Assess passive and active range of motion.
- **Assess ligamentous stability of knee joint.**
    - Assessment of varus & valgus stability at 0° and 30° (Fig. 10.2).
    - Anterior and Posterior drawer at 90° flexion (Fig. 10.3).
    - Lachman exam at 30° of flexion (Fig. 10.4).
- Additional functional tests.

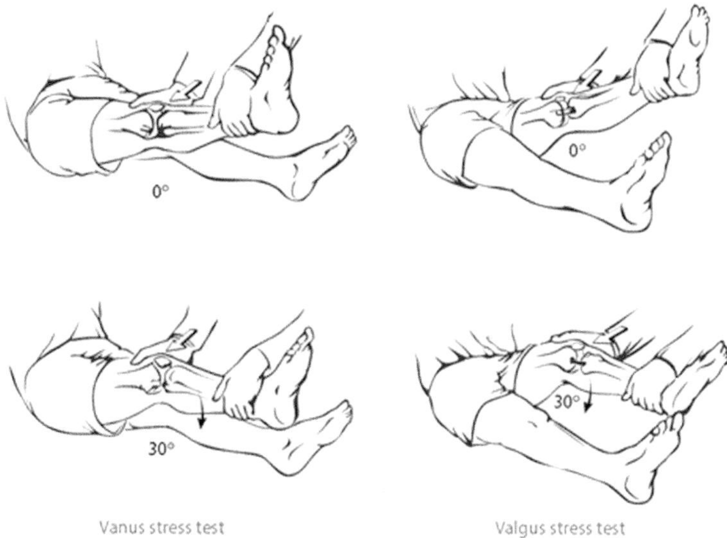

Fig. 10.2 Varus and valgus stress test

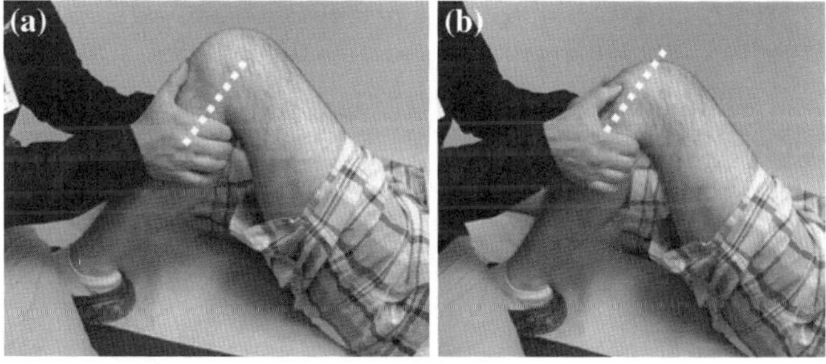

Fig. 10.3 Anterior drawer test: the patient lies supine with the hips 45° degrees and the knees flexed 90°. The physician sits on the patient's feet and grasps the upper part tibia and pulls it forward with both thumbs on the joint line to better assess the displacement of the tibia. If the tibia pulls forward or backward more than normal (compare to the contralateral side), the test is considered positive. (a) and (b) shows the forward translation of the tibia with the anterior drawer test (notice the position of the dotted line representing tibia) in relation to distal femur

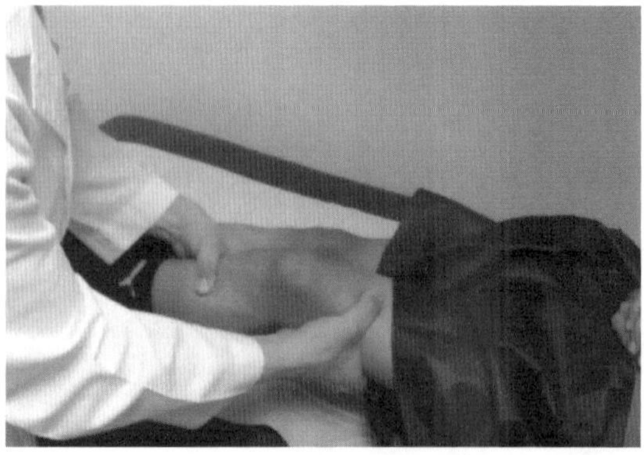

Fig. 10.4 Lachman test. Patient lies supine and the examiner keeps the knee in about 20° flexion. One hand stabilizes the lower thigh and the other hand holds the upper tibia and pushes it anterior and posterior in relation to the femur. The examined side should be compared to the normal side. Increased translation compared to the other side with abnormal 'soft' end point indicates ACL injury

- Assessment of meniscal pathology:
  - Apply Grinding test (see Chap. 7).
  - Mcmurray test: (see Chap. 7).
  - Deep knee bends or squats.
- Patellar apprehension (Fig. 10.5).
  - For assessment of lateral patellar subluxation or instability.

- Assess proximal and distal neurovascular status.
- Aspirate knee and obtain laboratory studies if suspicion of infection or inflammatory process.
  - CBC with differential, ESR, CRP.
  - Fluid analysis: cell count with differential, gram stain, crystals.

Imaging:

- Initial 4 view orthogonal knee radiographs.
  - AP, Lateral, 20° PA notch (for assessment of osteochondral lesions), and Skyline/Sunrise views (Fig. 10.6).

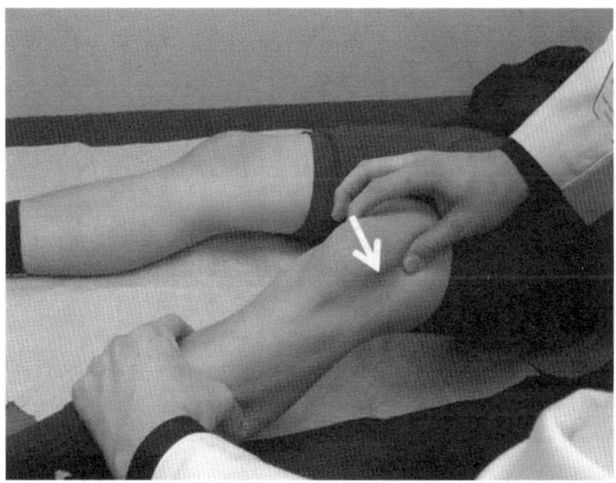

Fig. 10.5 Patellar apprehension test: The patient lies supine with the knee in about 30° degrees of flexion and the quadriceps muscle relaxed. The physician pushes the patella laterally observing the patient face for the apprehension look. A positive test is the presence of this reaction by the patient

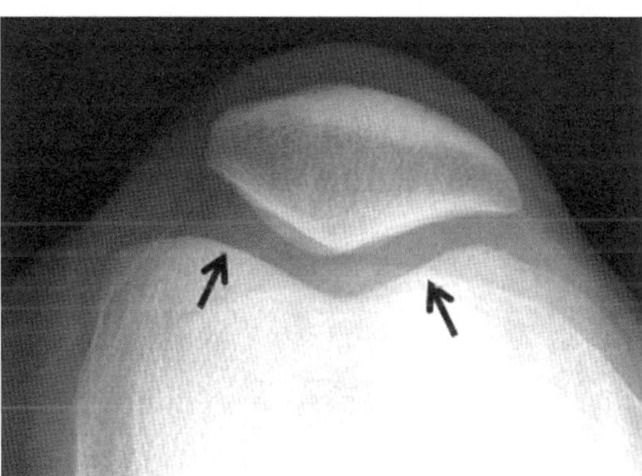

Fig. 10.6 Sunrise view. Tangential view for the patella to assess the alignment of the patellofemoral joint (position of the patella in the trochlear groove (*arrows*)

- Consider AP varus or valgus stress radiograph if suspecting injury to distal femoral physis or proximal tibial physis.
- CT or Ultrasound usually not warranted in acute setting.

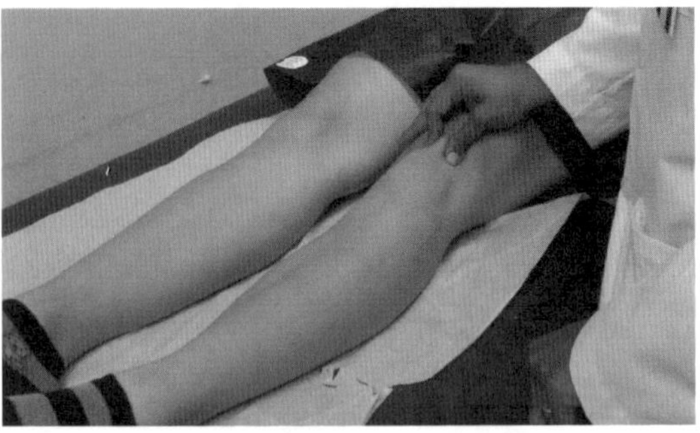

Fig. 10.7 Patellar grind test. With knee extended, the examiner pushes the patella distally into the trochlear groove of the femur. Patient tightens quadriceps to pull the patella proximally against the examiner movement. Pain with this manoeuvre indicates positive test

- MRI is helpful if there are concerns for soft tissue pathology, occult fracture or physeal injury, ligamentous instability, and intra-articular inflammatory process.

Patellofemoral Pain Syndrome (see also Chap. 7**)**

- Most common knee complaint presenting for evaluation; up to 30 % of all visits.
- Incidence of 7–10 % in young athletes.
- Etiology unclear, often secondary to overuse, decreased quadriceps flexibility, or extensor mechanism malalignment causing undue strain on patellofemoral joint.
- Old name was "chondromalacia patellae"; this was misnomer as cartilage of the patella in most cases is intact.

Clinical Presentation:

- Commonly complain of dull or achy anterior (retropatellar) knee pain.
- Pain worsened during and after sporting activity, prolonged sitting, stairs, or deep knee bends.
- Positive patellar grind test on exam (Fig. 10.7).
- Knee examination is usually normal:

- No soft tissue swelling.
- No joint line tenderness or ligamentous instability of knee.

■ May be associated with, miserable malalignment syndrome:

- Common rotational mal-alignment in adolescent females.
- It consist of the following three element (Fig. 7.24-knee):
    - □ Increased femoral anteversion (patella internally rotated).
    - □ External tibial torsion.
    - □ Pes planus (flat foot).

Imaging:

■ Radiographs: Normal.

Treatment:

■ **Patient reassurance and education**: the condition is typically self limiting.

■ Conservative management is the mainstay treatment; include Rest, Ice, activity modification, physical therapy for quadriceps stretching/flexibility, patellar taping, patellofemoral bracing, NSAIDs for pain.

Osteochondroses (see also Chap. 7):

■ Osgood-Schlatter Disease: Apophysitis of proximal tibial tuberosity at the insertion of patellar tendon.

■ Sinding-Larsen-Johansson Disease: Apophysitis of inferior patellar pole at the superior insertion of patellar tendon.

■ Jumper's knee: Inflammation of the patellar tendon. Not true osteochondroses, but have a similar clinical presentation.

Clinical Presentation

■ Common sport-related pathologies.

■ Commonly occur during adolescence growth spurt.

- Boys 13–14 years old; Girls 11–12 years old.
- Complaints of activity-related anterior knee pain.
- Occasional soft tissue swelling over anterior knee.
- Localized tenderness over tibial tubercle or inferior pole of patella.

- □ **Exacerbation with resisted knee extension, deep knee bends, or squatting**.

- Limited quadriceps flexibility.

Imaging:

- Radiographs obtained to exclude bony pathology;

  - Occasionally fragmentation or enlargement of inferior pole patellar or tibial tubercle.

Treatment:

- See Chap. 7.

Patellar Instability/Dislocation (**see also** Chap. 7):

- Spectrum of disease characterized by static and dynamic malalignment of the patella; range from acute instability due to trauma to chronic subluxation.
- **Occurs more commonly in female athletes.**
- Predisposing factors: see Chap. 7.

Clinical Presentation:

- Acute dislocation:

  - In most cases, reduction is done in the field by the trainer.
  - If no reduction is done: patella can be seen on the lateral aspect of the knee.
  - Rapidly developing knee effusion with severe pain and inability to bear weight.

- Recurrent dislocation/subluxation:

  - History of twisting moment or trauma about knee.
  - History of anterior knee pain, locking, giving away, or lateral displacement of patella.
  - On exam, effusion often noted along with medial parapatellar tenderness on palpation, **positive patellar apprehension test** (Fig. 10.5).

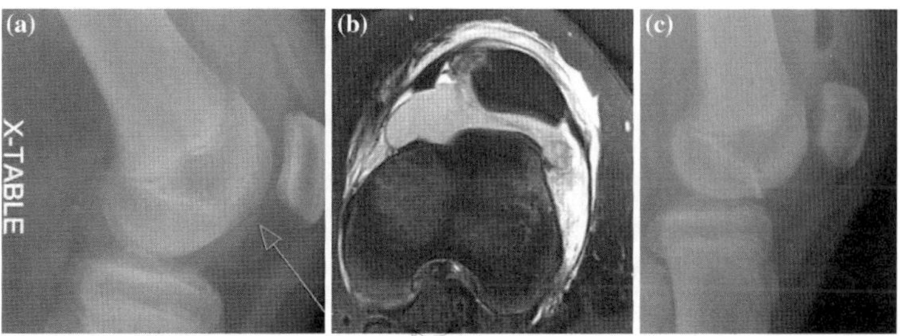

Fig. 10.8 Osteochondral fragment after patellar dislocation. A 12-year-old boy who sustained patellar dislocation while playing in physical education class. **a** Radiograph showed osteochondral fragment from the femoral condyle (arrow). **b** MRI shows effusion and disruption of the medial patellofemoral ligament. **c** The fragment was fixed by a screw

Imaging:

- AP, Lateral, and Sunrise view to rule out fracture and verify patellar position.
- MRI helpful to assess concomitant intra-articular chondral injuries or disruption of medial patellofemoral ligament (MPFL) (Fig. 10.8).

Treatment:

- Acute dislocation:
  - Acute patellar reduction if still dislocated; **gentle extension of knee with application of medial directed force to lateral patella**.
  - Immobilize in extension with knee immobilizer.
  - RICE: symptomatic treatment with rest, ice, compression, elevation.
  - NSAID's
  - Weight bearing is allowed in extension in a knee brace.
  - Consider physical therapy to strengthen VMO (vastus medialis obliqus) and patellofemoral knee bracing.
  - If associated with osteochondral fracture: orthopedic referral for fixation or excision of the fragment (Fig. 10.8).

- Recurrent dislocation/subluxation:
  - See Chap. 7.

OSTEOCHONDRITIS DISSECANS(SEE CHAP. 7)

Definition:

- Idiopathic lesion of subchondral bone with or without articular cartilage involvement.

Etiology:

- Proposed etiologies: acute trauma, repetitive micro trauma, vascular insufficiency or normal growth variant.

Clinical presentation:

- Typically occurs in adolescence, most commonly around the lateral aspect of medial femoral condyle(MFC).
- Lesion is bilateral in 20 %.
- Mild effusion, focal bony tenderness over MFC with palpation.
- Loss of extension or flexion if unstable lesion.
- If the lesion becomes detached from the underlying bone and loose in the knee, crepitus with passive joint motion.
- No ligamentous instability.

Imaging:

- AP, Lateral, 20° PA notch, and Sunrise views to evaluate for presence of bony lesion, subchondral fracture, subchondral separation, or loose body (Fig. 7.18 /knee).
- MRI may be helpful to characterize the extent of subchondral bone and overlying cartilage involvement.

Management (see Chap. 7**):**

- Initial treatment dependent on stage of lesion and skeletal maturity of patient;
- Immature patients (open physis) with intact non separated lesions can be treated by rest, activity modifications, weight bearing restriction, immobilization, NSAIDs.

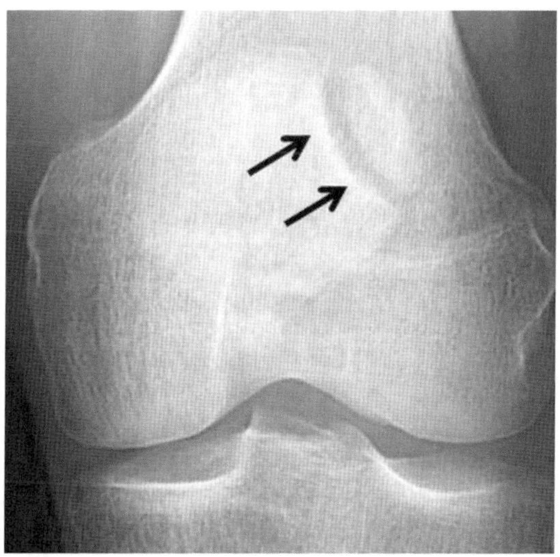

Fig. 10.9 Bipartite patella. A 14-year-old was playing soccer and twisted his knee. Radiograph showed bipartite patella (*arrows*) (accidental finding)

- Skeletally mature patient, presence of locked knee, or loose body require referral to orthopedics.

Bipartite patella:

- Patellar ossification occurs between 3–5 years of age with gradual fusion of multiple ossification centers.
- Failure of fusion leads to bipartite appearance; mimicking fracture.
- **Typical location is superolateral patella.**

Radiographs:

- Radiolucent area separating the patella into two segments (Fig. 10.9).
- Differentiated from fracture by:

- location of the radiolucent line (superolateral in bipartite patella, tansverse or longitudinal in fracture patella)
- smooth outline of the radiolucent line (while ragged in cases of fractures).

Clinical Presentation:

- Usually discovered as accidental finding when imaging the knee for a different reason.
- Rarely will cause anterior knee pain.
- No effusion or soft tissue swelling.

Treatment

- Most case can be managed without orthopedic referral. The condition responds well to conservative treatment: rest, activity modification, NSAID's, physical therapy for stretching/ strengthening.
- Failure to improve may require orthopedic referral for possible excision of symptomatic fragment.

SYNOVIAL PLICA

Definition:

- Remnant embryonic intra-articular synovial folds (Fig. 10.10).
- Thick bands of tissue that may become inflamed leading to mechanical irritation of the femoral condyles or patella.
- **Three main types of plicas are present:**
  - Medial shelf plica: is most common plica to cause knee pain.
  - Supra-patellar plica.
  - Infrapatellar plica.

Clinical Presentation:

- Medial knee pain with activities, squatting, deep knee bends, or stairs.
- Occasionally a palpable band can be felt along medial side of the knee.
- Snapping over medial condyle with joint motion.

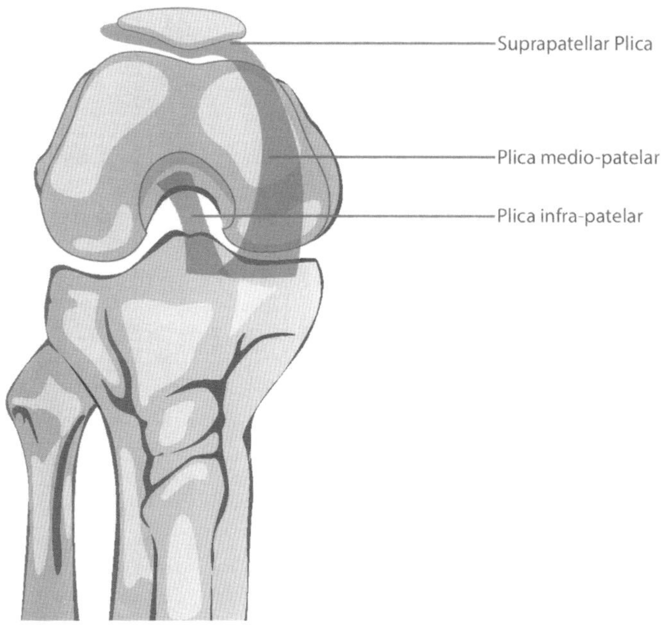

Fig. 10.10 Types of synovial plicas. Medial plica is the most clinically significant plica as a cause of knee pain

- No patellar or knee instability.

Imaging:

- Radiographs typically normal.
- MRI may reveal thickened fibrotic medial synovial band or reactive subchondral changes.

Management:

- Conservative: Rest, activity modification, NSAIDs, physical therapy for patellar mobilization and medial retinacular message.
- Failure to improve may require orthopedic referral for arthroscopic resection of plica.

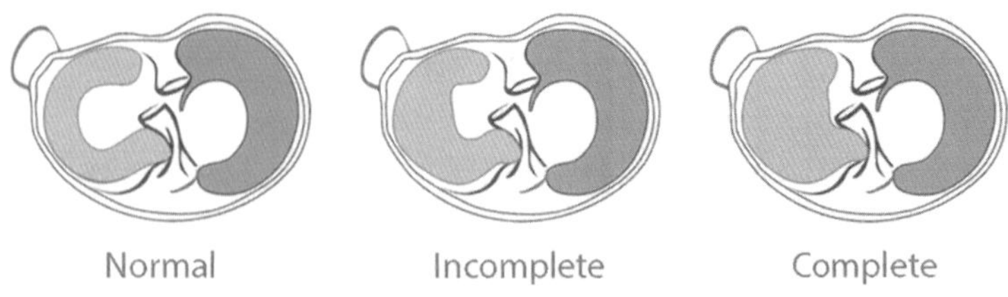

Fig. 10.11 Discoid meniscus. The condition commonly affect the lateral side. The shape of the meniscus becomes disc shaped rather than crescent

DISCOID MENISCUS

Definition:

- Congenital abnormality of knee Characterized by discoid shape meniscus (instead of the normal crescent shaped) (Fig. 10.11).
- Increased thickness leads to increase shearing forces and subsequent increased risk for tear.

Clinical Presentation:

- Incidence between 1–3 %.
- **Commonly involves lateral meniscus.**
- 20 % of cases are bilateral.
- The condition is usually asymptomatic.
- Complaints mimic meniscal tear: lateral joint pain, effusion, mechanical locking, catching, difficulty with squatting, or deep knee bends.

Imaging:

- Plain radiographs:
  - Lateral joint space widening, squaring of lateral condyle, cupping of lateral tibial plateau, and hypoplasia of lateral tibial spine.
- MRI:
  - modality of choice to visualize discoid meniscus

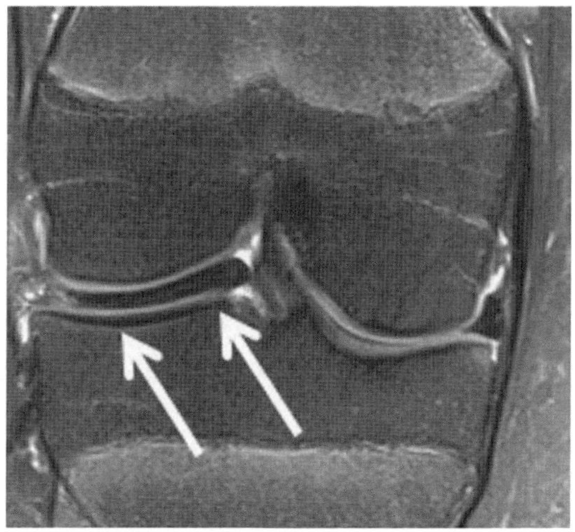

Fig. 10.12 MRI of a 12-year-old girl with pain in the lateral aspect of her knee with clicking. Lateral meniscus (*arrow*) has the shape of complete disc

- thickened meniscal appearance on three consecutive sequences (i.e., meniscal tissue connecting between the anterior and posterior horns of the meniscus rather than the normal separation between the two horns (Fig. 10.12).

Management.

- Treatment based on symptoms.
- Mild symptoms with no mechanical complaints:
  - Conservative management with rest, activity modifications, NSAIDs, physical therapy for stretching, and strengthening.
- Mechanical symptoms:
  - Orthopedic referral for arthroscopic reconstruction.

Anterior Cruciate Ligament (ACL) Injury (See Chap. 7)

- Anatomy: See Chap. 7.
- Most common ligamentous knee injury; in US there is 250,000 torn ACL per year.

- Increasing incidence in adolescent population due to increased sports participation at younger age.
- **Occurs in more commonly in adolescent female athletes compared to males.**
- **Sports associated with cutting movements (e.g., succor) have higher incidence of ACL injuries.**
- The injury occurs secondary to direct trauma to the knee, or non contact twisting or hyperextension injury to the knee.
- May be associated with injuries to medial and lateral collateral ligaments and menisci.

Clinical Presentation:

- Recent history of direct trauma, or twisting injury to the knee.
- In the acute setting:
    - The child will describe injury followed by "poping" of the knee and immediate swelling with inability to bear weight (this history is very characteristic of ACL injury)
    - Marked swelling (hemarthrosis)
    - Stressing the knee joint (Lachman and anterior drawer tests) cannot be performed in the acute setting because of pain.
- In the chronic setting:
    - Moderate effusion and diffuse knee pain with palpation
    - Joint tenderness
    - **Hallmark: positive provocative Lachman and anterior drawer tests** (Figs. 10.3 and 10.4).
- ACL tear in adolescents carries increased risk of recurrent injury and long term knee impairment.

Imaging:

- AP, Lateral, 20° tunnel, and Sunrise view to rule out fracture.
- MRI:
    - Diagnostic for ACL disruption (Fig. 10.13)
    - Also assess the integrity of menisci, collateral ligaments, and chondral surfaces.

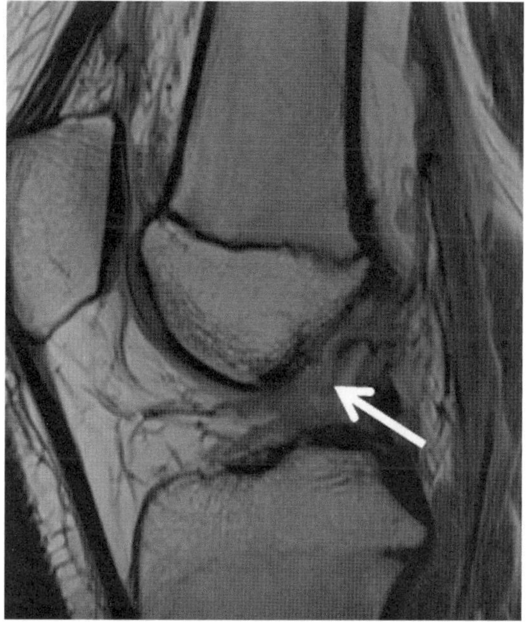

Fig. 10.13 MRI picture of ACL injury. A 15-year-old boy who had knee injury while playing soccer. MRI shows disruption of ACL fibers (arrow)

Management:

- Initial conservative management:
  - Rest, ice, activity modification, bracing, and physical therapy.
- **Early orthopedic referral for surgical consideration:**
  - Direct repair of the ACL is not possible.
  - Surgical reconstruction [by graft whether autograft (from the patient him/herself) or from donor (allograft)] is the standard of treatment if the patient wants to continue sport activity.
  - Reconstruction by graft requires drilling and passing tissues across the growth plate of the distal femur and proximal tibia which may affect these growth plates (see Chap. 16). This is of more concern in younger children.

- **In general the treatment of ACL in adolescent is:**
  - For skeletally mature and adolescent near skeletal maturity: surgical reconstruction if the patient wants to continue physical activity.
  - For skeletal immature children (less than 13 years old boy or 12 years old girl): non operative treatment (physical therapy for strengthening and change of physical activity) should be tried first. If this fails, risk and benefits of surgical treatment should be discussed with the family to allow them to take decision regarding surgical versus non surgical treatment.

Meniscal injury:

Anatomy of the menisci: see Chap. 7.

Pathology:

- Injury to the meniscus will result in tear to the meniscal tissue.
- More common in adolescent as a result of twisting injury to the knee.
- More common in the medial meniscus because it is less mobile (it can get caught between the tibia and femur).
- Can be associated with other ligament injuries like ACL injury.
- The tears are classified according to the shape and the site.

According to the shape

- The tear can be longitudinal (most common), radial, flap, or bucket handle tear (Fig. 10.14).

According to the site:

- Peripheral tear (red-red zone): in the peripheral one third of the meniscus near the capsule of the knee. It has the best healing potential as it has the best blood supply.
- Middle tear (red-white).
- Central (white-white): the tear is further away from the capsule. This part of the meniscus is Avascular. Has the least healing potential.

Clinical presentation

- Injury to the knee followed by pain and swelling

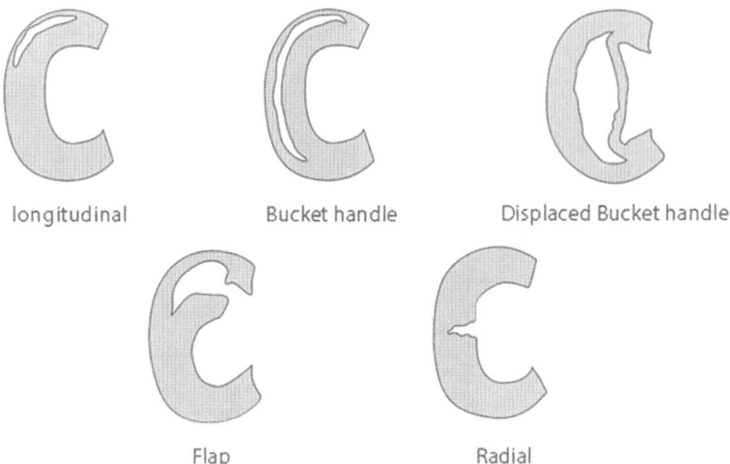

Fig. 10.14 Types of meniscal tears

- The swelling usually develop few hours after the injury (not immediately as in ACL injury)
- locking "catching" of the knee
- patient may complain of instability (giving away)
- Positive Mcmurry and Apply grinding test and deep squats (Fig 7.6 and 7.7).

Imaging:

- Plain radiographs (Anteroposterior, lateral, and sunrise) to exclude fractures or other bone pathology.
- MRI:
  - Can detect the meniscal tear (Fig. 10.15)
  - Can also show associated injuries (e.g., ACL injury).

Management:

- Most meniscal tears in adolescent are longitudinal peripheral tear that have good healing potential (in contrary to adults in which most tears have minimal healing potentials).
- Acute management: **RICE** (Rest, Ice, Compression, and Elevation).
- **Physical therapy** for range of motion (ROM) exercises and strengthening.

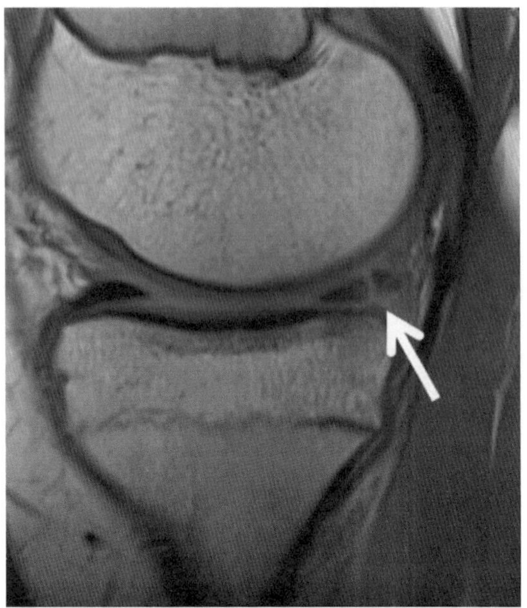

Fig. 10.15 A 16-year-old girl who twisted her knee while playing volleyball. MRI shows posterior horn medial meniscus injury

- **Return to sports:**
  - Full ROM (compared to the other knee) with no pain.
- **Indication for orthopedic referral:**
  - Failure of conservative therapy.
  - Bucket handle and flap tears.
  - Associated ACL injuries.

MEDIAL COLLATERAL LIGAMENT INJURY

Clinical presentation:

- Pain in the medial aspect of the knee following valgus injury.

- Instability of the knee on valgus stress (Fig. 10.2).

Radiograph:

- AP, Lat, and sun rise view to exclude fractures.
  - Salter Harris injury of the proximal tibia can have similar clinical presentation. The injury will show up in the radiographs as widening of the medial side of the proximal tibial physis.

MRI:

- Will show the injury to the medial collateral.

Management:

- Most medial collateral injuries can be treated conservative.
  - Acute management: **RICE** (Rest, Ice, Compression, and Elevation).
  - **Physical therapy** for range of motion (ROM) exercises and strengthening.
  - **Return to sports:**
    - Full ROM (compared to the other knee) with no pain.

Ankle injuries

Twisting inversion injuries of the ankle can lead to:

- Ankle sprain.
- Distal fibular Salter Hallis injury (see orthopedic trauma Chap. 16).
- 5th metatarsal base fracture (see orthopedic trauma Chap. 16).

Ankle sprain:

Definition

- Ankle sprain is a twisting injury of the foot and ankle followed by pain and swelling.
- The twisting injury in the majority of cases is "inversion type" (means that the ankle is in varus position at the time of injury (Fig. 10.16)).

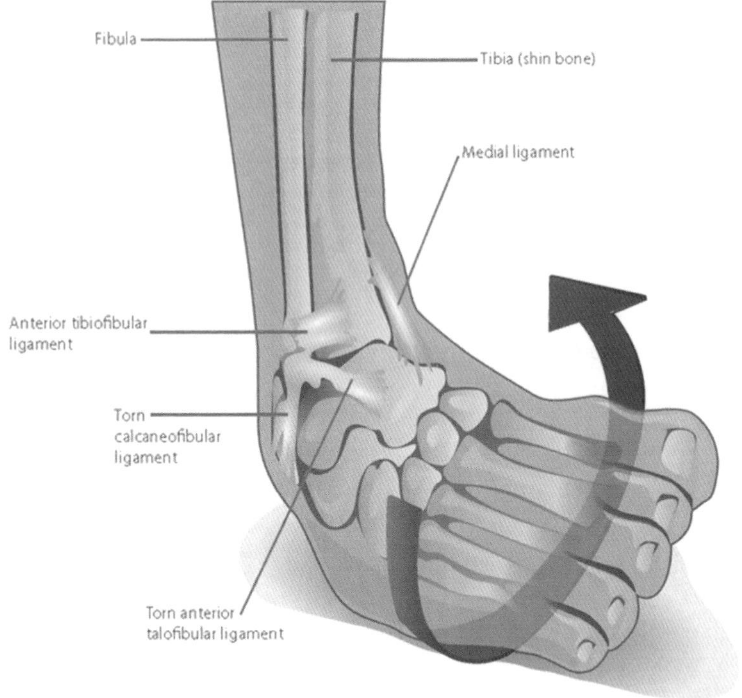

Fig. 10.16 Inversion type of ankle twisting injury. The ligaments affected are the anterior talofibular ligament (most common) and the calcaneofibular ligament

- **Inversion ankle sprain (most common):**
- **Pathophysiology:**
- Approximately 85 % of ankle sprains are inversion sprains of the lateral ligaments. This will cause injury to the lateral ankle ligament complex.
  - The lateral ankle ligament complex is composed of:
    1. anterior talofibular (ATFL)
    2. calcaneofibular
    3. posterior talofibular ligaments.
  - **The anterior talofibular ligament is the most commonly affected ligament in the lateral ankle ligament complex.**

- Eversion injuries (rare):
  - The ankle is in valgus position during twisting injury.
  - Injury to the deltoid (medial) ligament.
- Syndesmotic injuries (rare):
  - Syndesmotic injuries will cause disruption of the syndesmotic ligament between tibia and fibula (anterior and posterior tibiofibular ligaments).
  - These are usually referred to as "high sprain".

Ankle sprain classification:

- Ankle sprains are classified into the following 3 grades:
- **Grade 1**
  - Injuries involve a **stretch of the ligament with microscopic tearing.**
  - Swelling is usually minimal.
  - The joint is stable.
  - The patient is able to bear weight with minimal discomfort.
- **Grade 2**
  - Partial tearing of the ligament.
  - Moderate swelling and ecchymosis.
  - moderate joint instability.
  - Patients usually have difficulty in bearing weight.
- **Grade 3**
  - **Complete rupture of the ligament**.
  - Immediate and severe swelling and ecchymosis,
  - Inability to bear weight.
  - Severe instability of the joint.

Predisposing factors for recurrent ankle injuries:

- Poor proprioception (sense of position):
  - The peroneal muscle proprioception plays important role in stabilizing the ankle joint.

- Poor muscle tone.
- Obesity
- Connective tissue disorders (e.g., Ehler Danlos syndrome, Marfan syndrome)
- Tarsal collation:
  - Tarsal coalition is associated with recurrent ankle sprains.
  - The etiology may be related to abnormal mechanics of the foot by the fused bones.

Clinical presentation

- Depend on the degree of ankle sprain (see before).
- **Differentiate an ankle sprain from a fracture by:**
  - Palpate for any point bony tenderness in the following areas:
    - Medial malleolus.
    - Lateral malleolus.
    - Base of the fifth metatarsal.
    - Midfoot bones.
  - Any tenderness, bony deformity or crepitus, in one of those areas suggests the possible presence of a fracture.
- In lateral sprains (inversion injuries):
  - Passive inversion will reproduce pain.
  - Plantar flexion should also exacerbate the symptoms, because this motion stretches the ATFL to its maximum.
- The maximal points of tenderness for a lateral ankle sprain should be at the ATFL and/or calcaneofibular ligament areas.
- **Assessment of the stability of the ankle joint:**
  - Cannot be done in the acute setting because of pain.
  - Done in cases of recurrent ankle sprains or with persistence of pain few weeks after acute injury.
  - **Varus stress test** (Fig. 10.17).
    - The ankle is pushed into inversion (varus) and the movement of the talus is assessed and compare to the healthy side.

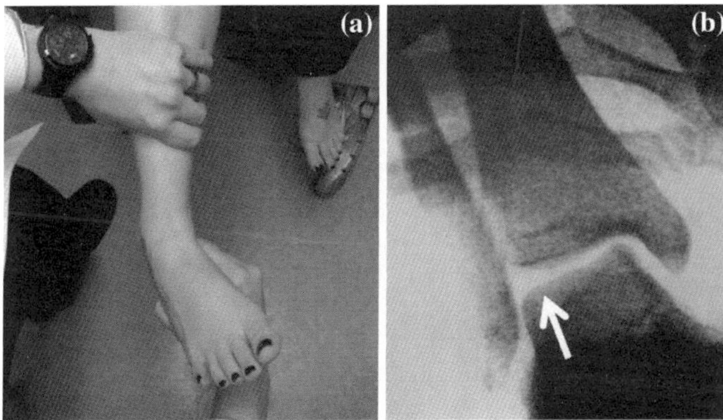

Fig. 10.17 Varus stress test. **a** The examiner stabilize the distal leg with one hand and the other hand pushes the ankle into inversion (varus) and the movement of the talus is assessed and compared to the healthy side. **b** Stress radiographs can be used for better assessment of the movement of the talus. Lateral gapping (*arrow*) indicate instability

  - May use stress radiographs to better assess the movement of the talus (Fig. 10.17).

- **Anterior drawer test:**
  - One hand holds the shaft of the tibia and the other hand pushes the heel forward while the ankle in equinus (Fig. 10.18)
  - The degree of movement of talus is compared to the normal side.
  - Assess the integrity of ATFL.

RADIOGRAPHY

Indication for X-ray:

- Bone tenderness at the posterior edge or tip of the lateral malleolus (i.e., the lower 6 cm of the fibula).
- Bone tenderness at the posterior edge or tip of the medial malleolus (i.e., the lower 6 cm of the tibia).

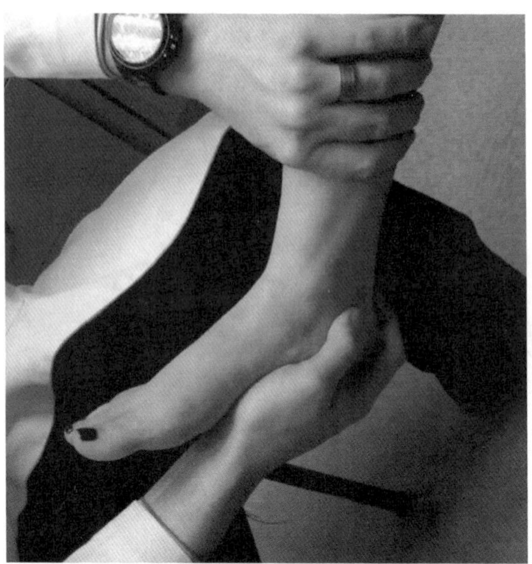

Fig. 10.18 Anterior drawer test ankle. One hand holds the shaft of the tibia and the other hand pushes the heel forward while the ankle in mild equinus. Assess movement of the talus in relation to the tibia

- Inability to bear weight immediately after the injury and in the emergency department.
- Bone tenderness at the base of the fifth metatarsal.
- Bone tenderness at the navicular bone.

Radiographic studies of the ankle should include the following views:

- An anteroposterior (AP) film with the ankle.
- A true lateral film.
- AP with the ankle in 20° internal rotation (mortise view).

MRI

- MRI may be useful when osteochondrosis is suspected or in patients with a history of recurrent ankle sprains and chronic pain.

Treatment

Conservative approach

- The acute phase of treatment lasts for 1–3 days after the injury.
- The goals of acute treatment are to control pain, minimize swelling, and maintain or regain ROM.
- **Rest, ice, compression, and elevation (i.e., RICE) are the mainstays of acute treatment.**
  - Ice is applied in the first 48 h for 20 min on the affected side 5–6 times/day.
- **Bracing or casting.**
  - Braces: multiple braces are available that can help stabilize the ankle (e.g., lace-up brace, air cast, cam boots).
  - Casting used rarely for ankle sprain nowadays, only with severe injuries in which patient is not able to bear weight with braces.
  - Discontinue the use of the brace when there is minimal swelling and pain at the site of injury.
- **Return to play:**
  - Patients can return to sports when they have normal painless range of motion.
- **Indication for physical therapy referral:**
  - If after 3 weeks the patient is still having pain or limited ROM of the ankle.
- **Indication for orthopedic referral:**
  - Acute or recurrent ankle sprains that do not improve with physical therapy.
  - Syndesmotic injuries with widening of the space between tibia and fibula in the radiographs.

OSTEOCHONDRITIS DISSECANS OF THE TALUS

Definition:

- Lesion of the subchondral bone of the talus resulting in weakening and possible separation of the overlying cartilage.

Etiology

- Unknown, may be related to repeated trauma.

Clinical presentation:

- Diffuse ankle pain.
- Repeated effusion.

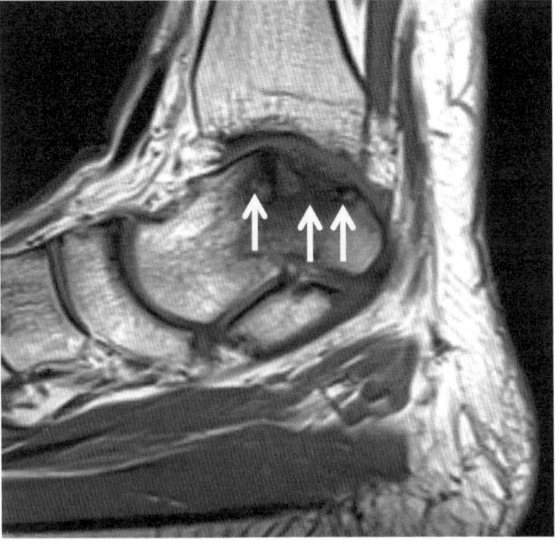

Fig. 10.19 A 16-year-old girl with few months history of ankle pain and recurrent ankle swelling. MRI showed osteochondral lesion in the postero-medial part of the talus with defect and fragmentation (*arrows*)

Radiograph:

- Can be normal in the early stage of disease. Later on will show the separated piece of bone.

MRI:

- Will show the marrow change and possible separation of the cartilage (Fig. 10.19).

Management

- Orthopedic referral.
- Management is similar to OCD of the knee:
  - If the lesion is stable (not separated): trial of physical therapy with decrease physical activity.
  - If there is failure of non operative management or there is separation of the cartilage, surgical treatment for excision or fixation of the fragment.

REFERENCES

Dowling S, Spooner CH, Liang Y, Dryden DM, Friesen C, Klassen TP, et al. Accuracy of Ottawa Ankle rules to exclude fractures of the ankle and midfoot in children: a meta-analysis. Acad Emerg Med. 2009;16:277–87.

DeLee JC, Drez D Jr, editors. Orthopaedic sports medicine: principles and practice, vol. 2. Philadelphia: WB Saunders; 1994. p. 1718–24.

Stanitski CL. Pediatric and adolescent sports injuries. Clin Sports Med. 1997;16(4):613–33.

Chapter 11

Sports Injuries: Upper Extremity

Justin M. Wright and Angel Garcia

INTRODUCTION

- Upper extremity injuries are common in pediatric sports.
- Due to the high stresses placed on individual joints, these athletes may present with acute or overuse injuries.
- As a result of skeletal immaturity, injury patterns in the pediatric athlete are different than their adult counterparts. Most pediatric upper extremity sports injuries respond well to conservative measures, including cessation of the offending activity and physical therapy.
- Identification of injuries requiring surgical intervention is key to preventing complications and returning these athletes to competition safely.

SHOULDER

- Anatomy
  - Bones (Fig. 11.1)
    - Clavicle
      - Subcutaneous bone that extends from the sternoclavicular joint medially to the acromioclavicular joint laterally
    - Scapula
      - A large, flat, and triangular bone that provides a framework for attachment of many of the major muscles about the shoulder
      - Components

A. Abdelgawad and O. Naga (eds.), *Pediatric Orthopedics*,
DOI: 10.1007/978-1-4614-7126-4_11,

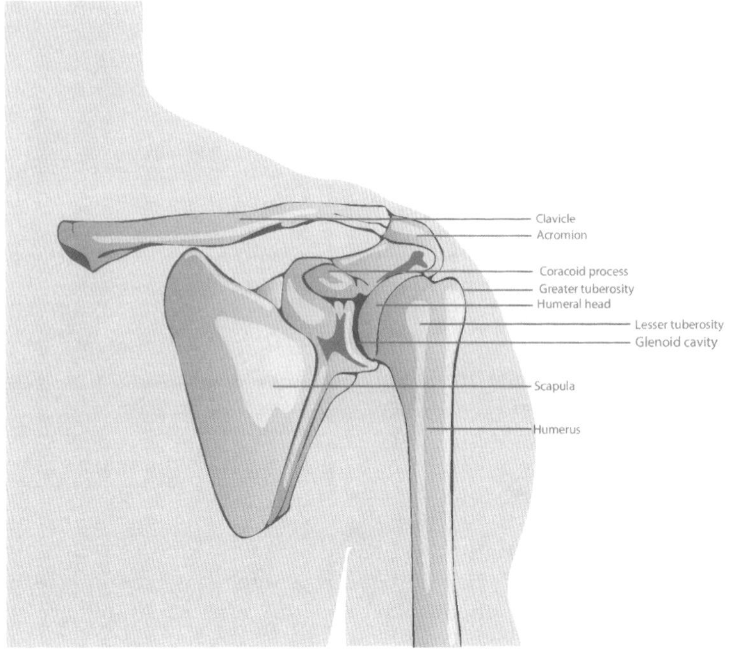

Fig. 11.1 Bony anatomy of the shoulder joint

- ◆ Glenoid—articulation site with the humerus
- ◆ Acromion—provides a roof over the shoulder joint
- ◆ Coracoid—attachment site for several muscles and ligaments that help to stabilize the acromioclavicular joint

□ Proximal Humerus

- ◆ Consists of humeral head, greater tuberosity, lesser tuberosity, and metaphyseal portion

- Articulations

  □ Glenohumeral (GH) joint

  ○ Most mobile major joint in the body

- The socket is deepened by glenoid labrum, a ring of cartilage outlining the glenoid
- Stabilized by glenohumeral ligaments and labrum statically, rotator cuff musculature dynamically

- Acromioclavicular (AC) joint
  - Between the distal end of clavicle and medial acromion
  - Stabilized by acromioclavicular ligaments and coracoclavicular ligaments, which are continuous with a thick periosteal tube around the distal clavicle
  - Moves up to 30° in elevation
- Sternoclavicular (SC) joint
  - Between the proximal end of clavicle, sternum, and first rib
  - Most clavicular motion occurs at SC joint
    - 30–35° of elevation, 35° of anterior-posterior glide, 45–50° of rotation
- Scapulothoracic articulation
  - Scapula glides over posterior thoracic wall
  - Provides mobile base to allow for full mobility of glenohumeral joint

- Musculature (Fig. 11.2)
  - Rotator cuff—provides dynamic stability for glenohumeral joint
    - Supraspinatus
      - Active in shoulder abduction
      - Depresses humeral head during abduction
    - Infraspinatus
      - Active in external rotation
    - Teres minor
      - Active in external rotation

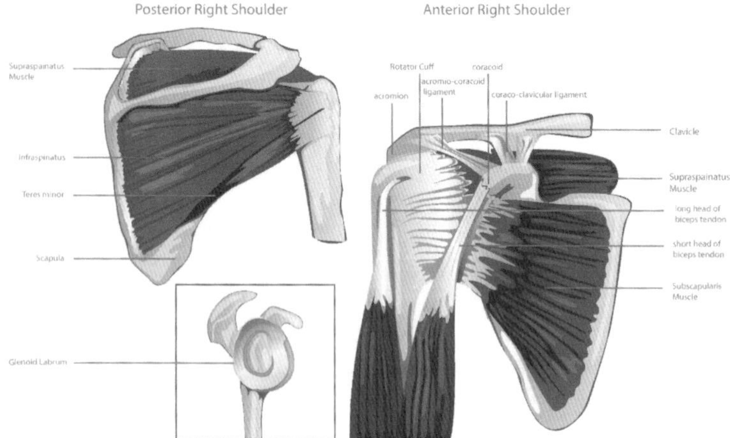

Fig. 11.2 Anatomy of the muscles of the shoulder joint

- ○ Subscapularis
  - ◆ Active in internal rotation
  - ◆ Stabilizes against anterior subluxation

□ Deltoid

- ○ Primary motor power for glenohumeral joint
- ○ Active in abduction and flexion

□ Pectoralis Major

- ○ Powerful adductor of the shoulder

□ Latissimus Dorsi

- ○ Extends, adducts, and rotates arm medially

□ Biceps Brachii

- ○ Has 2 proximal heads—Short head attaches at coracoid, long head crosses over humeral head and attaches to superior glenoid labrum
- ○ Primarily functions at elbow, but acts as humeral head depressor at the shoulder

- Examination
  - Inspection
    - The patient should either have his/her shirt removed or in a sports bra
    - Inspect for deformity, step-off
  - Palpation—assess for tenderness, crepitus, muscle tone changes, or bony deformity
    - Sternoclavicular joint
    - Clavicle
    - Acromioclavicular joint
    - Biceps tendon
    - Greater tuberosity of the humerus
  - Range of motion
    - Abduction
    - Flexion
    - Extension
    - External rotation
    - Internal rotation
  - Strength testing
    - Abduction—testing supraspinatus strength (Fig. 11.3)
    - External rotation—testing infraspinatus and teres minor strength (Fig. 11.4)
    - Internal rotation—testing subscapularis strength
      - Liftoff test (Fig. 11.5)
        - Positive test—the patient is unable to internally rotate enough to lift hand from the back
      - Belly press (Fig. 11.6)
        - Positive test—elbow drops to the patient's side as maximal internal rotation cannot be maintained.
  - Special tests
    - **Glenohumeral Instability**

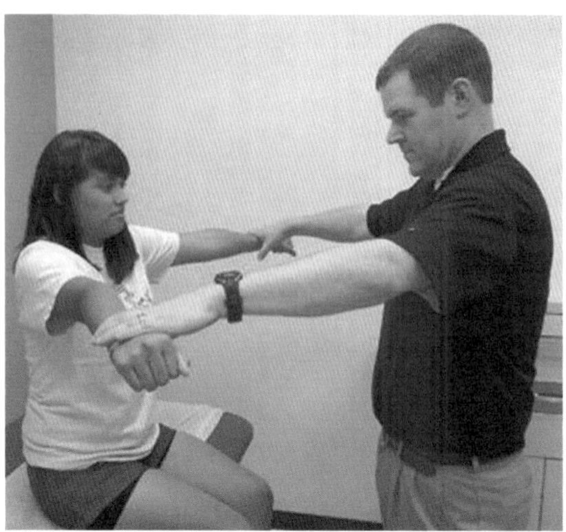

Fig. 11.3 Assessment of supraspinatus strength. Position of the patient: arms elevated to shoulder level, 30° angle anterior to coronal plane. Patient resists examiner's attempt to push *down*

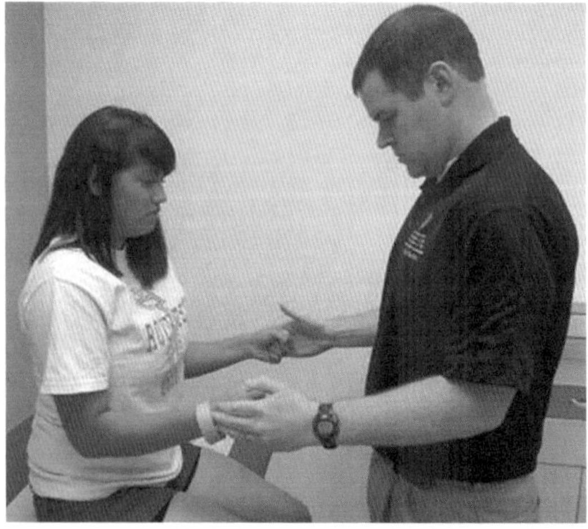

Fig. 11.4 Assessment of infraspinatus and teres minor strength. Position of the patient: arms *down* at side, elbow flexed 90° with arm pointing *forward*. Patient resists examiner's attempt to push toward *midline*

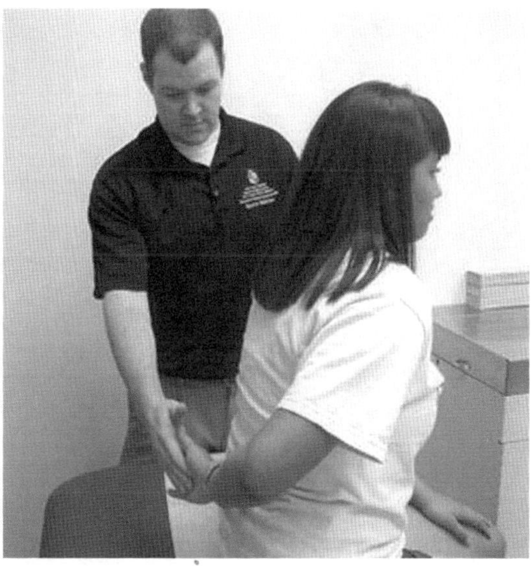

Fig. 11.5 Lift off test: Position of patient: patient's hand is placed on mid-lumbar region of back with the palm facing out. The patient is instructed to lift the hand away from the back

- Apprehension test—testing for anterior instability (Fig. 11.7)
  - Positive test—athlete experiences feeling of subluxation or dislocation and expresses discomfort (becomes 'apprehensive')
- Relocation test– confirmatory test (Fig. 11.8)
  - Positive test—athlete's apprehension is relieved and a greater amount of external rotation is achieved.
  - Examiner should return arm to neutral position prior to removing hand to avoid spontaneous dislocation.

Rotator cuff impingement

- Hawkin's (Fig. 11.9)
  - Position—shoulder flexed to 90°, elbow flexed to 90°. Examiner passively internally rotates arm

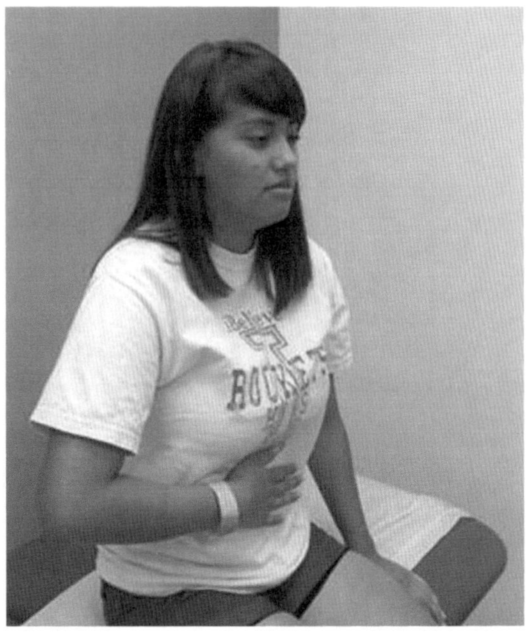

Fig. 11.6 Belly press. Position of the patient: patient actively presses on abdomen with the palm of the hand while attempting to keep the arm in maximal internal rotation, wrist in neutral flexion, and arm slightly abducted

- ◆ Positive test—pain with passive internal rotation
- ○ Neer's (Fig. 11.10)
  - ◆ Positive test—pain with passive shoulder flexion
- □ Labral tear
  - ○ O'Brien's (Active Compression Test) (Fig. 11.11)
    - ◆ Positive test—pain is elicited with arm internally rotated, relieved when externally rotated
- ■ Injuries
  - • Clavicle fracture

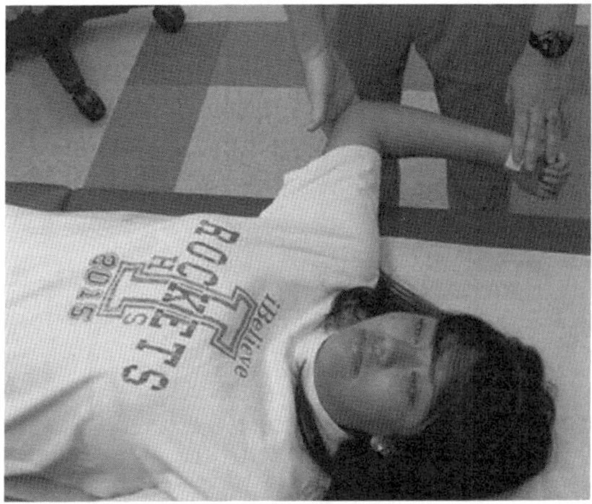

Fig. 11.7 Apprehension test. Position of the patient: with the athlete supine, arm abducted to 90°, and elbow flexed to 90°, the examiner applies an external rotation force, which forces the humeral head anteriorly. Notice the reaction on the patient's face

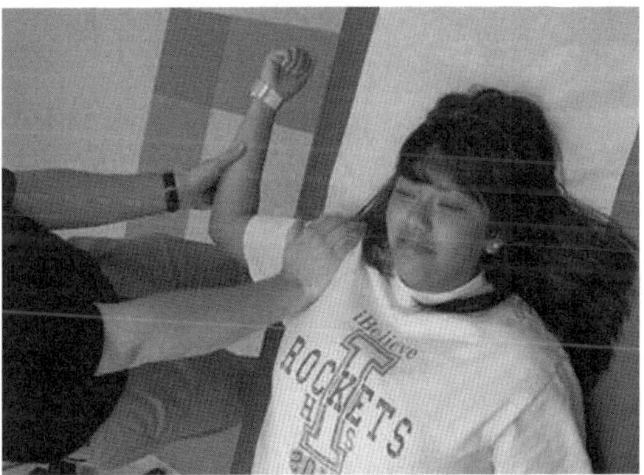

Fig. 11.8 Relocation test. Position of the patient: same as apprehension test, but while arm is externally rotated, a posteriorly directed force is applied to the anterior aspect of glenohumeral joint by examiner's palm

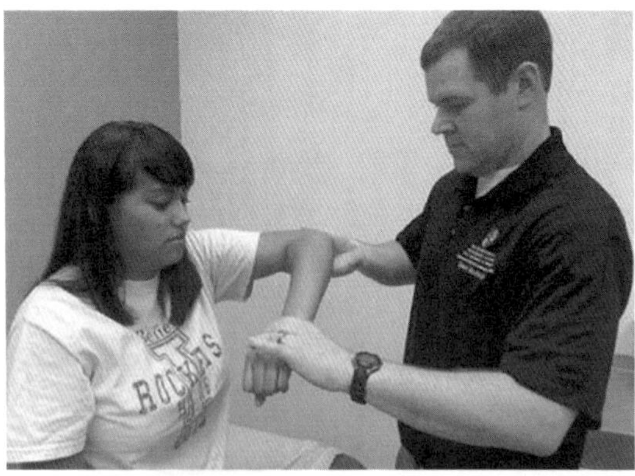

Fig. 11.9 Hawkin's maneuver. Position of the patient: shoulder flexed to 90°, elbow flexed to 90°. Examiner passively internally rotates the arm

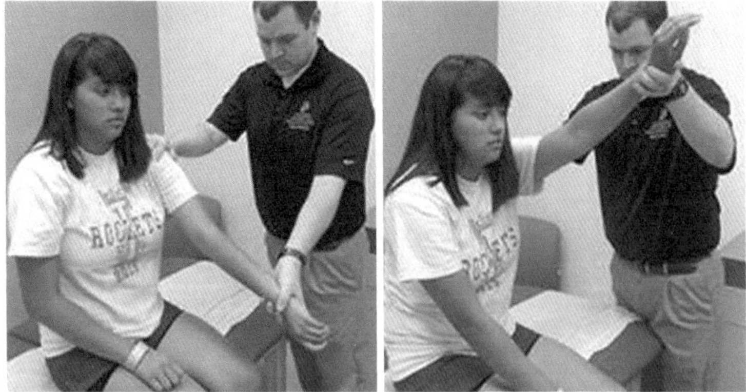

Fig. 11.10 Neer's maneuver: Position of the patient: starts with arm at the side and internally rotated. Examiner passively flexes arm at shoulder

- See orthopedic trauma.

- Acromioclavicular (AC) sprain
  - History

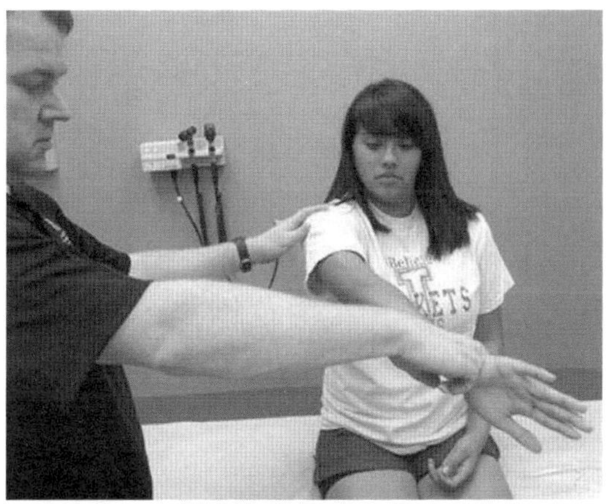

Fig. 11.11 O'Brien's (Active Compression Test) Position—arm flexed to 90° and internally rotated (*thumb down*), adducted slightly past *midline*. Examiner applies a *downward* and *outward* force. Test is repeated with arm externally rotated (*thumb up*)

- Occur after direct fall onto the point of the shoulder
- **In younger athletes, more likely to lead to lateral clavicle physeal or metaphyseal fracture**

- Exam
  - Swelling and tenderness over the affected AC joint
  - More severe injuries may show a deformity at the AC joint (Fig. 11.12)
  - Limited range of motion due to pain
  - Pain with cross-arm test: passive adduction of arm across body produces pain at the AC joint

- Diagnostic imaging
  - X-rays with AP, axillary, Zanca views
    - Zanca view—AP with 10 degree cephalic tilt focused on AC joint
    - Demonstrate widening and/or displacement of AC joint

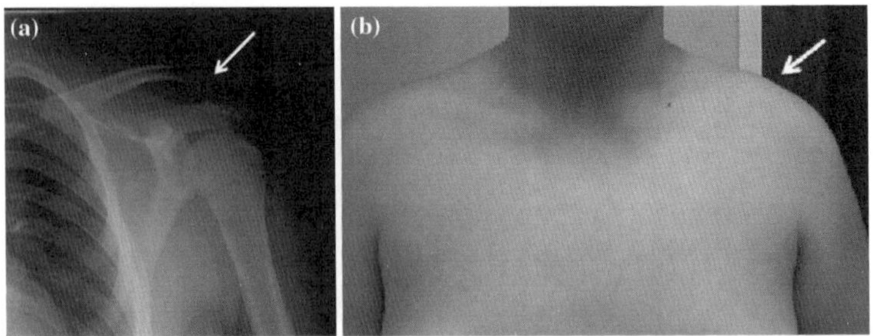

Fig. 11.12 A 13-years-old boy who fell down in football practice on his *left* shoulder. **a** Radiographs taken at the time of injury showed separation between the clavicle and acromion (*arrow*). **b** The patient had obvious deformity on the *left* shoulder (*arrow*) (compare to the right shoulder)

- Grading (Fig. 11.13)
  - Grade 1—mild sprain of acromioclavicular ligaments
  - Grade 2—disruption of AC ligaments with widening of AC joint, coracoclavicular ligaments intact
  - Grade 3—rupture of AC ligaments with 25–100% displacement of lateral aspect of clavicle
  - Grade 4—lateral clavicle displaced posteriorly into trapezius
  - Grade 5—more severe form of grade 3—lateral aspect of clavicle displaced more than 100%
  - Grade 6—displacement of the lateral clavicle inferior to the coracoid
- Treatment
  - Grades 1 and 2
    - Sling immobilization
    - Early range of motion—pendulum exercises as tolerated
      - The child bends forward at the waist, letting arm hang freely. Using momentum from body motion, allow the arm to swing in circles, passively moving at the glenohumeral joint

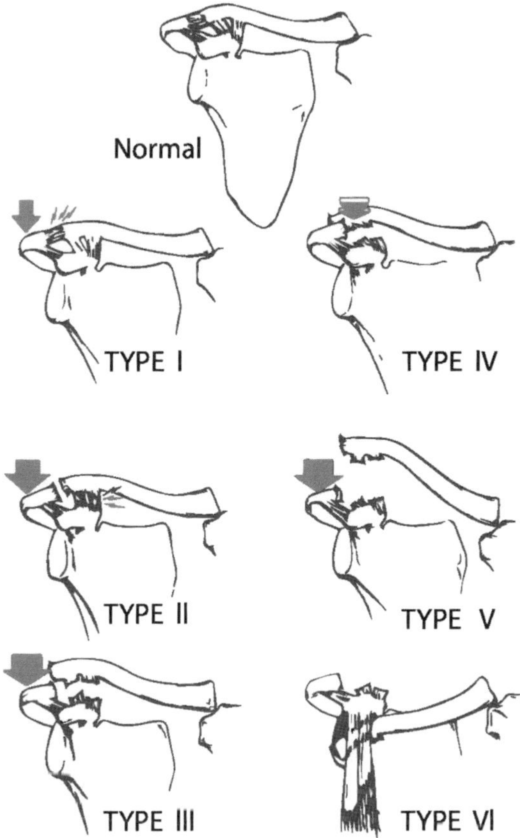

Fig. 11.13 Classification of the acromioclavicular joint disruption. In children, the injury disruption can occur by the periosteal sleeve rather than by disruption of the coracoclavicular ligaments

- ◆ Physical therapy for rotator cuff strengthening

- ○ Grade 3—controversial
  - ◆ Operative fixation may be appropriate in high-level athletes
- ○ Grades 4 to 6—operative repair

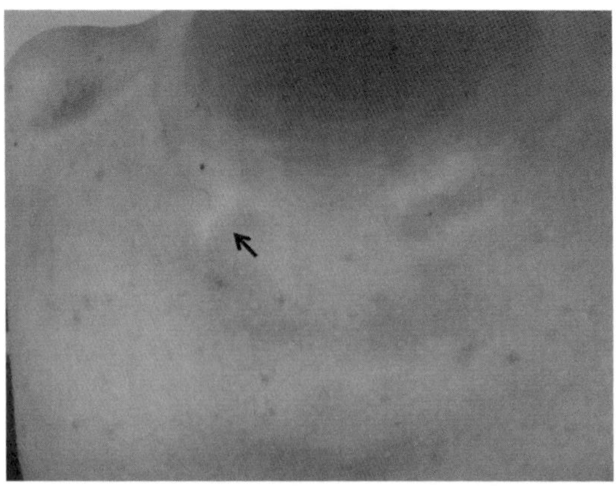

Fig. 11.14 A 17-year-old boy who sustained injury to his right shoulder which resulted in anterior sternoclavicular dislocation. Notice the deformity on the *right* side of the sternum (*arrow*) (compare to the left sternoclavicular joint)

STERNOCLAVICULAR (SC) JOINT INJURY

- Rare injury
- Important to identify posterior dislocation of the clavicle, as compression of mediastinal structures may occur
- Exam demonstrates tenderness and deformity over SC joint (Fig. 11.14)
- CT best to evaluate for physeal injury versus true posterior dislocation and potential mediastinal compromise
- Anterior dislocation is treated with observation. The child can return to full activity when pain subsides.
- Posterior dislocation requires emergent surgical consult for reduction with thoracic surgery backup

LITTLE LEAGUER'S SHOULDER (PROXIMAL HUMERAL EPIPHYSIOLYSIS)

- History
  - Pain in dominant (throwing) shoulder
  - Insidious onset, worsens over time
  - Increases with increased number and types of pitches
  - Lack of control and velocity in pitches

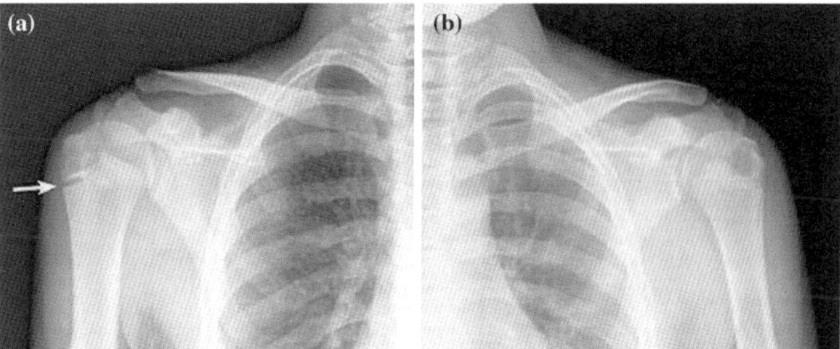

Fig. 11.15 Comparison radiographs of little leaguer's shoulder in a 15-year-old baseball player. Note the widening of the proximal humeral epiphysis in the *right shoulder* (*A*) compared with the *left shoulder* (*B*) (Reprinted with permission from the American Academy of Family Physicians)

- Exam
  - Focal tenderness over proximal humerus
  - Pain in proximal humerus with shoulder strength testing
- Diagnostic imaging
  - Obtain bilateral humerus X-rays for comparison (Fig. 11.15)
    - Affected shoulder shows widening of the proximal humeral physis
    - May also see metaphyseal sclerosis and demineralization or fragmentation of the proximal humeral physis
- Treatment
  - Immediate cessation of throwing activities
  - Avoidance of activities that may increase stress at shoulder
  - Physical therapy to focus on rotator cuff, periscapular, and core strengthening
  - Return to play—3 to 6 months after diagnosis
    - Full, pain-free range of motion of the shoulder
    - Gradual return to throwing
  - Prognosis—good with appropriate rest and rehabilitation

- Prevention
  - **Watch for signs of fatigue (decreased velocity, control, loss of mechanics). If present, discontinue pitching and allow to rest.**
  - **No overhead throwing of any kind for at least 2–3 months per year**
  - **Avoid pitching on multiple teams with overlapping seasons**
  - **Learn good throwing mechanics as soon as possible**
  - **A pitcher should not also be a catcher for his team**
  - **Follow recommended pitch counts for age** (Table 11.1)

Instability

- **Traumatic Instability**
  - Shoulder joint is one of the most mobile joints in the body, but comes at the expense of stability
  - **Anterior glenohumeral dislocation**
    - **Greater than 90 % of all dislocations**
    - History
      - Most commonly occurs after **f**all **o**n **o**ut**s**tretched **h**and (FOOSH) with arm abducted and externally rotated
      - The child often complain of 'dead arm' after dislocation
    - Exam
      - Obvious deformity—acromion prominent, humeral head may be seen anteriorly
      - Palpable defect inferior to acromion
      - The patient holds affected arm in abducted and externally rotated position
      - **Assess for axillary nerve compromise—sensation over lateral shoulder**
    - Diagnostic imaging
      - X-ray

TABLE 11.1 RECOMMENDED PITCH COUNTS FOR AGE

Age (years)	2010 Little League Baseball regulations
Daily limits	
17–18	105/day
13–16	95/day
11–12	85/day
9–10	75/day
7–8	50/day
Weekly limits	
7–18	21–35 pitches -> 1 day rest; 36–50 pitches -> 2 days rest; 51–65 pitches -> 3 days rest >66 pitches -> 4 days rest

Adapted with permission from the ASMI Position Statement on Youth Baseball Pitchers

- ◇ Pre-reduction (Fig. 11.16)
  - ▸ AP, axillary, and transscapular Y view to assess humeral position
- ◇ Post-reduction
  - ▸ AP, axillary, and transscapular Y view to confirm reduction and assess for associated fractures:
    - ▹ Hill-Sachs lesion—defect in posterior humeral head after impact with glenoid. Seen after repeated dislocations
    - ▹ Bony Bankart lesion—fracture of anterior glenoid after dislocation

◆ MRI

- ◇ Evaluate for associated labral, capsular, or rotator cuff injuries.
- ◇ Commonly done after the second dislocation, however some physicians perform the study after the first attack of dislocation.

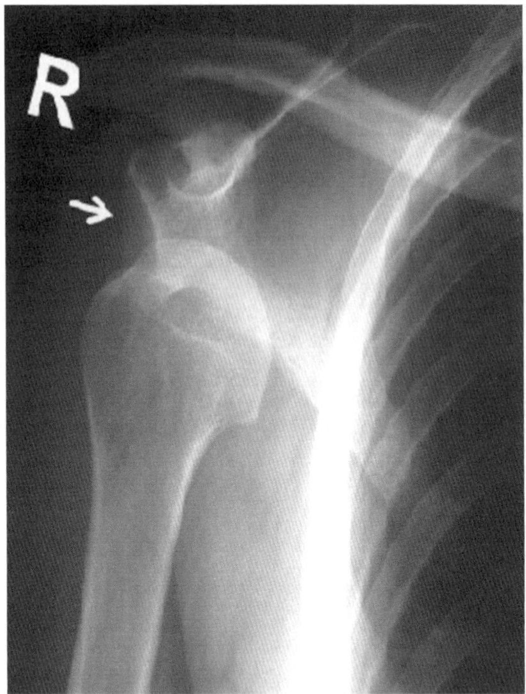

Fig. 11.16 A 15-year-old girl developed severe pain and deformity of her *right shoulder* after falling *down* playing volleyball. Radiograph of the shoulder shows anterior dislocation of the humeral head (notice the empty glenoid (*arrow*))

- Treatment
  - Acute—closed reduction should be accomplished as soon as possible before significant muscle spasm and pain develop
    - **Modified Kocher method** (Fig. 11.17)
      - Patient in supine position, body stabilized (may require countertraction)
      - Traction applied to humerus while arm is in an adducted, externally rotated, flexed position
      - Arm then internally rotated and further adducted

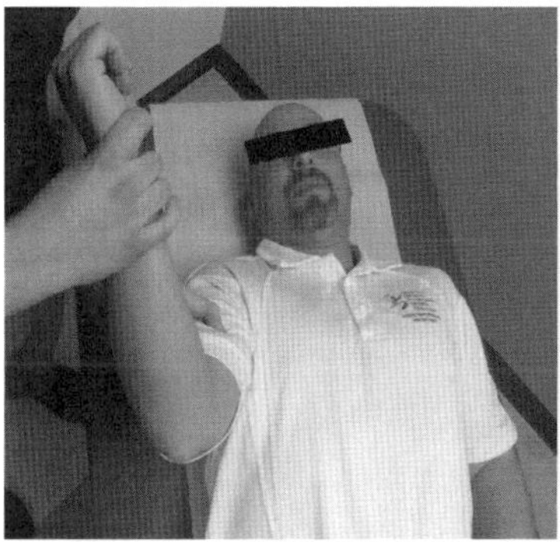 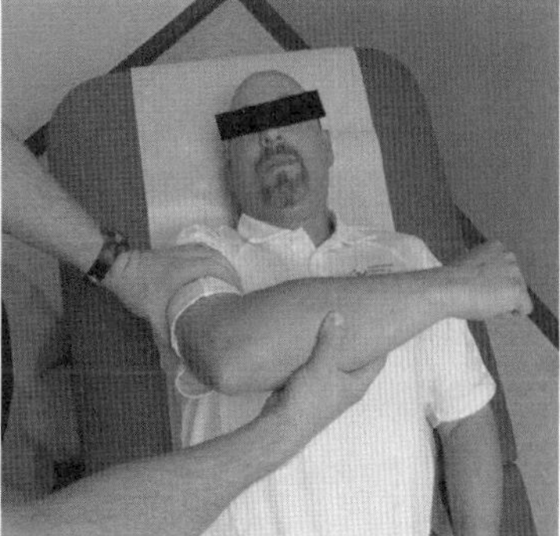

Fig. 11.17 Kocher maneuver

- ◇ **Stimson method**
  - ▸ Patient lies in prone position with arm hanging down below table
  - ▸ Weight is placed on arm
  - ▸ With aid of gravity, spontaneous reduction should occur in 5–15 min
- ◇ Post-reduction radiographs should be obtained and neurovascular exam should be performed
- ◇ Arm should be immobilized for 2–6 weeks in a sling
  - ▸ Immobilization in external rotation may reduce the risk of recurrent dislocation
- ◇ Gradual range of motion exercises and strengthening exercises as tolerated

◆ Return to Play

- ◇ Athlete must regain full range of motion and strength
- ◇ Good stability with overhead activities

◆ **Orthopedic referral for surgical treatment**

- ◇ Indications

- ▶ Recurrent dislocation or instability despite adequate course of rehabilitation

- ◇ Associated large bony Bankart and Hill-Sachs lesions
- ◇ Surgery after primary dislocation is controversial

  - ▶ Young athletes may benefit from surgical treatment after primary dislocation due to high rate of recurrence

- **Posterior glenohumeral dislocation**

  - Less than 5 % of all traumatic shoulder dislocations

    - **Commonly occurs as a result of seizures**
    - Fall on outstretched hand with shoulder in adduction and internal rotation
    - Direct anterior trauma to shoulder

  - History

    - Patient complains of pain in posterior shoulder

  - Exam

    - May not have obvious deformity
    - Arm held in adduction with slight internal rotation
    - **Limited external rotation**
    - Apprehension with posterior displacement of glenohumeral joint

  - Diagnostic imaging

    - X-rays with AP, transscapular Y, and axillary views

      - ◇ Demonstrate posterior displacement of humeral head
      - ◇ **AP view alone may not show the dislocation.**

  - Treatment

    - Orthopedic referral for closed reduction under general anesthesia.

- Chronic dislocation for more than 3 weeks may require open reduction.

- **Atraumatic Instability**
  - Multi-directional instability
    - **Generalized joint laxity**
    - History
      - No history of acute injury
      - Nonspecific shoulder pain
      - Feeling of subluxation or dislocation with overhead activities
      - Common in swimmers and gymnasts—increased flexibility and motion advantageous to competition
    - Exam
      - Generalized ligamentous laxity
      - Positive sulcus sign (presence of a subacromial sulcus with inferior traction of the arm)
      - Positive apprehension sign (abduction external rotation of the shoulder will cause the patient to feel the humeral joint is about to dislocate) (Fig 11.7).
      - Strength deficits localized to scapular stabilizers and rotator cuff muscles
    - Diagnostic imaging
      - Generally not indicated, unless predisposing acute injury suspected
    - Treatment
      - Rehabilitation
        - **Mainstay of treatment**
        - Rotator cuff and scapular stabilizer strengthening
      - Surgery
        - Rarely indicated

- **Rotator cuff tear**
  - Very rare in pediatric population—less than 1 % of all pediatric shoulder injuries
  - Causes
    - Acute traumatic event—fall onto outstretched arm or forcibly impacting an immoveable object
    - Secondary impingement due to poor muscular or proprioceptive control
      - Deficiency of humeral head stabilization leads to contact of the supraspinatus or subscapularis against the acromion or coracoacromial arch
    - Internal impingement due to tightness of posterior capsule
      - Leads to contact of the posterior supraspinatus and superior infraspinatus with the posterior glenoid rim, leading to partial tears of those tendons and glenoid labrum
  - History
    - Pain and weakness most common symptoms
    - Posterior shoulder pain with decreased pitching velocity and accuracy in patients with internal impingement
  - Exam
    - May have limited active range of motion, normal passive range of motion
    - Assess for abnormal scapular motion compared to unaffected side
      - With patient facing away from examiner, both arms are abducted fully, then are slowly lowered back down to the side. The examiner evaluates for equal and smooth scapular motion throughout the movement. Asymmetric positioning and a lack of fluidity are signs of abnormal scapular motion (scapular dyskinesis)

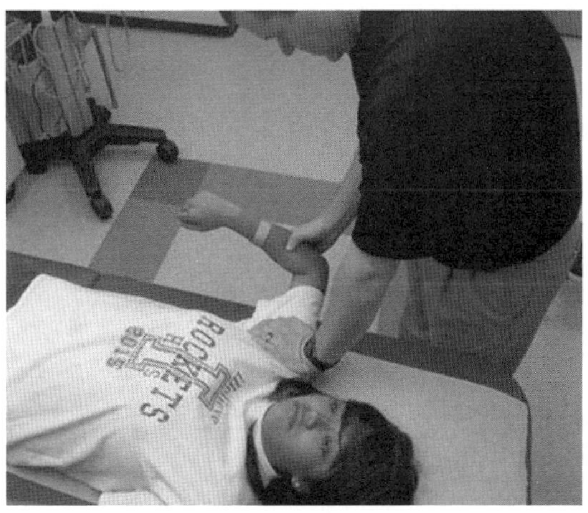

Fig. 11.18 Assessment of posterior capsular tightness with the patient supine, abduct the arm 90° with the elbow flexed 90°. Pin the shoulder against the exam table to restrict scapular motion. Internally rotate arm until it cannot move without the scapula moving, and compare rotation to unaffected side

  - Assess posterior capsule tightness by isolating glenohumeral internal rotation compared to unaffected side (Fig. 11.18)
  - Tenderness to anterior and lateral shoulder
  - May have strength deficits in abduction and external rotation
  - Hawkin's (flexion internal rotation of the arm with the elbow flexed), Neer's (flexion of the shoulder with the arm internally rotated and the elbow extended) tests may be positive Fig 11.9 and 11.10

- Diagnostic imaging
  - X-ray often normal, but may see calcifications with chronic rotator cuff tear
  - MRI or ultrasound of the shoulder to identify location and extent of tear

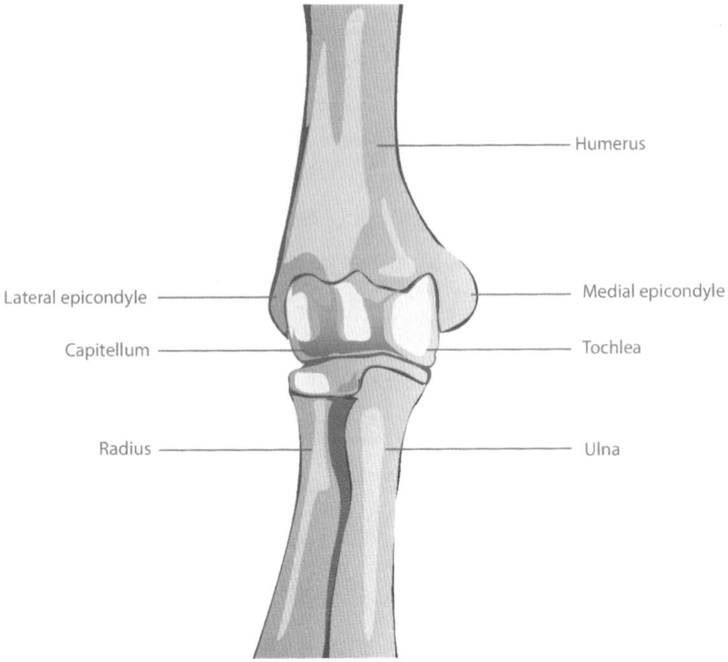

Humerus
Lateral epicondyle
Medial epicondyle
Capitellum
Tochlea
Radius
Ulna

Fig. 11.19 Elbow anatomy

Lateral collateral ligament complex
medial collateral ligament complex
Radial collateral ligament
Lateral ulnar collateral ligament
Annular ligament
Anterior oblique
Posterior oblique
transverse
View from lateral side
View from medial side

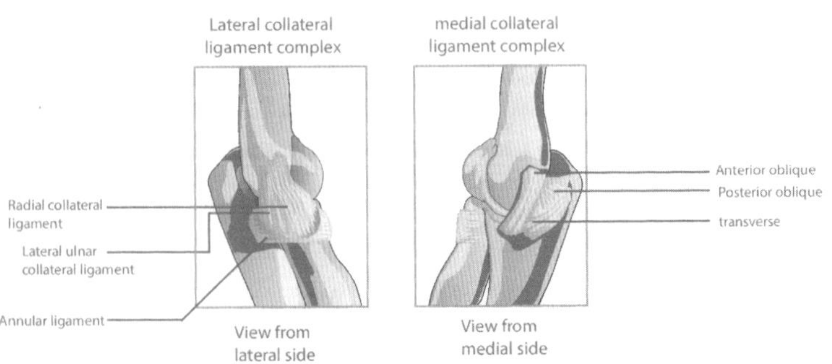

Fig. 11.20 Elbow ligaments

- Treatment
  - Conservative management includes cessation of offending activity and focused physical therapy program
    - Strengthening of scapular stabilizers and rotator cuff muscles
  - Surgical repair reserved for full thickness tears with significant disability and those who fail to improve with conservative measures

- **Glenoid labrum injury**
  - Overview
    - Consequence of glenohumeral dislocation (anterior labrum) or chronic overuse with abnormal mechanics (SLAP tear—Superior Labrum Anterior Posterior)
    - **SLAP tear**—2 common mechanisms
      - Peel back mechanism—torsional force at superior labrum with maximal abduction and external rotation during overhead activity (e.g., pitching, tennis serve)
      - Secondary to posterior capsule tightness, leading to glenohumeral internal rotation deficit (GIRD)—glenohumeral motion shifts in posterosuperior direction, increasing shear forces across labrum
  - History
    - Insidious onset of nonspecific shoulder pain
    - May complain of mechanical symptoms (clicking, popping)
    - Decrease in pitching velocity
    - May complain of "dead arm" feeling after throwing
  - Exam
    - Examine for abnormal scapular motion
    - Atrophy of supraspinatus and infraspinatus muscles may be sign of suprascapular nerve compression and indicate presence of a paralabral cyst

- Range of motion usually normal
- Examine for signs of instability
  - Apprehension, sulcus sign
- O'Brien's (active compression test) often positive in SLAP tears (Fig. 11.11)

- Diagnostic imaging
  - X-rays often normal
  - MR arthrogram most sensitive for detection of SLAP tears

- Treatment
  - Initial conservative treatment—discontinue offending activity and start physical therapy
    - Posterior capsule stretching and rotator cuff strengthening
  - Surgical intervention indicated for persistent symptoms lasting greater than 3 months despite rest and rehabilitation

ELBOW

- Overview
  - **In athletes, the elbow is highly susceptible to overuse injury, particularly in overhead throwing sports, making it the most commonly injured joint in pediatric baseball players.**
  - The mechanics of overhead throwing place high tensile forces on the medial aspect, compressive forces on the lateral aspect, and shearing forces on the posterior aspect of the elbow that predispose young athletes to a spectrum of overuse injuries.
- Anatomy (Fig. 11.19)

- Bones
  - Humerus
    - Medial epicondyle
      - Attachment site for wrist flexors, ulnar collateral ligament
    - Lateral epicondyle
      - Attachment site for wrist extensors, radial collateral ligament
    - Trochlea
      - Articulates with olecranon of ulna to allow for flexion and extension
    - Capitellum
      - Articulates with radial head.
  - Ulna
    - Olecranon
      - Articulates with trochlea of humerus to allow for flexion and extension
    - Coronoid
      - Stabilizes anterior humeroulnar joint
  - Radius
    - Radial head—articulates with capitellum
  - Ossification centers of the elbow: See growth and development chapter
- Articulations
  - Humeroulnar joint
    - Modified hinge joint
    - Allows for flexion and extension

- Humeroradial (radiocapitellar) joint
  - Hinge and pivot joint
  - Allows for flexion, extension, and rotation of the radial head during supination/pronation.
- Radioulnar joint
  - Pivot joint which allows for supination/pronation

- Musculature
  - Flexors
    - Brachialis
    - Biceps
    - Brachioradialis
  - Extensors
    - Triceps
    - Anconeus
  - Supinators
    - Biceps
    - Supinator
  - Pronators
    - Pronator quadratus
    - Pronator teres
    - Flexor carpi radialis
  - Ligaments (Fig. 11.20)
  - Ulnar collateral (medial) ligament complex (UCL) (Fig. 11.20)
    - Provides valgus stability to the elbow
    - Composed of three bundles
      - Anterior oblique
        - Originates from medial epicondyle and inserts into coronoid process

      - ◇ Major ligamentous support of the medial elbow

    - ◆ Posterior oblique
    - ◆ Transverse

  - □ Lateral collateral ligament complex (Fig. 11.20)

    - ○ Provides primarily varus with some rotatory stability
    - ○ Composed of:

      - ◆ Radial collateral ligament
      - ◆ Lateral UCL ligament

        - ◇ Primary restraint to posterolateral rotatory instability

      - ◆ Annular ligament

        - ◇ Stabilizes radius within the radial notch
        - ◇ Contributes to varus stability

- • Nerves (Fig. 11.21)

  - □ Median

    - ○ Traverses antecubital fossa

  - □ Ulnar

    - ○ Runs posterior to medial epicondyle in cubital tunnel

  - □ Radial

    - ○ Traverses anterior to the lateral condyle of the humerus.

- ■ Examination

  - • Inspection for erythema, swelling, ecchymosis, obvious deformity
  - • Palpation

    - □ Palpate all bony landmarks (distal humerus, medial and lateral epicondyles, radial head, proximal ulna and olecranon) for area of maximal tenderness and for any crepitus

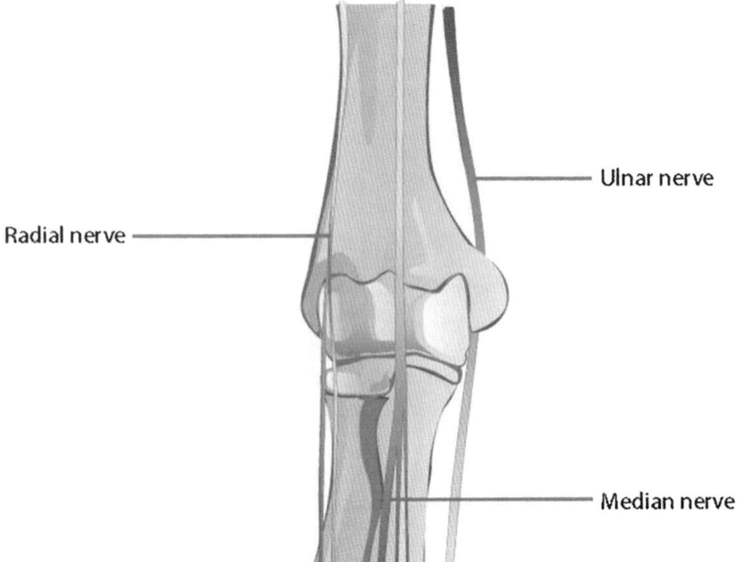

Fig. 11.21 Nerves around the elbow joint. On the medial side, the ulnar nerve passes behind the medial epicondyle. On the lateral side, the radial nerve passes in front of lateral condyle. The median nerve passes front of the *middle* of the elbow

- Neurovascular assessment
  - Assess distal pulses along with sensory and motor function
- Range of motion (ROM)
  - Normal values variable, should be compared to unaffected side
    - Extension: 0–(-)15°
    - Flexion: 0–150°
    - Supination: 0–85°
    - Pronation: 0–80°
  - Active and passive ROM

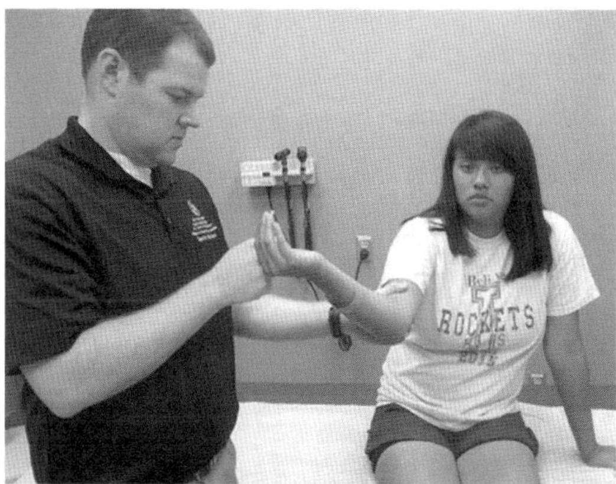

Fig. 11.22 Valgus stress test (Milking Maneuver): Flex elbow to 20° to free olecranon from olecranon fossa then supinate forearm. Support distal arm with one hand, while the opposite hand supports elbow and applies a medially directed force

- Active tested first—if there is any limitation, the examiner passively tests motion
- Muscular and/or tendinous injury suspected if passive ROM better than active ROM
- Feel for crepitus and/or locking as this maybe suggestive of intra-articular pathology or fracture

- Strength testing-compare to unaffected side
  - Flexion
  - Extension
  - Pronation
  - Supination
- Provocative maneuvers to assess for ligamentous injury and joint stability
  - Valgus stress test (Milking Maneuver) (Fig. 11.22)
    - Assesses medial joint stability
    - May have some laxity, but should be symmetrical with unaffected side and have good end point

- Positive if athlete experiences pain and/or increased laxity

- Varus stress test

  - Assesses lateral joint stability

    - Flex elbow to 20° to free olecranon from olecranon fossa
    - Pronate forearm
    - Support distal arm with one hand, while the opposite hand supports elbow and applies a laterally directed force

  - May have some laxity, but should be symmetrical with unaffected side and have good end point
  - Positive if athlete experiences pain and/or increased laxity

Little Leaguer's Elbow (Medial Epicondyle Apophysitis)

- Overuse-related apophyseal injury to medial epicondyle

  - Not seen in children after closure of apophysis.
  - Usually affects children **between 9 and 12 years** of age who participate in overhead throwing sports.

- History

  - Insidious onset of medial elbow pain while throwing. May progress to pain after activity or at rest if athlete continues to throw without period of rest.
  - Loss of pitching control and velocity
  - May play on multiple teams throughout the year without a true 'off-season' to rest

- Exam

  - Initially, symptoms may not be reproducible on exam
  - As injury progresses may show:

    - **Focal medial epicondyle tenderness**
    - May have localized swelling

      - Loss of range of motion demonstrated by slight flexion contracture
      - May have pain with application of valgus stress
         - Re-creates mechanism of injury
         - Unstable joint upon valgus stress indicative of other pathology (i.e., medial epicondyle avulsion fracture, UCL tear)

- Diagnostic imaging
   - X-ray with AP, lateral, and oblique views
      - Used to rule out other pathology
      - Usually normal (85 %) but may demonstrate medial epicondyle hypertrophy
   - Valgus and varus stress views indicated if joint stability is in question
      - Should be compared with unaffected joint

- Treatment
   - **Responsive to conservative management**
      - No throwing for 4–6 weeks
      - Ice
      - NSAIDs or acetaminophen for pain
         - Pain medication should not be used in order to allow for game participation
         - If the athlete requires medication in order to play, he or she is not ready for participation
      - Athlete should continue aerobic conditioning
      - Physical therapy
         - Core (trunk) strengthening
         - General stretching
         - Correction of body mechanics
      - After initial rest period, may begin with gradual throwing program and progress as tolerated over 6–8 weeks

- Indication for orthopedic referral
    - Failure of conservative management
    - Displaced avulsion fractures or other abnormal findings on x-ray
- **Best treatment is prevention**
    - **Teaching proper body mechanics**
        - **Early trunk rotation increase tensile forces on medial epicondyle**
    - **Core strengthening**
    - **Adhering to published pitching counts and rest periods (see table 11.1)**

- **Medial Epicondyle Avulsion fracture**
    - See orthopedic trauma

ULNAR COLLATERAL (MEDIAL) LIGAMENT COMPLEX (UCL) TEAR

- Rare injury until fusion of medial epicondyle has occurred
- Usually a chronic overuse injury, though can be acute
    - Acute injuries associated with rupture of ligament
    - Chronic injuries usually have micro-tears

- History
    - Athletes with chronic injuries present with progressive medial elbow pain, particularly while pitching, decreased pitch control and velocity
    - Athletes with acute injuries present with sudden medial elbow pain during pitching/forceful throwing, may state they felt a pop
    - May complain of distal paresthesias in the ulnar nerve distribution

- Exam
  - Tenderness along medial aspect of elbow
    - Focal maximal tenderness at medial epicondyle maybe indicative of medial epicondyle fracture
  - Varying degrees of swelling/ecchymosis depending on injury acuity
  - Pain with varying degrees of laxity on valgus stress (Fig. 11.22)
    - Acute ruptures will not have a firm endpoint if tear is complete
    - Chronic injuries may just have pain
    - Compare with unaffected side
  - Evidence of ulnar nerve involvement
- Diagnostic imaging
  - X-ray with anteroposterior, lateral, and oblique views
    - Used to rule out other pathology, particularly fractures of medial epicondyle
  - MR arthrogram study of choice to evaluate for UCL tears
- Treatment
  - Chronic injuries without complete tear likely to respond to conservative management
    - 2–3 month period free from throwing
    - Physical therapy
      - Core strengthening
      - Shoulder and scapular strengthening
      - Correction of body mechanics
    - Graduated throwing program initiated once athlete is pain-free
  - Indication for orthopedic referral

  - Persistence of symptoms after conservative management
  - Athletes with acute UCL ruptures

- Prevention is key
  - Educating athlete on proper body mechanics
  - Adhering to suggested pitch counts (see table 11.1 above)

Panner's Disease

- An idiopathic, self-limited, osteochondrosis of the capitellum occurring in children 4–12 years of age.
- **Most common cause of lateral elbow pain in children less than 10 years old.**
- History
  - Insidious onset of lateral elbow pain, which is vague in nature and associated with stiffness
- Exam
  - No focal tenderness to lateral aspect of elbow
  - Usually swollen
  - May have limitation in extension
- Diagnostic imaging
  - X-rays with AP, lateral, and oblique
    - Demonstrate capitellar pathology of varying degree, from decrease in size to fragmentation, which improves in 2 years
- Treatment
  - Rest, ice, immobilization, and NSAIDS for 3–4 weeks
  - Graduated return to activities as pain tolerates
  - Indication for orthopedic referral
    - Rarely needed, unless loose bodies are present

Osteochondritis dissecans (OCD) of capitellum

- Results from injury to the articular cartilage and subchondral bone through repetitive compressive force from valgus stress
- Seen predominantly in throwing sports, particularly baseball, and gymnastics in athletes **12–16** years of age (main distinguishing feature from Panner's disease)
- History
  - Present with lateral elbow pain which is dull, diffuse, and aggravated by activity
  - May also complain of mechanical symptoms
    - Clicking, catching, or locking
- Exam
  - Tenderness over the radiocapitellar joint on lateral aspect of elbow
  - Decreased extension
  - Mild swelling over affected area and feel crepitus or catching during ROM
- Diagnostic imaging
  - X-rays with AP, Lateral, and Oblique
    - Demonstrate radiolucency of the capitellum with flattening of the articular surface and areas of subchondral sclerosis. May also see loose bodies depending on severity of injury
  - MRI
    - Is diagnostic
    - Provides better characterization of articular surface and loose bodies if present
  - Grading
    - Stage 1—intact articular cartilage
    - Stage 2—disruption of articular cartilage
    - Stage 3—loose bodies present

- Treatment
  - Good prognostic factors
    - Open physis
    - Minimal sclerosis
  - Stage 1
    - Conservative treatment with activity restriction for 3–6 weeks followed by physical therapy
    - At 3 months may begin graduated return to activity as tolerated
    - Requires serial X-rays to monitor progression of lesion
  - Indication for orthopedic referral
    - Stage 1—if pain persists or lesion progresses
    - Stage 2 or Stage 3 lesions

Olecranon Impingement Syndrome (Valgus Extension Overload)

- Result of the posterior shear forces involved in overhead throwing or repetitive overload of the elbow while in extension (gymnasts, football linemen)
  - Leads to compression of the olecranon against the olecranon fossa at terminal extension
  - May be associated with UCL injury
- History
  - Athletes complain of posteromedial elbow pain and decreased extension
    - May complain of catching, locking, or clicking
    - Overhead throwers may also complain of loss of ball control and velocity depending on severity of injury and concomitant UCL involvement
- Exam
  - Loss of extension compared to unaffected side

- Reproduction of symptoms with elbow extension and valgus stress
- Possible findings of UCL laxity or tear

- Diagnostic imaging
  - X-ray
    - Findings vary
      - May see osteophytes in olecranon fossa, calcification of UCL, and loose bodies
  - MRI maybe indicated depending on other associated injuries or x-ray findings (suspicion of UCL tear, loose bodies)
- Treatment
  - Isolated olecranon impingement usually responds to conservative management
    - Rest, activity modification
    - NSAIDs
    - Physical therapy
  - Indication for orthopedic referral
    - Failure of conservative management or concomitant UCL injury

Elbow dislocation

- Result from FOOSH injury
- **Posterior dislocations are most common**
  - Proximal ulna becomes posterior in relation to the humerus.
- Exam
  - Obvious deformity
  - Pain
  - Swelling of the elbow
  - **Examine for neurovascular deficits**

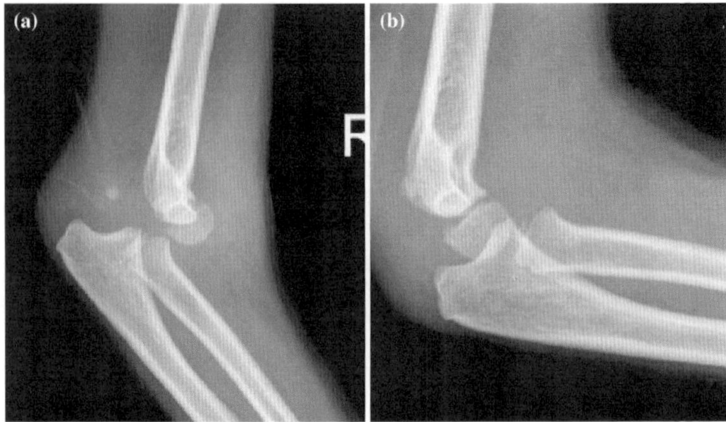

Fig. 11.23 4-years-old boy fall down from sling and presented with right elbow pain and deformity. (**a**) Radiograph showed posterior elbow dislocation (olecranon is posterior to the humerus). (**b**) Closed reduction was applied and post-reduction radiograph showed good alignment

- Diagnostic imaging
  - X-ray with AP, lateral, and oblique (Fig. 11.23)
  - May show isolated dislocation of olecranon from olecranon fossa or associated fractures (e.g., coronoid process, medial epicondyle)
- Treatment
  - Immediate reduction
    - Traction applied to arm
    - Elbow is flexed while providing pressure to olecranon
  - Stable reductions should be placed in posterior splint for 1–2 weeks with subsequent gradual ROM exercises
    - Return to activity once pain has resolved and ROM and strength are at baseline

- Indication for orthopedic referral
  - Reductions with persistent neurovascular findings merit emergent referral
  - Unstable reductions or irreducible dislocations may have associated fracture
  - If the medial epicondyle is entrapped in the joint space.(see trauma chapter) (Fig. 16.30/trauma)

Olecranon stress fracture

- Overuse injury that results from repeated tensile forces on proximal ulna
- Seen in adolescent throwers
- History
  - Gradual onset of pain that is initially present during throwing
  - May have pain at rest as injury progresses
- Exam
  - Minimal to no swelling
  - Pinpoint tenderness over posterior aspect of olecranon
- Diagnostic imaging
  - X-rays with AP, lateral, and oblique
    - Initially negative—may show frank fracture line for more advanced injuries
  - MRI demonstrates bone marrow edema (stress reaction) early in injury.
- Treatment
  - Immediate cessation of activity
  - Avoid weight-bearing loads
  - Gradual progression in activity level once pain and focal tenderness resolve
    - May need 3–4 months before returning to pre-injury competition level

- Indication for orthopedic referral
  - As there is debate to whether surgical or conservative management is best initial treatment for this injury, orthopedic referral is recommended

DISTAL FOREARM AND WRIST

- Anatomy (Fig. 11.24)
  - Bones
    - Distal forearm
      - Radius
      - Ulna
    - Wrist
      - Proximal row (radial to ulnar)
        - Scaphoid
          - Links distal and proximal carpal row
          - Principal bony block to excessive extension—susceptible to fracture
          - Blood supply arises distally and proceed proximally
        - Lunate
        - Triquetrum
        - Pisiform
      - Distal row (radial to ulnar)
        - Trapezium
        - Trapezoid
        - Capitate
        - Hamate
  - Articulations
    - Wrist joint: joint between the distal radius and the carpal bone

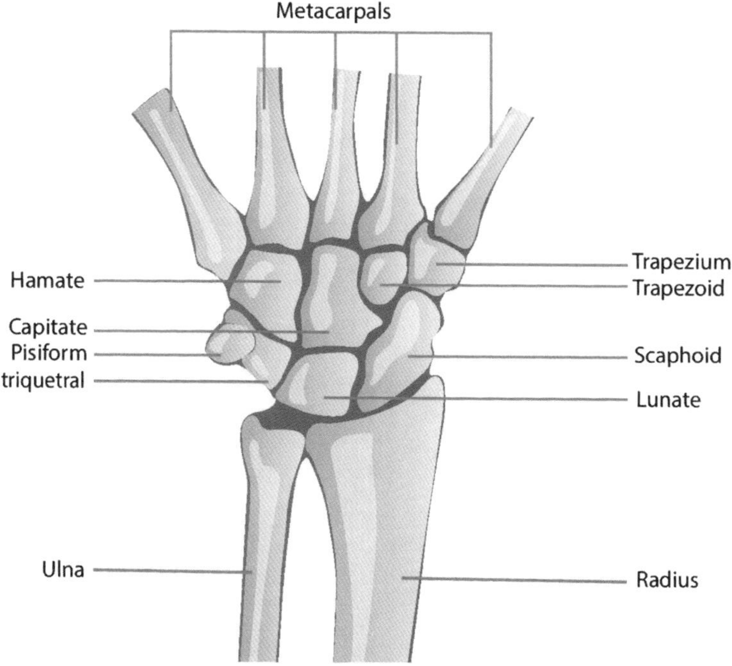

Fig. 11.24 Anatomy of the wrist

- Distal radioulnar joint (DRUJ): articulation between the distal radius and distal ulna
- Numerous articulations among the carpal bones

- Ligaments
  - Triangular fibrocartilage complex (TFCC)
    - Primary stabilizer of DRUJ
  - Scapholunate Ligament
    - Important for carpal row stability

- Ligamentous injury extremely rare in skeletally immature athletes

- Nerves

  - Median

    - Travels through carpal tunnel
    - Supplies sensation to palmar aspect of thumb, index, middle, and ulnar half of ring finger
    - Allows for fine control of pincer grasp

  - Ulnar

    - Travels through Guyon's canal

      - Bony tunnel formed by hook of hamate and pisiform

    - Supplies sensation to palmar aspect of little and radial half of ring finger
    - Provides power grip

  - Radial

    - Located on posterior aspect of wrist
    - Supplies sensation to posterior aspect of hand and fingers
    - Accounts for wrist and finger extension
    - Subject to entrapment proximally at the radial head

- Examination

  - Inspection for erythema, swelling, ecchymosis, obvious deformity, muscular atrophy
  - Palpation

    - Bony landmarks

      - Distal radius
      - Ulnar styloid
      - Starting with the **scaphoid (anatomical snuff box**), palpate all carpal bones in a systemic fashion (radial to ulnar, proximal to distal)

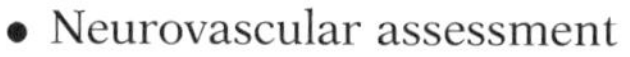

- Neurovascular assessment
  - □ Radial pulse and capillary refill distally
  - □ Gross sensation to median, ulnar, and radial nerve distributions
- Range Of Motion (ROM):
  - □ Normal values variable, should be compared to unaffected side
    - ○ Extension: 70°
    - ○ Flexion: 70°
    - ○ Radial deviation 20°
    - ○ Ulnar deviation 40°
    - ○ Forearm Supination: 80–85°
    - ○ Forearm Pronation: 75–80°
- Strength testing-compare to unaffected side

■ Gymnast's wrist (Radial epiphysitis)

- Chronic overuse injury in skeletally immature athletes secondary to repetitive compression of the distal radial physis
- Mechanism—repeated axial loads on hyperextended wrist
- Most commonly reported physeal stress injury, particularly in gymnasts who participate in floor exercises and pommel horse
- History
  - □ Achy dorsal wrist pain aggravated by activities that compress the distal radius physis
  - □ As injury progresses may have pain without weight-bearing activity, which could indicate stress reaction or fracture
- Exam
  - □ Tenderness over distal radial physis
  - □ May have decreased extension
  - □ Pain with reproduction of mechanism

- Diagnostic imaging
  - X-rays with Posteroanterior (PA), lateral, and oblique views
    - Widening or irregularity of physis
    - Findings may be subtle, so comparison with unaffected limb recommended
  - MRI more sensitive for physeal widening or irregularity
    - Evaluate for concomitant osseus stress reaction
- Treatment
  - Discontinuing weight bearing exercises until pain-free, followed by gradual return to weight bearing activities
    - Consider wrist braces which limit hyperextension
  - Indication for orthopedic referral
    - Progression to stress fracture
    - Failure of conservative management

Scaphoid Fracture

- High risk fracture due to pattern of blood supply.
  - Blood supply to scaphoid pass from distal part of the bone to proximal part.
  - Fractures can result in disruption of the blood supply to the bone resulting in avascular necrosis and collapse of the bone.
- Most common carpal fracture in pediatric athletes
  - Peak incidence at 15 years of age
  - Rare in those younger than 8
- FOOSH injury
- History
  - Dull pain to radial aspect of wrist
  - Exacerbated by clenching fist

- Exam
  - May note some swelling and ecchymosis to radial aspect of wrist
  - Limited ROM secondary to pain
  - **Most sensitive exam is anatomic snuff box tenderness**
  - Most specific exam is tenderness to scaphoid tubercle on volar aspect of wrist
- Diagnostic imaging
  - X-ray with PA, lateral, oblique and scaphoid views (Fig. 11.25)
    - High false negative rate initially
    - High index of suspicion required for early diagnosis
  - MRI of wrist warranted if X-rays are negative and clinical suspicion is high
    - Demonstrates fracture line and evaluate for avascular necrosis
- Treatment
  - Initial suspicion of fracture with negative X-rays
    - **Treat as though scaphoid fracture is present**
    - Place the child in short thumb spica splint for 1–2 weeks
    - X-rays repeated after 2 weeks
      - If repeat X-rays are negative and athlete's exam is unchanged, then immobilization should continue with thumb spica cast and MRI should be obtained
      - If repeat X-rays are negative and athlete is pain-free then likelihood of fracture is low and immobilization can be discontinued
    - If X-rays are positive for fracture
      - Nondisplaced fracture
        - Treatment with thumb spica cast for 6–8 weeks
        - X-rays repeated every 2 weeks to assess healing

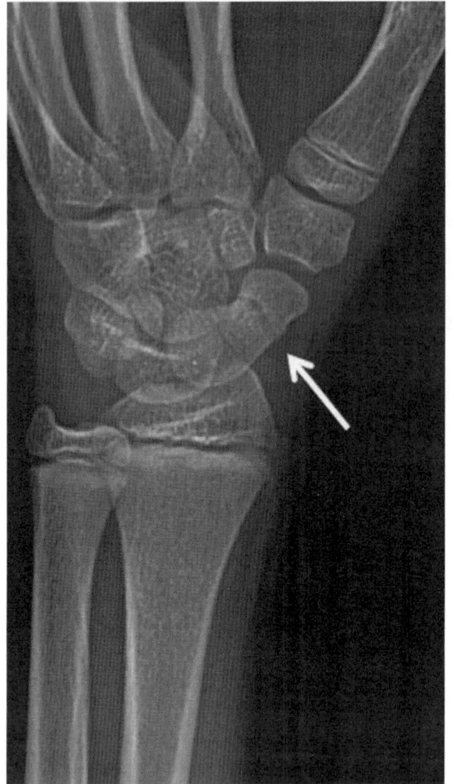

Fig. 11.25 Scaphoid fracture. A 13-year-old child fell down while playing football. The patient had pain at the wrist centered over the anatomical snuff box. Oblique radiograph shows fracture of the scaphoid

- ◆ Indication for surgery
  - ◇ Displaced fracture
  - ◇ Presence of nonunion or avascular necrosis

■ Hook of Hamate fracture

- Secondary to blunt trauma to hypothenar region (ulnar aspect) of the hand, usually from the end of a baseball bat at terminal swing or golf club when contact is made with the ground during golf swing

- History
  - Complain of sudden onset of pain to ulnar aspect of hand proximal to 5th digit, pain is usually well localized
  - May have paresthesias in the ulnar nerve distribution
- Exam
  - Variable degree of swelling
  - If present acutely, will have focal tenderness to hypothenar region
  - Chronic injuries have vague discomfort to hypothenar region
  - Assess integrity of flexor tendon of 5th digit as well as neurovascular status
- Diagnostic imaging
  - X-ray with PA, lateral, oblique, and carpal tunnel views
    - Usually demonstrate fracture
  - In the setting of high clinical suspicion and negative X-rays, CT of the wrist should be obtained
- Treatment
  - Acutely should be placed in volar splint
  - **Usually requires surgical resection of avulsed fragment**
  - Urgent referral is necessary if neurovascular deficits or flexor tendon injury noted on exam

- **Distal radial/ulnar fractures**
  - See orthopedic trauma
- **Physeal fractures**
  - See orthopedic trauma

HAND AND FINGERS

- Anatomy
  - Bones (Fig. 11.26)
    - Metacarpals
      - Physis located proximally on thumb metacarpal, distally on other 4 metacarpals
      - Metacarpals articulate with the proximal phalanx at the metacarpophalangeal (MCP) joint
    - Fingers
      - The thumb contains two phalanges, which articulate at the interphalangeal (IP) joint
      - Remaining four fingers contain three phalanges; the proximal and middle articulate at the proximal interphalangeal (PIP) joint and the middle and distal articulate at the distal interphalangeal (DIP) joint
      - Physis located at the base of each phalanx
  - Tendons
    - The flexor digitorum profundus inserts onto the distal phalanx, and the flexor digitorum superficialis inserts onto the middle phalanx
    - Extensor tendons insert onto the epiphyses of the terminal phalanges
  - Ligaments
    - Collateral ligaments insert onto the metaphysis and epiphysis of the respective bones at the interphalangeal joints
      - Exception is proximal phalanx—collateral ligaments insert into epiphysis only
    - Also insert into the volar plate—a soft tissue structure that functions to stabilize the joint against hyperextension forces.

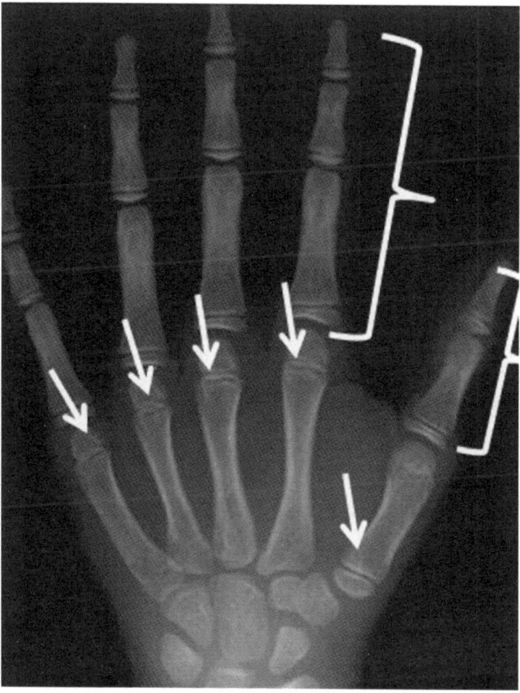

Fig. 11.26 Antero-posterior radiograph of 6-years-old girl. Notice the growth plates (*physis*) of the thumb metacarpal is in the proximal part of the metacarpal while in the rest of the fingers it is in the distal part of the metacarpal (*arrows*). The thumb has 2 phalanges while the rest of the fingers have 3 phalanges (*brackets*)

- Examination
  - Inspection for any swelling or deformity
  - Active and passive range of motion of the affected part
  - To evaluate for malrotation, have the patient make a loose fist, flexing at the MCP and PIP joint, keeping the DIP joint extended. In this position, all fingers should point to the scaphoid (Fig. 11.27)
  - Neurovascular status should be documented

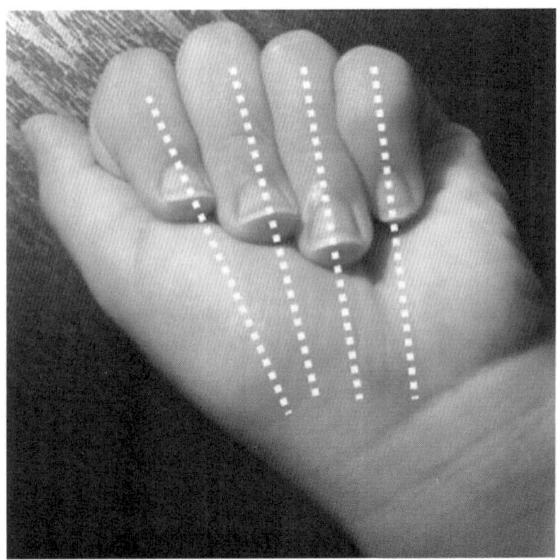

Fig. 11.27 Normal rotation of the digits. When the patient makes a loose fist all fingers should point to the scaphoid

■ Injuries

• Hand

□ Metacarpal fractures

○ Thumb metacarpal

- ◆ Most common—Salter Harris II fracture at the ulnar aspect
- ◆ Usually minimally displaced
- ◆ Pain and swelling at thenar eminence, decreased thumb range of motion
- ◆ Treatment
  - ◇ Thumb spica splint or cast for 4 weeks
  - ◇ Repeat X-rays every 2 weeks to document healing

- **Indication for orthopedic referral**
  - Intra-articular injuries (Salter Harris III (Bennett's) and IV fractures)

- **Metacarpal shaft fracture**
  - Occurs in older children
  - Mechanism—torsional force to finger that leads to spiral or oblique fracture of metacarpal
  - Assess rotation of the digit (see before, Fig. 11.27)
  - Treatment
    - Closed reduction and placement in dorsal and volar splints with wrist slightly extended and MCP joint in maximal flexion for 3–4 weeks
    - Repeat X-rays in 5–7 days to ensure reduction, then every 2 weeks to document healing
  - Indication for orthopedic referral
    - Unstable fractures, irreducible fractures, or multiple metacarpal fractures

- **Distal metacarpal neck ("Boxer's") fracture**
  - **Most commonly at 5th metacarpal**
  - Result of direct axial force, usually from punching a solid object (Fig. 11.28)
  - Treatment
    - Placement in ulnar gutter splint with wrist in slight extension, MCP joint in full flexion, and PIP and DIP joints extended for 3 weeks
    - Repeat X-rays in 5–7 days to ensure reduction, then every 2 weeks to document healing
  - Indication for orthopedic referral
    - **Rarely indicated**
    - Irreducible fractures, angulated, or displaced fractures of the 2nd or 3rd metacarpals.

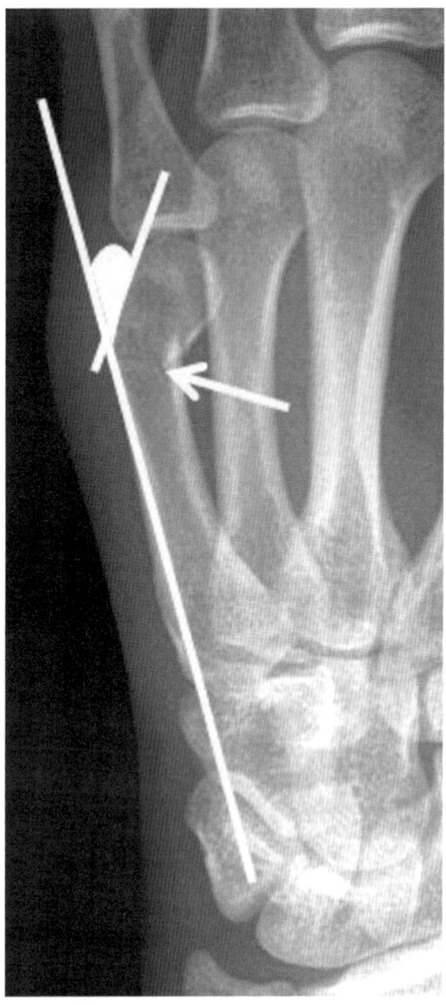

Fig. 11.28 Boxer's fracture. A 16-year-old boy who 'punched' the wall. Patient presented with left hand pain and swelling at the base of the small finger. Radiograph shows fracture of the neck of the fifth metacarpal (*arrow*) with about 30° angulation (the measured angle)

- **Metacarpophalangeal dislocation**
  - Occurs after fall with hyperextension of the MCP joint
  - Direction determined by relative position of proximal phalanx to metacarpal
  - Dorsal dislocation is most common
  - Treatment
    - Closed reduction by hyperextending the joint, then pushing the base of the phalanx over metacarpal head and into place. Avoid pulling traction to prevent volar plate from entering the joint.
    - Splint in 60° of flexion for 7–10 days, then transition to buddy taping and range of motion exercises
  - **Indication for orthopedic referral**
    - Irreducible dislocations (>2 attempts), volar dislocations, fracture dislocations, and open dislocations

- Finger
  - **Phalanx fractures**
    - Distal phalanx
      - Most common mechanism is crush injury
      - Salter Harris II fractures occur frequently
      - Commonly associated with nail bed injury
      - Treatment
        - Splinting of DIP joint for 2–3 weeks
        - In case of nail plate avulsion, attempt to reattach the nail in order to provide coverage and stability to the fracture
      - Indication for orthopedic referral (rarely indicated)
        - Open fractures, or entrapment of the mail matrix between the fracture ends.
    - **Mallet finger**
      - Avulsion of the distal extensor mechanism from its insertion at the proximal portion of the distal phalanx.

- ◆ In children, most commonly results in Salter Harris fracture (Fig. 11.29).
- ◆ Mechanism- forced flexion of an extended finger
- ◆ History
  - ◇ History consistent with forced flexion
  - ◇ **Catching a ball in a wrong way**, jamming against hard object unexpectedly
- ◆ Exam
  - ◇ Pain and swelling at the DIP joint
  - ◇ Inability to actively extend at the DIP joint
- ◆ Diagnostic imaging
  - ◇ Plain films—AP, lateral, and oblique views
  - ◇ May show avulsion fracture of distal phalanx (Fig. 11.29)
- ◆ Treatment
  - ◇ Placement in hyperextension splint for 3–4 weeks (Fig. 11.30).
- ◆ Indication for orthopedic referral:
  - ◇ Volar subluxation, inability to extend DIP passively, and fracture involvement of >30 % of the articular surface

○ **Proximal phalanx fracture**

- ◆ Caused by lateral deviation combined with twisting or rotational forces
- ◆ Most common fractures are Salter Harris II of the small finger ('extra octave' fracture at proximal physis with compression on one side and tension on the other)
- ◆ The finger has angular deformity (abduction and extension) (Fig. 11.31)
- ◆ Treatment
  - ◇ Closed reduction by traction, flexion of metacarpophalngeal joint, and adduction of the digit.

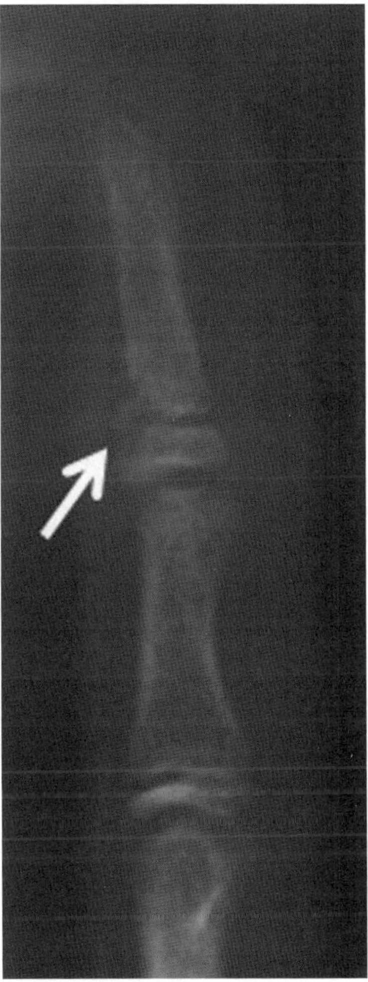

Fig. 11.29 Mallet fracture. A 10-year-old was hit by a basketball. Lateral radiograph of the index finger shows avulsion of the dorsal proximal part of the distal phalanx (*arrow*) (bony mallet lesion)

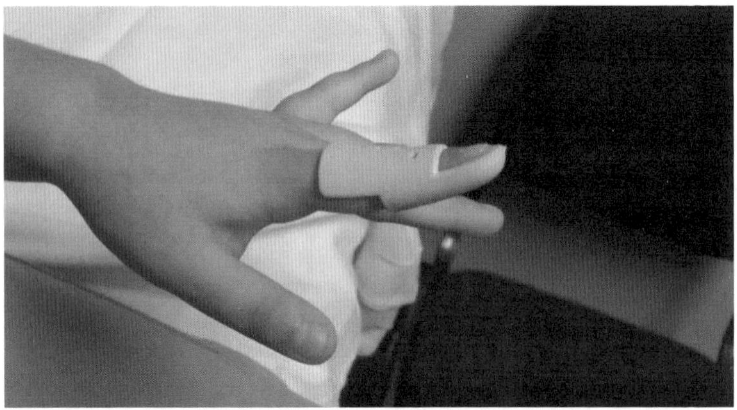

Fig. 11.30 Hyperextension splint

- ◇ Splint in ulnar gutter splint with wrist extended 30°, MCP joints fully flexed, and PIP and DIP joints in full extension for 3–4 weeks

- ◆ Indication for orthopedic referral
  - ◇ Inability to obtain adequate reduction.

- ○ **Proximal interphalangeal (PIP) joint dislocation**
  - ◆ Classified by relative position of middle phalanx to proximal phalanx
  - ◆ Dorsal dislocation
    - ◇ Most common direction of PIP joint dislocation
    - ◇ Result from an axial load to the finger
    - ◇ Likely will be reduced prior to evaluation
    - ◇ X-rays should be obtained to evaluate for fracture of base of middle phalanx
    - ◇ Treatment
      - ▶ Reduction by applying traction, hyperextending the PIP, then pulling the PIP into flexion.
      - ▶ Assess for active PIP extension to evaluate for central slip integrity
      - ▶ Buddy tape to adjacent finger for 3–6 weeks

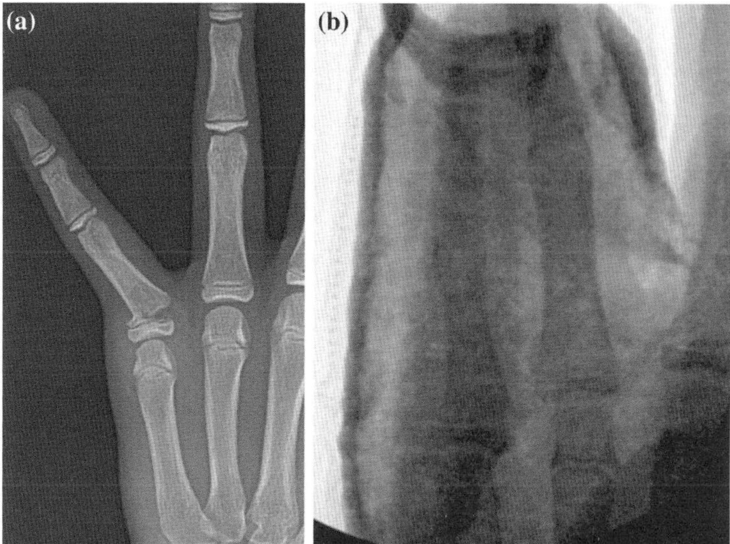

Fig. 11.31 Extra octave fracture. **a** Fracture of the base of the small finger (Salter Harris type II) with lateral angulation in an 8-year-old boy who had his finger caught in a table at school. **b** Closed reduction was applied with restoration of alignment and application of ulnar gutter splint

- ◇ Indication for orthopedic referral
  - ▸ Irreducible joint dislocations, fracture dislocations, bayonet dislocations (dorsal dislocation combined with either radial or ulnar dislocation), and open dislocations.

- □ **Jersey finger**
  - ○ Avulsion of the flexor digitorum profundus (FDP) tendon from distal phalanx, resulting in retraction of the flexor tendon
  - ○ Most commonly occurs in ring finger
  - ○ Mechanism
    - ◆ Forced extension of a flexed finger
    - ◆ Grabbing a flag or jersey while opposing player runs away

- Exam
  - Swelling and ecchymosis
  - Assessment of FDP integrity
    - Isolate the FDP by stabilizing the PIP joint in extension and asking the patient to flex the DIP
    - Inability to flex the DIP is consistent with FDP injury
  - End of retracted tendon may be palpated proximal to the avulsion site
- Diagnostic imaging
  - X-rays with lateral and oblique views
  - May identify an avulsed fracture fragment
- Treatment
  - **Early identification and urgent referral for surgical correction**
  - Injured finger should be splinted in slight flexion at DIP and PIP joints while waiting for evaluation

REFERENCES

Curtis RJ. Shoulder: Anatomy and biomechanics: 2. Anatomy, biomechanics, and Kinesiology of the Child's shoulder. In: DeLee JC, Drez D, Miller MD, editors. DeLee and Drez's Orthopaedic sports medicine. 3rd ed. Philadelphia: Elsevier Saunders; 2009. p. 779–91.

Babatunde OM, Kim HM, Desandis BA, Rogers CE, Levine WN. A physician's guide to the physical examination of the shoulder. Phys Sportsmed. 2012;40(1):91–101. Epub 2012/04/18.

Flynn JM, Nagda S. Upper extremity injuries. In: Dormans JP, editor. Pediatric orthopaedics and sports medicine: requisites. 1st ed. St. Louis: Elsevier Mosby; 2004. p. 21–48.

Mariscalco MW, Saluan P. Upper extremity injuries in the adolescent athlete. Sports Med Arthrosc. 2011;19(1):17–26. Epub 2011/02/05.

Eiff MP. Clavicle and Scapula fractures. In: Eiff MP, Hatch R, editors. Fracture management for primary care. 3rd ed. Philadelphia: Elsevier Saunders; 2012. p. 175–86.

Bishop JY, Flatow EL. Pediatric shoulder trauma. Clin Orthop Relat Res. 2005(432):41–8. Epub 2005/03/02.

Brennan BW, Kelly MJ. Little Leaguer's shoulder. Clin Pediatr (Phila). 2011;50(5):462–3. Epub 2010/09/15.

Frush TJ, Lindenfeld TN. Peri-epiphyseal and Overuse injuries in Adolescent athletes. Sports Health: A Multidisciplinary Approach. 2012;1(3):201–11.

American Sports Medicine Institute. Postition Statement for Youth Baseball Pitchers. 2012 (cited July 7, 2012); Available from: http://www.asmi.org/asmiweb/position_statement.htm.

Carson S, Woolridge DP, Colletti J, Kilgore K. Pediatric upper extremity injuries. Pediatr Clin North Am. 2006;53(1):41–67, v. Epub 2006/02/21.

Krabak BJ, Alexander E, Henning T. Shoulder and elbow injuries in the adolescent athlete. Phys Med Rehabil Clin N Am. 2008;19(2):271–85, viii. Epub 2008/04/09.

Curtis RJJ. Shoulder: Glenohumeral instabilities: 2. Glenohumeral instabilities in the child. In: DeLee JC, Drez D, Miller MD, editors. DeLee and Drez's Orthopaedic sports medicine. 3rd ed. Philadelphia: Elsevier Saunders; 2009.

Paul J, Buchmann S, Beitzel K, Solovyova O, Imhoff AB. Posterior shoulder dislocation: systematic review and treatment algorithm. Arthroscopy. 2011;27(11):1562–72. Epub 2011/09/06.

Tarkin IS, Morganti CM, Zillmer DA, McFarland EG, Giangarra CE. Rotator cuff tears in adolescent athletes. Am J Sports Med. 2005;33(4):596–601. Epub 2005/02/22.

Keener JD, Brophy RH. Superior labral tears of the shoulder: pathogenesis, evaluation, and treatment. J Am Acad Orthop Surg. 2009;17(10):627–37. Epub 2009/10/02.

Cassas KJ, Cassettari-Wayhs A. Childhood and adolescent sports-related overuse injuries. Am Fam Phys. 2006;73(6):1014–22. Epub 2006/03/31.

Chumbley EM, O'Connor FG, Nirschl RP. Evaluation of overuse elbow injuries. Am Fam Phys. 2000;61(3):691–700. Epub 2000/03/01.

Cheng JC, Wing-Man K, Shen WY, Yurianto H, Xia G, Lau JT, et al. A new look at the sequential development of elbow-ossification centers in children. J Pediatr Orthop. 1998;18(2):161–7. Epub 1998/04/08.

Patel B, Reed M, Patel S. Gender-specific pattern differences of the ossification centers in the pediatric elbow. Pediatr Radiol. 2009;39(3):226–31. Epub 2009/01/07.

Benjamin HJ, Briner WW, Jr. Little league elbow. Clin J Sport Med. 2005;15(1):37–40. Epub 2005/01/18.

Bradley JP, Petrie RS, Tejwani SG. Elbow and Forearm: 2. Elbow Injuries in Children and Adolescents. In: DeLee JC, Drez D, Miller MD, editors. DeLee and Drez's Orthopaedic Sports Medicine. 3rd ed. Philadelphia: Elsevier Saunders; 2009. p. 1227–40.

Mostofi SB. Elbow. In: Mostofi SB, editor. Rapid orthopedic diagnosis. 1st ed. London: Springer; 2009. p. 39–59.

Carlisle JC, Gerlach DJ, Wright RW. Elbow Injuries. In: Madden CC, Putukian M, Young CC, McCarty EC, editors. Netter's sports medicine. Philadelphia: Elsevier Saunders; 2010. p. 360–7.

Forman TA, Forman SK, Rose NE. A clinical approach to diagnosing wrist pain. Am Fam Phys. 2005;72(9):1753–8. Epub 2005/11/23.

Atanda A, Jr., Shah SA, O'Brien K. Osteochondrosis: common causes of pain in growing bones. Am Fam Phys. 2011;83(3):285–91. Epub 2011/02/10.

Daniels JM, 2nd, Zook EG, Lynch JM. Hand and wrist injuries: Part I. Nonemergent evaluation. Am Fam Physician. 2004;69(8):1941–8. Epub 2004/05/01.

O'Brien ET. Wrist: 2. Wrist Injuries in the Child. In: Delee JC, Drez D, Miller MD, editors. DeLee and Drez's Orthopaedic Sports Medicine. 3rd ed. Philadelphia: Elsevier Saunders; 2009. p. 1363–78.

Petering RC. Carpal fractures. In: Eiff MP, Hatch R, editors. Fracture management for primary care. 3rd ed. Philadelphia: Elsevier Saunders; 2012a. p. 84–101.

Poletto ED, Pollock AN. Radial epiphysitis (aka gymnast wrist). Pediatr Emerg Care. 2012;28(5):484–5. Epub 2012/05/09.

Caine D, DiFiori J, Maffulli N. Physeal injuries in children's and youth sports: reasons for concern? Br J Sports Med. 2006;40(9):749–60. Epub 2006/06/30.

DiFiori JP, Caine DJ, Malina RM. Wrist pain, distal radial physeal injury, and ulnar variance in the young gymnast. Am J Sports Med. 2006;34(5):840–9. Epub 2006/02/24.

Overlin AJF, Hect S. Gymnastics. In: Madden CC, Putukian M, Young CC, McCarty EC, editors. Netter's sports medicine. Philadelphia: Elsevier Saunders; 2010. p. 565–70.

Phillips TG, Reibach AM, Slomiany WP. Diagnosis and management of scaphoid fractures. Am Fam Phys. 2004;70(5):879–84. Epub 2004/09/17.

Prawer A. Radius and Ulna fractures. In: Eiff MP, Hatch R, editors. Fracture management for primary care. 3rd ed. Philadelphia: Elsevier Saunders; 2012. p. 102–29.

Shepler T. Hand: 2. The pediatric hand. In: DeLee JC, Drez D, Miller MD, editors. DeLee and Drez's Orthopaedic Sports Medicine. 3rd ed. Philadelphia: Elsevier Saunders; 2009. p. 1404–30.

Webb CW. Metacarpal fractures. In: Eiff MP, Hatch R, editors. Fracture management for primary care. 3rd ed. Philadelphia: Elsevier Saunders; 2012. p. 63–83.

Petering RC. Finger fractures. In: Eiff MP, Hatch R, editors. Fracture management for primary care. 3rd ed. Philadelphia: Elsevier Saunders; 2012b. p. 36–62.

Chapter 12

Management of Pediatric Orthopedic Patients During the Postoperative Period

Indu Pathak and Michael Lee

- Orthopedic patients admitted in the hospital wards needs special care to ensure adequate pre operative and post operative management.
- Severity of injury, including soft tissue and neurovascular injury as well as surgical technique and internal fixation stability should be assessed.

Assessments of patients in the immediate postoperative period
Assessment in the immediate postoperative period should include the following:

- Assessment of airway
- Vital signs
- Level of consciousness/sedation
- Evaluation of the surgical site for circulation and sensation
- Patency/rate of intravenous fluids
- Pain status
- Assessment of bowel function
- **Assessment of the neurovascular bundle distal to the surgical site**
- **Assessment of softness/hardness of compartments at the surgical site**

Re-establishing oral intake in the immediate postoperative period

- Assess the patient's neurological status, patency of airway, coordination of swallowing mechanism as well as signs of postoperative ileus prior to initiating a diet (especially in spine surgery).

A. Abdelgawad and O. Naga (eds.), *Pediatric Orthopedics*,
DOI: 10.1007/978-1-4614-7126-4_12,

- After satisfactory return of bowel function, a clear liquid diet can be started.
- Diet should be advanced to regular appropriate diet for age as tolerated because clear liquid diet fails to provide adequate nutrients to the postsurgical patient.
- Surgeries on the spine (scoliosis surgery) are more prone to cause bowel dysfunction.

Postoperative nausea and vomiting (PONV)

- Common postoperative complication which can lead to increased recovery room time as well as length of stays
- Risk factors include: female sex, history of PONV/motion sickness, use of volatile anesthetics, use of intra-operative and postoperative opioids and duration of surgery
- Rare in children less than 2 years old. Risk increases with age, decreasing after puberty
- After keeping patient nothing by mouth or Nil Per Os (NPO), a bedside evaluation is required to exclude medication or mechanical factors
- Ondansetron 50–100 microg/kg up to 4 mg can be used in patients with PONV
- Patients in whom ondansetron is not effective, dexamethasone 150 microg/kg or perphenazine 70 microg/kg can be added

Postoperative fever

- Body temperature >38 C (100.4 F) can be common in the first few days in the postoperative period and is a poor predictor of complications
- Can be caused by inflammatory stimulus and resolves spontaneously but also can be a manifestation of postoperative complications
- **Causes in immediate postoperative period (0–3 days) include:**
  - Cytokine release due to trauma.
  - Reactions to medications or blood products.
  - Infections present prior to surgery.
  - Rarely malignant hyperthermia.

- **Causes within the first week (3–7 days) include:**
  - Surgical site infection
  - Pneumonia or UTI.
  - IV catheter infection.
  - Bowel ischemia.

Management:

Evaluation should include detailed physical examination with laboratory studies as indicated (CBC, blood cultures, CRP, procalcitonin, urinalysis, urine culture, gram stain, culture of catheter port, chest X-ray, etc.)

- Empiric antibiotics should be avoided unless indicated
- Recent literature suggests that the association between atelectasis and postoperative fever is controversial but atelectasis should be considered in the differential diagnosis of postoperative fever. Deep breathing exercises with incentive spirometry, early ambulation, and physiotherapy can be used postoperatively to reduce the incidence of atelectasis

Analgesia in the immediate postoperative period

- Pain is to be expected during the postoperative period.
- The amount of analgesics necessary will depend on the personality and pain tolerance of the patient
- An assessment/rating of the patient's mental status in conjunction with the pain scale may help avoid excess use of analgesics during the postoperative period.
- Depending on the patient's age, a numerical scale (0–10), descriptive (excellent-poor), or faces (smiling-sad) may be used to quantify/document the level of pain experienced by the patient.
- A description of the quality of pain should be documented if possible (burning, spastic, shooting, stabbing…etc.).

Evaluation of pain in nonverbal patients

- Infants, toddlers, and patients with developmental delay present a unique challenge
- Often lack the cognitive skills necessary to report and describe pain

- The evaluation should include the following
  - Careful search for potential causes of pain or discomfort
  - Assessment by caretaker/parent
  - Observation of patient behaviors: Facial expression, body activity, crying/verbalization, **and** posture change
  - **Changes in vital signs including heart rate**

Postoperative analgesia with opioids

- Opioids are the mainstay of postoperative analgesia.
- As needed (PRN) IM/IV dosing are suboptimal in the management of severe postoperative pain due to the wide variations in plasma opioid levels as well as periods of analgesia followed by prolonged periods of no pain relief.
- Around the clock (ATC) is the preferred method of administration.
- Once PO tolerant, oral dosing of opioids should be established.
- Codeine and hydrocodone are commonly used in conjunction with NSAIDs.
- Narcotics side effects include mood changes, nausea, vomiting, constipation, dizziness, pruritus as well as ileus, and respiratory depression in cases of overdoses.

Postoperative analgesia with NSAIDs

- NSAIDs (alone or in conjunction with opioids) are the medications of choice in managing postoperative pain.
- Use of NSAIDs postoperatively may decrease the use of postoperative opioids by 20–40 % while maintaining the same degree of analgesia.
- It is better to use NSAIDs around the clock (ATC) rather than PRN because ATC use of NSAIDs provides more consistent and constant analgesia (by more inhibition of the cytokines cascade).
- Inflammatory mechanisms play an important part in the pathogenesis of postoperative pain; therefore the use of NSAIDs is appropriate in the postoperative setting. Their side effects such as platelet dysfunction, gastritis, and acute renal dysfunction should be noted.
- Effect of NSAIDs on fracture healing:

- Inflammation is a stage of bone healing (inflammation, granulation tissue, soft callus, hard callus, remodeling)
- **Theoretical concern for NSAIDs use is inhibition of inflammation which can lead to delayed healing.**
- **This had never been shown in clinical studies in children.**
- Most pediatric orthopedic surgeon thinks that a short-duration NSAID regimen is a safe and effective supplement to other modes of post-fracture pain.
- For soft tissue procedures (e.g., muscle release or reduction of dislocated hip) use of NSAIDs should not be of any concern
- **Communication with the surgeon is important to know his opinion for the use of NSAIDs after surgeries that requires bone healing:**
  - fracture fixation
  - lengthening of bone
  - osteotomies
  - spinal fusion
  - arthrodesis

Antibiotic management

- Indicated for all contaminated and open wounds
- Check tetanus immunization or treat with toxoid as appropriate
- Cephalosporins are drug of choice
- Vancomycin or clindamycin can be used in penicillin and cephalosporin allergy
- Aminoglycoside should be added if there marked wound contamination.
- **preoperative and post operative prophylactic antibiotic**:
  - First generation cephalosporins (e.g., cefazolin) (50–100 mg/kg/day divided q6–8 h. Max dose 6 g in 24 h) **within one hour before the incision**, then continue with the same antibiotic 24 h (3 more doses).
  - If the child has penicillin allergy: Use Clindamycin (10–30 mg/kg/day divided q6–8 h. Max dose 1.8 g in 24 h)

Range of motion (ROM) exercises

- Early rehabilitation in the postoperative period is beneficial and can lead to more rapid attainment of short-term functional milestones
- Patients should avoid load bearing and active ROM exercises in the immediate postoperative period
- Passive ROM exercises can be initiated on the affected extremity within 24–48 h
- Active ROM exercises can be started in non affected extremity in the immediate postoperative period.
- A splint or brace should be used if immobilization of the affected extremity is required
- Rehabilitation after fractures should be progressed in stepwise manner. Different protocols exist depending on the body part involved and the extent of the injury and repair
- **The plan for rehabilitation and advancement of activity should be discussed with both the surgeon and therapist.**

Specific orthopedic examination for inpatients with orthopedic conditions:

In addition to the general examination, the following should be assessed in orthopedic patients

- **Neurovascular status distal to the site of trauma or surgery.**
  - Detailed examination of the **pulses** and the **nerves** is very important after trauma or orthopedic surgeries.
  - all the nerves distal to fracture/surgery have to be assessed (see orthopedic trauma for sings of nerve injury)
- **Sign and symptoms of compartment syndrome**
  - **Increase in the pain level**
  - **Increase in the narcotic requirement**
  - **Pain on passive extension of the fingers or toes**
  - **Numbness of the extremity**
  - **Signs of ischemia (pulseless, pallor) are late and may never occur**
- Neurological exam of the extremities for the patients who underwent spine surgery.

- Assessment of adequate gastrointestinal function for patients who underwent spica cast, shoulder cast or body cast application.
- Signs of tight cast (see Chap. 18)
- Assessment of the wound condition:
  - The following are sings of early deep wound infection:
    - Redness
    - Increased discharge from the wound
    - Increased tenderness around the wound area
    - Induration around the wound.

Postoperative complications

Post operative compartment syndrome:

- **Definition and clinical presentation:**
  - **see orthopedic trauma chapter and sign and symptoms of compartment syndrome in the previous section.**
  - **Fixation of fractures and osteotomies** in the lower leg and forearm are procedures most commonly associated with compartment syndrome.
  - Patients with post operative epidural analgesia or other regional nerve block may not have excessive pain with compartment syndrome and more close monitoring for the tightness of their compartment is needed.
- **Management**
  - Medical emergency requiring immediate surgical treatment, (i.e., fasciotomy) to allow the pressure to return to normal.
  - Immediate surgical consult should be done in patients when compartment syndrome is suspected.

Vascular injuries

- **Background**
  - Commonly result from penetrating or blunt trauma as well as iatrogenic causes.
  - Signs include pulselessness, pallor, paresthesias, pain, paralysis, poikilothermy, bleeding, rapidly expanding hematoma, palpable thrill, audible bruit.

- **Diagnosis and management**
  - Duplex ultrasonography, arterial pressure index, or angiogram can confirm clinical suspicion (Fig. 12.1a–c).
  - **Urgent Surgical consults indicated if suspecting postoperative vascular injury**.

Nerve injuries

- **Background**
  - **see also nerve injuries** in Chap. 16
  - Most closed traumatic nerve injuries are initially treated by observation
- Neuropraxia: stretching of the nerve. Recovery is usually complete.
- Axonotemesis (crushing): injury of the nerve axon with intact neural sheath.
- Neurotemesis: (transaction) injury to both the nerve axon and neural sheath. Worst prognosis
  - Complete transactions are rare. Most likely the nerve is injured during pin insertion or stretched by injury or intraoperative traction.

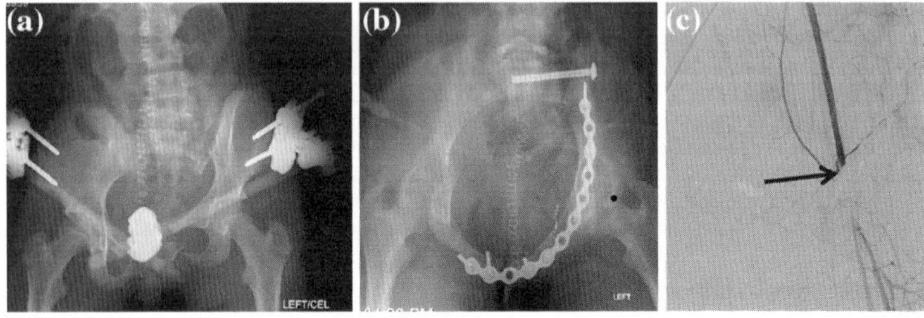

Fig. 12.1 **a**, A 14-year-old girl with pelvic fracture. **b** Patient had surgery for fixation of the fracture by plate and screws. Postoperatively, no pulses were felt in her left lower extremity. **c** The patient had an angiogram, which showed intimal tear of her external iliac artery with complete obstruction of blood flow (*arrow*). A stent was applied and blood flow was re-established in the extremity (Courtesy of Dr. Kanlic)

- **Diagnosis and management**
  - Quick assessment of major nerves
    - Radial, median, ulnar—Have patient extend thumb IP (interphalangeal) joint, flex and spread the fingers respectively
    - Posterior tibial and peroneal—Have patient flex and extend toes and ankle respectively
    - Release of flexion (stop contraction of flexors) should be differentiated from active extension. Active extension means that the child is able to move the finger or the toe up from neutral position.
  - If a neurologic impairment is present, it is often relieved by reduction of the fracture or dislocation.
  - If a neurologic impairment persists following the reduction, it is usually treated by simple observation and exercises to prevent contractures.
  - Adequate documentation of the nerve (distal to surgery or fracture) condition should be done.

Important aspects for inpatient with certain orthopedic conditions:

Child abuse

- See also non accidental trauma chapter (Chap. 15).
- History
  - Should include timing and mechanism of injury
  - Witness accounts (if available)
  - Timing of events
  - Family history of underlying conditions, child's developmental ability, risk factors for child abuse.
  - Parental/caregiver response and attitude should be documented.
- Physical examination
  - Document locations, size and number of bruises, welts, abrasions, lacerations, scars, burns.
  - Neurological status examination.

- Management
  - Place the child in a safe, protected environment
  - Notify social worker and child protective services
  - Imaging: Radiographic study of acute injury, Skeletal survey, CT—Head, Spine, Abdomen (As indicated)
  - Laboratory evaluation can include CBC, amylase, lipase, liver function tests, urinalysis, fecal occult blood, coagulation studies, urine toxicology, calcium, phosphorous, basic metabolic profile (As indicated)
  - Special considerations
    - Abdominal injury: Urinalysis (hematuria), fecal occult blood (melena), amylase, and liver function test (pancreatic and hepatic injury)
    - Malnourishment/neglect: CBC (anemia), bone density (osteopenia)
    - Metabolic and genetic diseases should be ruled out

Osteogenesis Imerfecta:
For patients with Osteogenesis imerfecta who are admitted with fractures:

- Can continue (or initiate) oral bisphosphonate (was found not to delay fracture healing)
- Parenteral bisphoshonate should be delayed unit the fracture had completely healed.

Cerebral palsy

- **See neurological chapter and spasticity chapter.**
- **Management**
  - For fracture patients: the goal of treatment is to restore the child to pre-fracture level of function.
  - The patient's spasticity and inability to communicate may predispose to skin problems/decubitus ulcers.
  - Physical therapy should be started in the immediate postoperative period to avoid osteopenia, joint stiffness, and deconditioning.

- Post operative pain in these children can cause increased spasticity and muscle spasm which can lead to more pain and vicious cycle
  - □ Diazepam 0.2 mg/Kg every 8 h oral or 0.1 mg/kg every 8 h IV will control the patient spasms and pain

■ **Postoperative complications associated with cerebral palsy**

- Higher incidence of dysphagia, gastroesophageal reflux, and reduced bowel motility
- Gastric rupture is uncommon but often fatal
  - □ Early signs include gastric distention, decreased PO tolerance, and signs of sepsis

Muscular dystrophy

■ **see neurology**

- The goal of orthopedic management is to preserve or prolong patients' ambulatory status for as long as possible.
- Fracture care methods should allow children to be ambulatory as soon as possible.
- Physical therapy should be started in the immediate postoperative period.
- Patients with Duschenne muscular dystrophy have more tendency to bleed intraoperative, close post operative monitoring of hemoglobin should be done.

Slipped capital femoral epiphysis (SCFE)

■ **see** Chap. 6

- SCFE is more common in children with underlying metabolic and endocrine disorders such as hypothyroidism, hypopituitarism, and renal osteodystrophies
  - □ Measurements of Free T4, TSH, vitamin D, calcium, cortisol, growth hormone, FSH, and LH should be determined if underlying pathologies are suspected
  - □ Treatment includes hospitalization with immediate bed rest, pain management, and surgical correction by in situ

pinning with cannulated screw to prevent further progression.
- Obesity has been identified as a common clinical presentation. If indicated, lifestyle modifications such as avoidance of sedentary lifestyle and dietary modifications should be discussed with the patient and parents.

Legg-Calve-Perthes disease (LCPD)

- Treatment should include limitation of activities, pain management, physical therapy to preserve ROM, traction, and surgical management.
- Surgical management with various osteotomy of proximal femur is the most common procedure preformed for these patients.
- Goal of treatment is preservation of femoral head and range of motion
- Sickle cell anemia, Factor V leiden mutation, protein C and S deficiency and presence of lupus anticoagulants, anticardiolipin antibodies, antitrypsin, and plasminogen activator may lead to abnormal coagulation which may lead to increased risk of developing Legg-Calve-Perthes disease
- Children with thrombophilic disorders are at increased risk of developing deep venous thrombosis. Discussions about use of oral estrogen based contraceptives, promotion of lifestyle modifications (avoidance of smoking, sedentary lifestyle, obesity) should be discussed with the patient and parents
- Children with sickle cell disease are more prone to develop microvascular ischemia, splenic sequestration, acute chest syndrome, renal disease, and neurological complications.
- In cases of inherited thrombophilic disorders, consultation with hematologist should be started. The parents should be informed of the results and testing 'if indicated' should be offered to family members

REFERENCES

Browner BD, Jupiter JB, Levine AM, Trafton PG, Krettek C. Skeletal trauma: Basic science, management, and reconstruction, volume 1, 4th ed. Philadelphia, PA: Saunders Elsevier; 2009.

Beaty JH, Kasser JR. Rockwood and Wilkin's Fractures in children, 7th ed. Philadelphia, PA: Lippincott, William & Wilkins; 2010.

Egol KA, Koval KJ, Zuckerman JD. Handbook of fractures, 4th ed. Philadelphia, PA: Lippincott Williams & Wilkins; 2010.

Arendt EA, Bhandari MM, Buss ODD, Clohisy D, et al. Manual of orthopaedics. 6th ed. Philadelphia, PA: Lippincott, Williams & Wilkins; 2006.

Young WD. Slipped capital femoral epiphysis. Avaliable at: http://emedicine.medscape.com/article/91596-overview. Aug 11, 2011.

Ramachandran S, Gellman SH. Osteogenesis Imerfecta. Avaliable at: http://emedicine.medscape.com/article/1256726-overview. Jun 15, 2012.

Harris, Lavernia. Legg-calve-perthes disease. Available at: http://emedicine.medscape.com/article/1248267-overview. May 4, 2011.

Kovac AL. Management of postoperative nausea and vomiting in children. Paediatr Drugs. 2007;9(1):47–69.

Bone healing in children with osteogenesis imerfecta treated with bisphosphonates.

Pizones J, Plotkin H, Parra-Garcia JI, Alvarez P, Gutierrez P, Bueno A, Fernandez-Arroyo A. J Pediatr Orthop. 2005 May-Jun;25(3):332–5.

Eldridge J, Dilley A, Austin H, EL-Jamil M, Wolstein L, Doris J, Hooper WC, Meehan PL, Evatt B. The role of protein C, protein S, and resistance to activated protein C in Legg-Perthes disease. Pediatrics. 2001 Jun;107(6):1329–34.

Chapter 13
Tumors and Tumor-Like Conditions

Ayman Bassiony

GENERAL PATHOLOGICAL CONSIDERATIONS

Bone Tumors can be divided into **primary and secondary**.

- **Primary bone tumor** can be benign or malignant
- **Secondary tumors** (all malignant) can be further subdivided into:
  - Metastatic tumors
  - Tumors resulting from contiguous spread of adjacent soft tissue neoplasms
  - Tumors representing malignant transformation of the pre-existing benign lesions.

Metastatic cancers:

- **Metastases are the most frequent malignant tumors found in bone.**
- Predominant occurrence in two age groups: adults over 40 years of age and children in the first decade of life.
- Characterized by: **multifocality and predilection for the hematopoietic marrow sites** in the axial skeleton (vertebrae, pelvis, ribs, and cranium) and proximal long bones.
- ***Most common malignancies producing skeletal metastases in pediatric age group are:***
  - Neuroblastoma,
  - Rhabdomyosarcoma,
  - Retinoblastoma

A. Abdelgawad and O. Naga (eds.), *Pediatric Orthopedics*,
DOI: 10.1007/978-1-4614-7126-4_13,

Primary bone tumors are characterized by the following:

- Predominant occurrence in the first three decades of life (during the ages of the greatest skeletal growth activity).
- **The commonest sites for many primary tumors, both benign and malignant, are in the distal femur and proximal tibia, the bones with the highest growth rate.**
- Relatively specific radiographic presentations. In some cases, the diagnosis can be confidently made based on the radiographic features alone.
- **Benign tumors are by far more common than malignant ones**. Some of them are not true neoplasms, but rather represent hamartomas (e.g., osteochondroma).
- **The most common benign tumors in the pediatric age group are osteochondroma, non-ossifying fibroma, and enchondroma**.
- **The most common primary malignant neoplasms in the pediatric age group are** osteosarcoma and Ewing's sarcoma.

CLASSIFICATION OF BONE TUMORS

Secondary:

Secondary bone tumors are the most common malignant bone tumors

Primary:

Classified according to the tissue of origin

I. OSTEOGENIC BONE TUMORS (OSTEOBLASTIC ORIGIN)

Benign:

- Osteoid osteoma

Malignant:

- Osteosarcoma

II. CHONDROGENIC BONE TUMORS (CARTILAGINOUS ORIGIN):

Benign:

- Enchondroma

Malignant:

- Chondrosarcoma

III. COLLAGENIC BONE TUMORS (FIBROUS ORIGIN)

Benign:

- Non-ossifying fibroma
- Subperiosteal fibrous cortical defect (Metaphyseal cortical defect)

Malignant:

- Fibrosarcoma
- Malignant fibrous histiocytoma

IV. MYELOGENIC BONE TUMORS (MARROW ORIGIN):

ALL are malignant

- Ewing's sarcoma
- Multiple myeloma

V. BONE TUMORS OF VASCULAR AND LYMPHATIC ORIGIN

Benign:

- Hemangioma
- Lymphangioma

Malignant:

- Hemangiosarcoma
- Lymphangiosarcoma

CLINICAL PRESENTATION OF BONE TUMORS

- Patients may present with:
  - Pain
  - Mass
  - Abnormal radiographic finding detected during the evaluation of an unrelated problem
- History:
  - Sex:
    - This is rarely of diagnostic significance.
  - Family history:
    - Occasionally can be helpful, as in cases of multiple hereditary exostosis and neurofibromatosis.
  - Age
    - Age is the most important information obtained in the history because most musculoskeletal neoplasms, both benign and malignant, occur with in specific age range.

- ***Primary osteosarcoma and Ewing's sarcoma are tumors of children and young adults.***

INVESTIGATIONS FOR BONE TUMORS

Biopsy of bone tumors: (Fig. 13.1)

- Open biopsy is performed when the pathologic diagnosis either is inconclusive or does not correlate with the clinical presentation and radiologic findings.

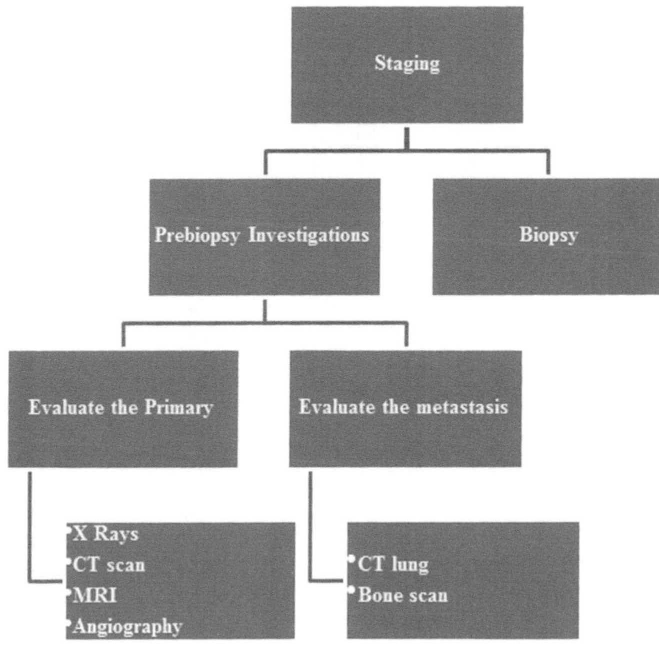

Fig. 13.1 Algorithm for investigation of bone tumors

- Bone biopsies, using a core needle biopsy (CNB), should be performed under CT or fluoroscopy guidance, and multiple cores should be obtained.
- Biopsy of a deep seated or pelvic soft-tissue tumors is performed under CT guidance.
- CT guided biopsy is a trustable mean for diagnosis of pure cellular tumors like Ewing sarcoma.

Radiologic Features of Bone Tumors

X ray should answer the following:

- **Site:**
  - Some tumors has predilection to certain sites (Table 13.1).

TABLE 13.1 SOME BONE TUMORS WITH THEIR SITE PREDILECTION

Adamantinoma:	Tibia
Chordoma	Sacrum
Osteosarcoma	Knee
Giant cell tumor	Knee
Enchondroma	Metatarsal, metacarpals, and phalanges

- **Localization:**
  - Diaphyseal:
    - Ewing's sarcoma
    - Adamantinoma
    - Osteoid osteoma
    - Fibrous dysplasia
  - Metaphyseal
    - Chondromyxoid fibroma
    - Non-ossifying fibroma
    - Bone cyst, Osteoblastoma
    - Osteochondroma
    - Osteosarcoma
    - Enchondroma, Chondrosarcoma
  - Epiphyseal
    - Chondroblastoma
- **Pattern of bone destruction**
- **Periosteal reaction**
- **Cortical erosion, penetration, and expansion**
- **Internal or external trabeculation**
- **Presence and nature of visible tumor matrix** :
  - Chondroid matrix stippled pattern
  - Osteoid matrix with fluffy cotton appearance
- **Soft tissue mass.**

Review of common Bone tumors in children:

Benign tumors:

Osteochondroma

- **Osteochondroma is the most common benign bone tumor.** They account for approximately 35 % of benign bone tumors
- These tumors are often diagnosed as an incidental finding in radiographs taken for other reasons.
- Osteochondromas may be
  - Solitary
  - Multiple: Associated with the autosomal dominant syndrome, hereditary multiple exostoses (HME).
- The osteochondroma may have a stalk (pedunculated) or it may have a broad base of attachment (sessile).
- Whether sessile or pedunculated, **the medullary canal of the stalk and the bone are in continuity**.
- **Pathology**
  - Osteochondromas can occur in any bone that ossify in cartilage.
  - It is most commonly found around the knee and the proximal humerus; however, it can occur in any bone.
  - It arises from the metaphysis near the epiphyseal cartilage.
  - By definition, the medullary canal of the affected bone and the canal of the tumor are connected.
- **Clinical picture:**
  - Osteochondromas are most commonly diagnosed incidentally based on a radiograph obtained for some other reason (Fig. 13.2).
  - The second most common presenting symptom is a mass, which may or may not be associated with pain.
  - Most of these lesions do not need to be treated, and asymptomatic lesions can be safely ignored.
    - **No orthopedic referral is needed for asymptomatic lesions.**
  - When painful, however, they need to be properly evaluated.

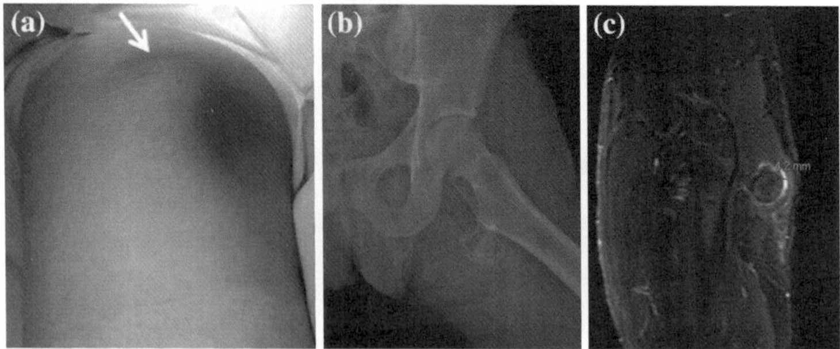

Fig. 13.2 A 15-year-old boy presents with mass in the posterolateral part of the left gluteal area (*arrow*). Radiograph showed osteochondroma (pedunculated). MRI assessed the thickness of the cartilaginous cap (4 mm)

- **Radiograph:**
  - Radiographs (Fig. 13.2) will show the **bony part** of the osteochondroma.
  - Classically the lesion will be oriented away from the physis.
  - The cortex of the lesion will be continuous with the cortex of the host bone and medulla of the lesion will be continuous with the medulla of the host bone.
- **MRI:**
  - To evaluate the thickness of cartilaginous cap. Cartilaginous cap thicker than 1 cm may be an indication of malignant transformation.
- **Causes of pain in osteochondroma**:

1. A direct mass effect on the overlying soft tissue.
2. An associated bursitis over the exostosis.
3. Irritation of surrounding tendons, muscles, or nerves can result in pain.
4. Pain can also be a result of the stalk of the osteochondroma fracturing with direct trauma.
5. The bony cap of the stalk may infarct or undergo ischemic necrosis.
6. Malignant transformation.

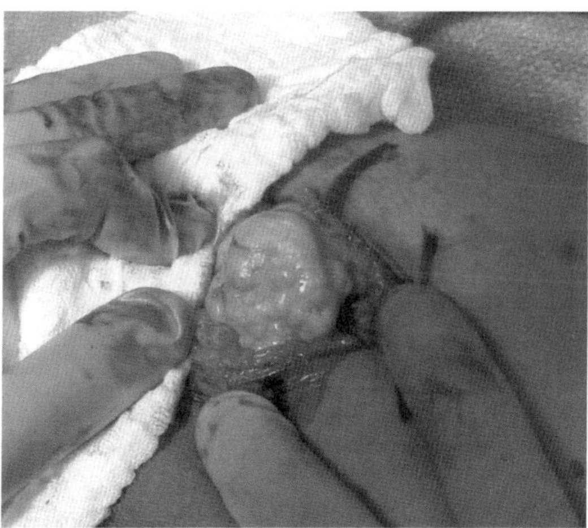

Fig. 13.3 The lesion in Fig. 13.2 was removed because it was causing pain during sitting from direct irritation and direct mass effect, notice the shape of the cartilaginous cap

- **Indications For Excision (Indication for orthopedic referral)**

1. Development of painful lesion (Fig. 13.3).
2. Location that subjects tumor to recurrent injury.
3. Significant cosmetic deformity.
4. Clinical or radiographic suspicion that malignant degeneration has occurred.

Multiple hereditary exostoses (MHE)

- Most cases are inherited as an autosomal dominant trait, about 10 % of cases occur as new spontaneous mutations.
- MHE lesions show significant variability in size, number, and distribution.
- The three most common locations for involvement are the forearm, the ankle, and the knee (Fig. 13.4).

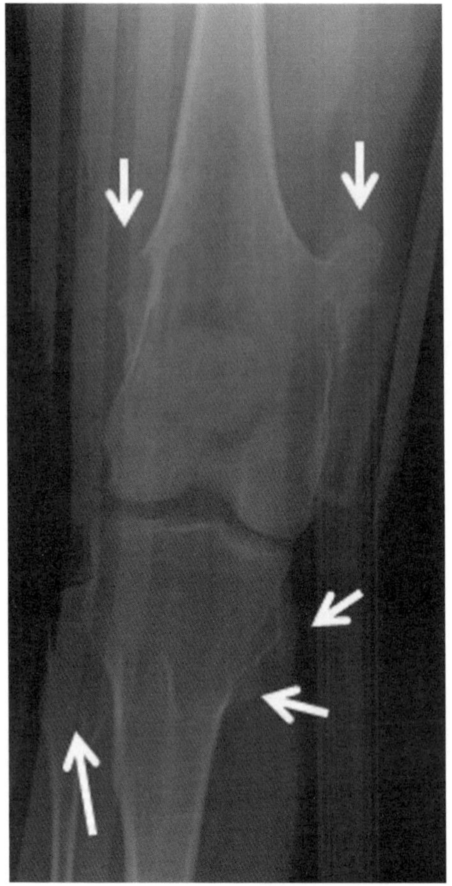

Fig. 13.4 Multiple hereditary exostosis (*MHE*). Multiple osteochondromas can be detected in the distal femur, proximal tibia, and fibula (*arrows*). Some of the lesions are sessile and some are pedunculated

- **Clinical presentation:**
- **Deformity**:
  - The forearm is the most commonly affected part, resulting in ulnar deviation of the wrist associated with relative ulna

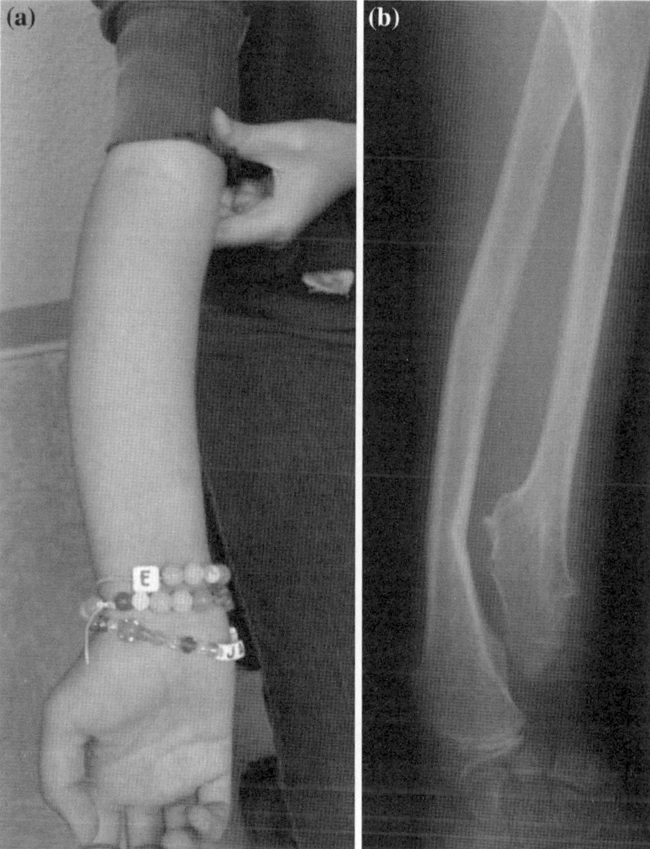

Fig. 13.5 Forearm deformity in MHE. A 9-year-old girl with MHE and forearm deformity (**a**). Notice the short ulna, ulnar deviation of the wrist, and bowing of both the ulna and the radius (**b**)

shortening, bowing of both the ulna and the radius, and late dislocation of the radial head (Fig. 13.5).

- These deformities usually progress, leading to functional impairment and cosmetic deformity.

- **Contracture:**
  - Knee, ankle, and finger contractures can occur from compression of the tendon by the lesion.
- **Limb length discrepancy:**
  - From affection of the growth plate by the tumor.
- **Malignant transformation:**
  - The incidence of malignant transformation of the MHE ranges from 1–5 %. The cartilage part of the tumor will change to chondrosarcoma.
- **Management:**
  - Only symptomatic lesion needs to be excised.
  - If there is deformity, limb length discrepancy or contractures: orthopedic referral.

Enchondroma

- It is a developmental disorder rather than a true tumor. An island of cartilage cells persists in the medulla of the bone.

Age:

- Common between 10–30 years.

Sex:

- Equal among males and females.

Clinical Picture:

- In most cases, the condition is asymptomatic.
- The main presentation is pathological fracture.
- Less commonly, the patient present with swelling or mild discomfort.

Radiographs:

- Well circumscribed radiolucent cystic like lesion within the bone (Fig. 13.6).
- Bony expansion.

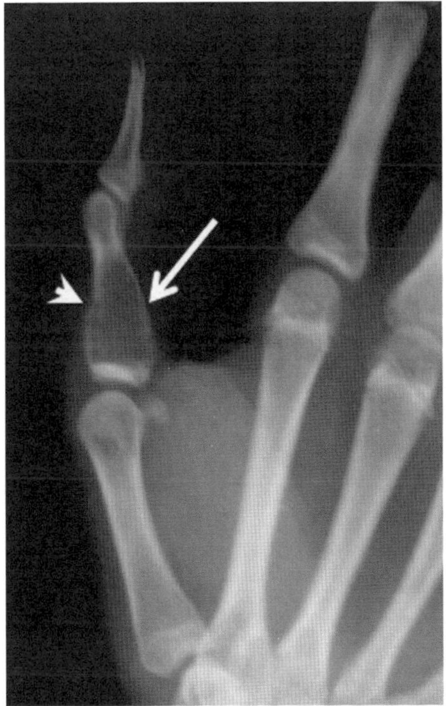

Fig. 13.6 Enchondroma. A 10-year-old girl with pain and swelling of the left thumb. Radiographs showed enchondroma of the proximal phalanx (*arrow*) with pathological fracture (*arrow head*)

- Stippling calcification (pathognomonic).
- There may be a pathological fracture.

Complications:

- Pathological fracture.
- Recurrence after excision.
- Malignant (sarcomatous) change.

Treatment:

- Asymptomatic enchondromas can be observed.
- Orthopedic referral for removal of symptomatic lesions.

- Thorough curettage with a rim of normal tissue.
- Bone graft.

When to suspect malignancy?

- When the lesion starts to grow after years of quiescence.
- If the lesion suddenly became painful.

Ollier's disease (Multiple Enchondromatosis)

- A rare, non-hereditary disorder characterized by multifocal proliferation of dysplastic cartilage.
- It is usually diagnosed in children and adolescents between 10 and 20 years of age.
- The risk of malignant transformation (usually to chondrosarcoma) is very high (20–30 %).
- **Maffucci syndrome**: presence of multiple enchondromatosis with multiple hemangiomas. Associated with risk of CNS, pancreatic, and ovarian malignancies.

CHONDROBLASTOMA

Definition:

- It is a benign tumor usually affecting long bones arising from chondroblasts.

Age:

- common between 10–20 years.

Sex:

- more common in males.

Site and Localization

Epiphyseal, especially proximal humerus, proximal femur and proximal tibia (Fig. 13.7).

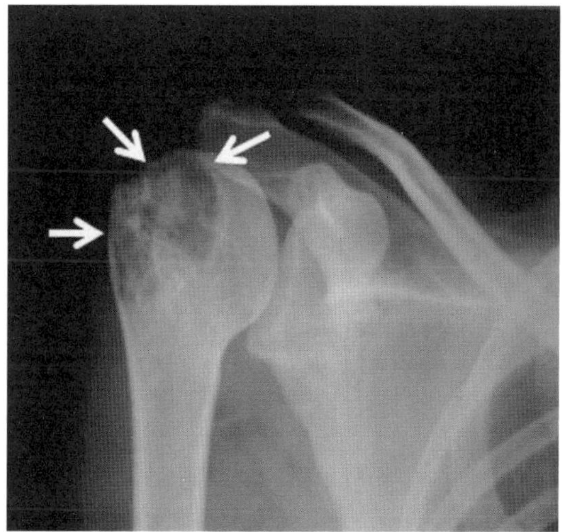

Fig. 13.7 Chondroblastoma. A 16-year-old boy with right shoulder pain. Radiograph of the shoulder showed well-circumscribed epiphyseal eccentric radiolucent lesion with calcification of the proximal humerus (*arrows*)

Clinical picture

- Pain in the affected joint.
- Firm swelling can be felt in some cases.
- Muscle stiffness and wasting secondary to interference with function.

X rays

- Well-circumscribed epiphyseal eccentric radiolucent lesion.
- With a surrounding rim of reactive bone (Sclerosis).
- Intralesional calcification.

Prognosis

- Malignant change is very rare.
- Recurrence occurs in 10-20 % of cases.

Treatment

- Orthopedic referral for surgery (thorough curettage with bone graft).

OSTEOID OSTEOMA

Definition:

- Osteoid osteoma is a benign tumor consisting of a well-demarcated bone-forming lesion called a nidus, surrounded by a radiodense, reactive zone of host bone.

Incidence:

- It is most commonly seen in the second and third decades
- More commonly affects males in an incidence of 2: 1.

Site:

- The most common skeletal sites are the diaphysis of long bones.
- Can affect the spine resulting in painful scoliosis.

Clinical picture:

- The most important clinical characteristic of osteoid osteoma is **pain**.
- Characters of pain in osteoid osteoma:
  - Increased at night with congestion.
  - Relieved by aspirin and other NSAID.
  - Early it is vague.
  - Later increases in severity and becomes aching in character.
  - It is not relieved by rest.

X-rays:

- A small defect less than 1.5 cm in diameter and is associated with a variable degree of cortical and endosteal sclerosis.
- In most cases, the defect cannot be seen and surrounding sclerosis is the only finding in the radiograph (Fig. 13.8).

Treatment:

- Excision of the lesion: complete surgical resection which must include the nidus will provide cure.

- CT-guided Percutaneous radiofrequency ablation of the nidus can lead to complete resolution of symptoms.
- The technique involves introducing a radiofrequency probe over a biopsy needle, placed under CT control.

FIBROUS CORTICAL DEFECT (FCD) AND NONOSSIFYING FIBROMA (NOF)

Definition:

- Fibrous cortical defect (FCD) and Nonossifying fibroma (NOF) are nonaggressive fibrous lesions of bone that are distinguished from one another by their size and natural history.
- Both are considered developmental defects and nonaggressive.
- This benign lesion is the most common bony lesion in children.

Age:

- Peak occurrence is in those aged 10–15 years.

Site:

- Occurs most commonly in the metaphysis of long bones (femur, tibia) in children.
- The lesion is eccentric in position.

Clinical Features:

- Most fibrous cortical defects are completely asymptomatic and are accidentally discovered during evaluation for another complaint.
- Pain is rare and, if present, is usually associated with a fracture.
- Larger lesions may be associated with a pathologic fracture.

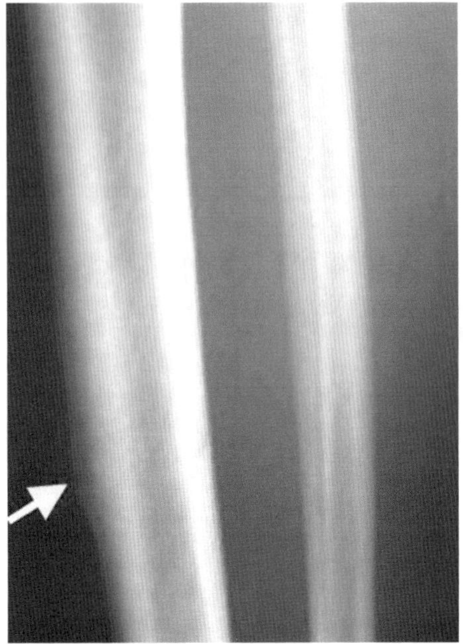

Fig. 13.8 Osteoid osteoma. A 14-year-old boy with right leg pain, more at night. Radiograph shows cortical thickening of the tibia (*arrow*), notice that the tumor itself cannot be seen because of the surrounding sclerosis

X-rays:

Fibrous Cortical Defects (FCD)

- Fibrous cortical defects are well-delineated, circular, or oval lesions with smooth or lobulated edges.
- The adjacent bone is typically sclerotic

Nonossifying fibroma (NOF)

- The nonossifying fibromas are more elongated and multiloculated. They frequently exhibit slight bony expansion and cortical thinning (Fig. 13.9).
- Can be associated with pathological fracture.

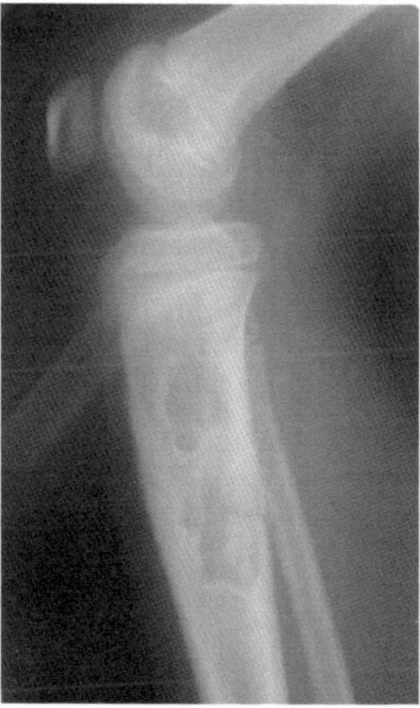

Fig. 13.9 Non-ossifying fibroma (NOF). An 8-year-old girl presenting with left leg pain after ground level fall. Radiographs showed well-delineated, multi-lobulated eccentric lesion with pathological fracture (*arrow*)

Treatment:

- **No treatment needed for accidentally discovered lesion.**
- For symptomatic lesions (pain or pathological fractures): orthopedic referral: Curettage and bone grafting is the treatment of choice with possibility of internal fixation.

Malignant Tumors:

- Osteosarcoma and Ewing's sarcoma are the most common malignancies of bone in children.

- Osteosarcoma, the more common of the two types, usually presents in bones around the knee.
- Ewing's sarcoma may affect bones of the pelvis, thigh, upper arm, or ribs.

Osteosarcoma:

- Osteosarcoma is a primary malignant tumor of bone **with malignant osteoid formation** arising from bone-forming mesenchymal cells.
- Two suppressor genes, p53 and Rb (Retinoblastoma), have major roles in tumorigenesis in osteosarcoma.
- The strongest genetic predisposition to osteosarcoma is found in patients with hereditary retinoblastoma. In hereditary retinoblastoma, mutations of the RB1 gene are common.

Types of Osteosarcoma:

A. **Conventional (classic) osteosarcoma (75–85 %):**

- Conventional osteosarcoma is the commonest primary malignant bone tumor below 20 years (75–85 % of all osteosarcoma).

B. **Osteosarcoma Variants:**

- Examples include Parosteal osteosarcoma (juxta cortical sarcoma), Periosteal osteosarcoma, High grade periosteal (High Grade Surface), Central low grade osteosarcoma, and telangiectatic Osteosarcoma.

Conventional (classic) osteosarcoma

Site and Localization:

- Metaphysis of long bones.
- 70 % of classis osteosarcomas occur around the Knee.

Clinical picture

- ***Pain:***
  - **Is the first and most common symptom,** constant, severe.
  - Increased at night due to venous congestion

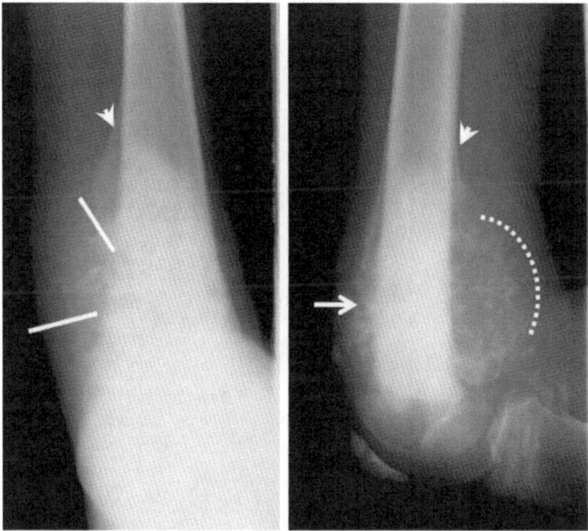

Fig. 13.10 Osteosarcoma. Anteroposterior (A) and lateral (B) views of right knee showing signs of osteosarcoma: Sun ray appearance (*arrow*), Codman's triangle (*arrow head*), cortical erosion (*line*), and soft tissue shadow (*dotted line*)

- ***Swelling*** usually preceded by pain.
- ***Pathological fracture***
- Rare except in central low grade and telangiectatic Osteosarcoma

Imaging

X-rays:

- **Skeletally immature patient with an osteolytic lesion which is metaphyseal, eccentric, and having ill-defined edges.**.
- Reactive bone formation:
  - Codman's reactive triangle (new bone formation at an angle to the shaft secondary to elevated periosteum).
  - Sun ray appearance (new bone formation along stretched periosteal vessels that pass perpendicular to the cortex) (Fig. 13.10).
- Erosion of the cortex.
- Soft tissue shadow.

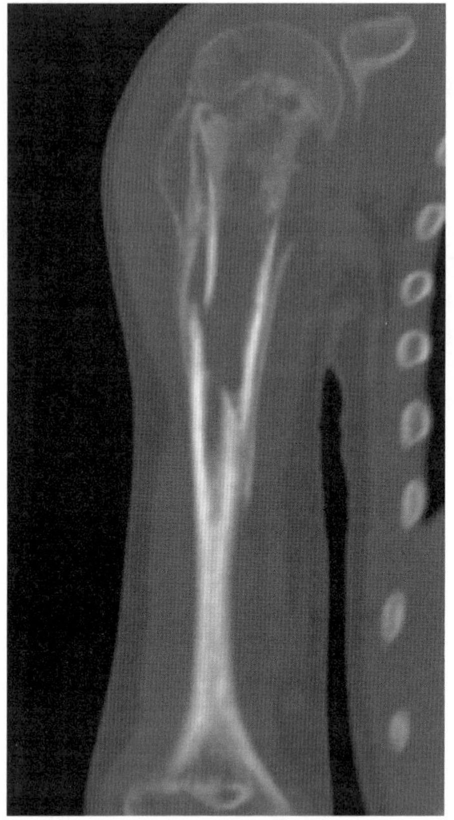

Fig. 13.11 A 12-year-old boy with osteosarcoma of the proximal humerus. CT scan shows the extent of bone destruction and reactive new bone formation

CT:

- Better assessment of bone destruction (Fig. 13.11).

MRI:

- Better assessment of soft tissue mass, invasion of nearby neurovascular bundle and satellite lesions (skip lesions in the same bone).

Treatment:

- Requires cooperation between the orthopedic surgeon and the oncologist.
- Treatment and prognosis depends on the subtype and grade of the tumor.
  - Low grade tumors: are surgically removed and usually not treated with chemotherapy; 85 % of the patients should expect a 5 year event-free survival.
  - Intermediate and high grade tumors: are treated with both surgery and chemotherapy.
- Osteosarcomas do not respond to radiation therapy.
- Removal of the tumor is by either:
  - Amputation of the extremity Or
  - Removal of the tumor and replacing the bone with a bone graft or prosthesis (limb preservation surgery).
- Commonly used drugs in chemotherapy are ifosfamide, cisplatin, methotrexate, and doxorubicin.

EWING'S SARCOMA

Definition:

- It is a primary malignant bone tumor that arises from the medullary tissue mostly from the lining cells of the medullary blood or lymphatic channels.
- **It is a round cell sarcoma**.

Incidence:

- It is the second most common primary malignant tumor after osteosarcoma in patients less than 30 years old.
- It is the most common primary malignant tumor in patients less than 10 years old.
- It represents about 6 % of the primary total bone malignancy.

Age and Sex:

- It occurs more commonly in males in the first two decades of life.

Site and Localization:

- Although any bone in the skeleton may be affected, it usually involves the long bones of the lower limb.
- It occurs in **diaphysis** of the long bones.

Clinical Picture:

- Pain and tenderness over the involved area.
  - early: the pain is intermittent (remissions and exacerbations).
  - later it becomes persistent and severe.
- Swelling
  - characterized by being: slowly growing, warm, tender, ill-defined, hard, diaphyseal, and fusiform with smooth surface.
- Fever, Anorexia, headache, and malaise may be the presenting symptoms (clinical presentation may be similar to osteomyelitis).

X-rays (Fig 13.12):

- Medullary destruction: mottled areas of intermediate density replacing the bone trabeculae.
- Soft tissue mass.
- Reactive new bone formation.
  - Onion peel appearance (most classic, rare): The elevated periosteum produces one or more layers of bone, then these layers are perforated by the tumor which continues to grow, so the periosteum lays another layers of new bone.
  - Codman's reactive triangle.
  - Sun ray appearance: Differs from osteosarcoma as it occurs in diaphysis and in younger age.

Treatment:

- Chemotherapy
- Radiotherapy
- Excision of the tumor
  - Amputation or limb salvage

BONE CYSTS

Unicameral Bone Cyst (Simple Bone Cyst)

- The unicameral bone cyst is probably not a true neoplasm.
- The pathogenesis of simple bone cysts is unknown.
- Age:
  - 5–15 years.
- Sex:
  - Males predominate (2:1)
- localization:
  - Simple bone cysts are found in tubular bones.
  - Within the long bones, most simple bone cysts are situated in the proximal metaphysis.
- Site:
  - Most cases are in the proximal humerus and upper femur.
- Clinical presentation:
  - Because the solitary bone cyst develops very slowly, it rarely causes pain.
  - Pathological fracture: pain after minor trauma due pathological fracture of the affected bone.
  - Occasionally, a bone cyst is discovered in radiographic surveys done for another reason.

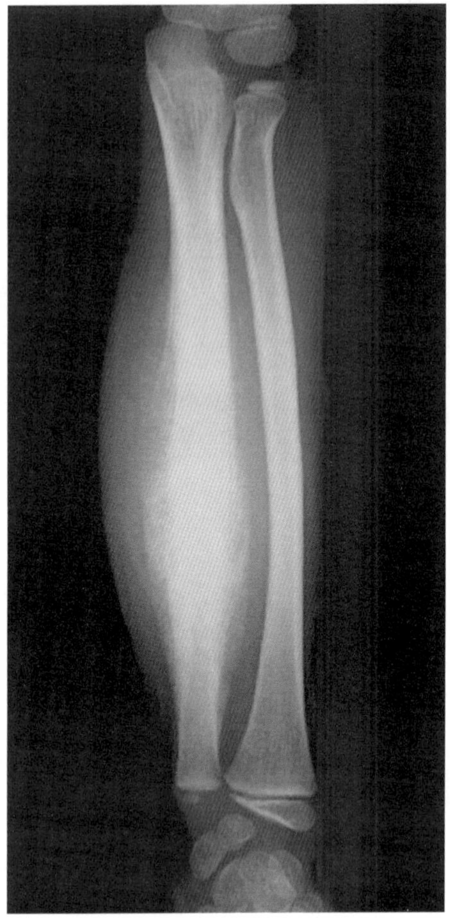

Fig. 13.12 Ewing's sarcoma. An 8-year-old boy with left forearm pain and swelling. Radiograph showed Ewing's sarcoma of the ulnar diaphysis. Notice the location of the lesion (diaphysis) and the periosteal new bone formation

X-rays:

- A well-defined, geographic lesions with narrow transition zones (Fig. 13.13).
- A thin sclerotic margin is a typical finding.
- Simple bone cysts usually are situated in the intramedullary metaphyseal region immediately adjacent to the physis.

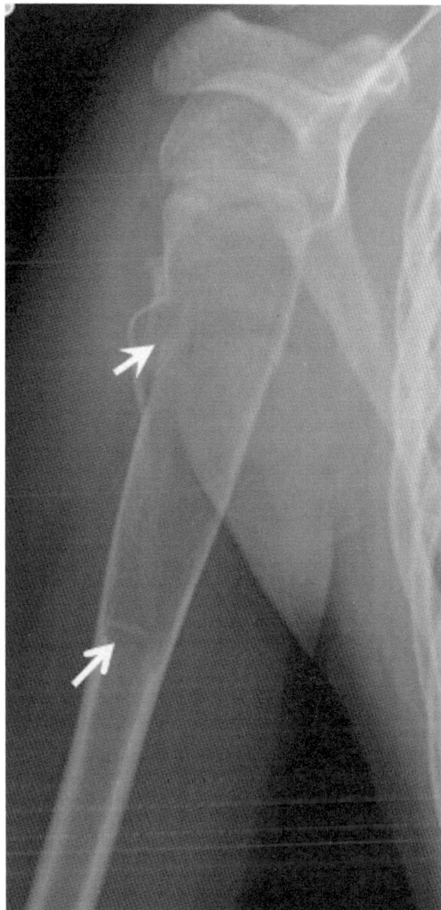

Fig. 13.13 Simple bone cyst with pathological fracture. An 8-year-old boy who fell down while playing on the slide and developed right shoulder pain. Radiographs showed simple bone cyst of the proximal humerus with pathological fracture (*arrow head*). Notice the fallen leaf sign pathognomonic for simple bone cyst (arrow)

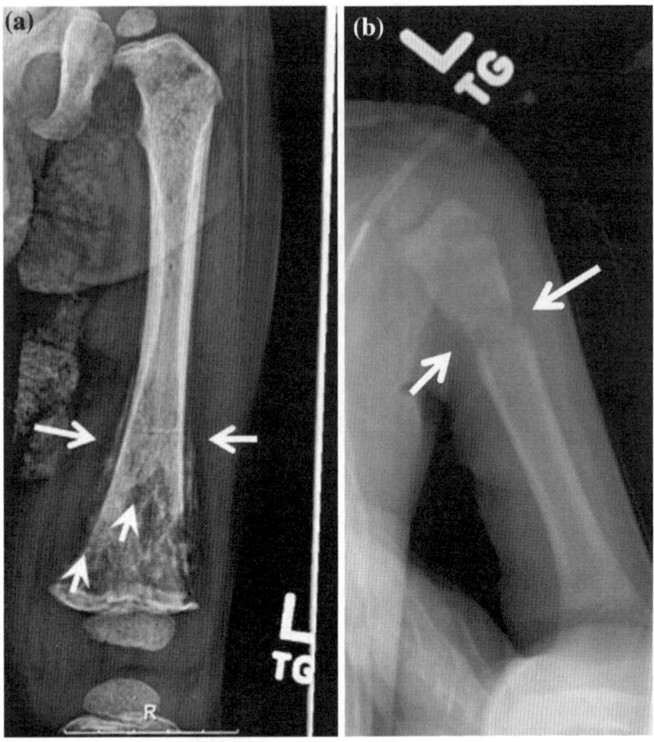

Fig. 13.14 Leukemic affection of the bone. A 2-year-old boy with leukemia and skeletal manifestations. **a** Notice in the left femur, the presence of periosteal new bone formation (*arrows*) and bone erosion in the distal metaphyseal area (*arrow head*). **b** Left humerus shows pathological fracture at the upper diaphysis with bone destruction (arrows)

- **A fallen fragment (fallen leaf) sign is pathognomonic of a simple bone cyst**

Treatment:

- If the lesion is symptomatic, orthopedic referral.
  - The traditional method of treating unicameral cysts had been curettage and grafting.
  - Successful healing has been reported by injecting methylprednisolone acetate (200 mg) into the cyst cavity.

ANEURYSMAL BONE CYST

- The aneurysmal bone cyst (ABC) is an expansile cystic lesion.
- The true etiology is unknown. Most believe that ABCs are the result of a vascular malformation within the bone.
- ABCs most commonly affect long tubular bones, followed by the spine and flat bones.
- The gross appearance of the ABC is that of a blood-soaked sponge. A thin subperiosteal shell of new bone surrounds the structure and contains cystic blood-filled cavities.
- **Clinical presentation:**
  - Pain
  - Mass and swelling
  - Pathologic fracture

Radiographs:

- An eccentric or, less commonly, a central or subperiosteal lesion that appears cystic or lytic.
- Images may show expansion of the surrounding bone with a blown-out, ballooned, or soap-bubble appearance with an eggshell-appearing bony rim surrounding the lesion.
- Treatment:
  - Orthopedic referral:
    - Can be treated with intralesional curettage and bone grafting or wide excision.

BONE MANIFESTATIONS IN ACUTE LEUKEMIA

- The skeletal manifestations of acute leukemia are important to recognize, as they may be the presenting signs and symptoms and may be first seen by an orthopedist

- Musculoskeletal pain is a common symptom early in the course of acute leukemia, and is a presenting complaint in about half of patients
- Gait abnormalities or refusal to walk at presentation is present in about half of the patients
- Pain and swelling in the joints, resembling juvenile rheumatoid arthritis, is present in about 10% of patients with ALL at presentation, Typically, more than one joint is involved, with knees, ankles, and elbows being most commonly affected
- An increased risk of fracture is seen in leukemia, and is likely related to osteoporosis

Radiographs (Fig. 13.14):

- Osteopenia
- Bone osteolystic lesions (leukemic infiltrate)
- Radiolucent metaphyseal bands (represent abnormal mineralization rather than infiltration of leukemia cells)
- Diaphyseal periosteal new bone formation
- Pathological fractures

Management:

- For any child presenting with vague musculoskeletal pain together with general constitutional symptoms, (with or without positive radiological findings), an oncologic consultation should be obtained.

REFERENCES

Springfield DS, Gebhardt MC. Bone and soft tissue tumors. In: Morrissy RT, Weinstein SL, editors. Lovell and Winter's pediatric orthopaedics. 6th ed. Philadelphia: Lippincott Williams and Wilkins; 2005. p. 494–549.

Cornwall R, Dormans J. Diseases of the hematopoietic system. In: Morrissy RT, Weinstein SL, editors. Lovell and Winter's pediatric orthopaedics. 6th ed. Philadelphia: Lippincott Williams and Wilkins; 2005. p. 358–404.

Conrad C. Tumors. In: Staheli LT, editor. Practice of pediatric orthopedics. 2nd ed. Philadelphia: Lippincott Williams and Wilkins; 2006. p. 366–84.

Weber KL, Sim FH. Malignant bone tumors. In: Chapman MW, editor. Chapman's orthopaedic surgery. 3rd ed. Philadelphia: Lippincott Williams and Wilkins; 2001. p. 3418–49.

Gereige R, Kumar M. Bone lesions: benign and malignant. Pediatr Rev. 2010;31(9):355–62.

Chapter 14
Spasticity and Gait

Mahmoud A. Mahran and Walid Abdel Ghany

Cerebral Palsy:

Cerebral Palsy is the most common pediatric neurologic disorder, with an incidence of 3.6 per 1,000 live births.

Characteristics of Cerebral Palsy (See also Cerebral Palsy in Chap. 20).

By definition it is:

- A static encephalopathy.
- A motor disability.
- Disorder of movement and posture.
- Non-progressive.
- Present before 2 years of age.
- Secondary to a variety of etiologies (see Chap. 20).

What is Tone and what is Hypertonia?

- ***Tone*** is the continuous and passive partial contraction of the muscles at rest.
- ***Hypertonia*** is the increase in muscle's resistance to passive stretch during resting state.

Abnormal tone in Cerebral Palsy children:

- Abnormal muscle tone is a diagnostic feature of cerebral palsy.
- Types of abnormal tone:

1. **Hypertonia** (the most frequent):

   a. Spasticity.
   b. Dystonia.
   c. Rigidity.
   d. Mixed Type.

A. Abdelgawad and O. Naga (eds.), *Pediatric Orthopedics*,
DOI: 10.1007/978-1-4614-7126-4_14,

2. Hypotonia
3. Combined hypotonia-hypertonia

Spasticity:

- **The most common tone abnormality in Cerebral Palsy children**.
- It is defined as: resistance to externally imposed movement increases with increasing speed of stretch and varies with the direction of joint movement (i.e., velocity dependent and length dependent).
- Clonus is a common associated feature.
- Seen as a common consequence of injury to the white matter of the brain.
- Further subclassified anatomically into

  - **Diplegic** (Fig. 14.1):

    - Lower extremities are more affected than the upper extremities.
    - Hypoxic encephalopathy remains the most common identifiable cause of Cerebral Palsy, leading to periventricular leukomalacia. Fibers of the pyramidal system controlling lower limbs are the most affected track in this area**, so spastic diplegia is the most common form of spasticity in Cerebral Palsy**.

  - Hemiplegic:

    - Affection of one side of the body more than the other.
    - The upper extremity is affected more than the lower extremity.

  - Quadriplegic cerebral palsy (Fig. 14.2):

    - All four extremities are profoundly affected.

Dystonia:

- Many children with Cerebral Palsy will have dystonia. The second most common type of tone abnormality after spastic cerebral palsy.
- Failure to respond to anti-spasticity treatments indicates underlying dystonia.

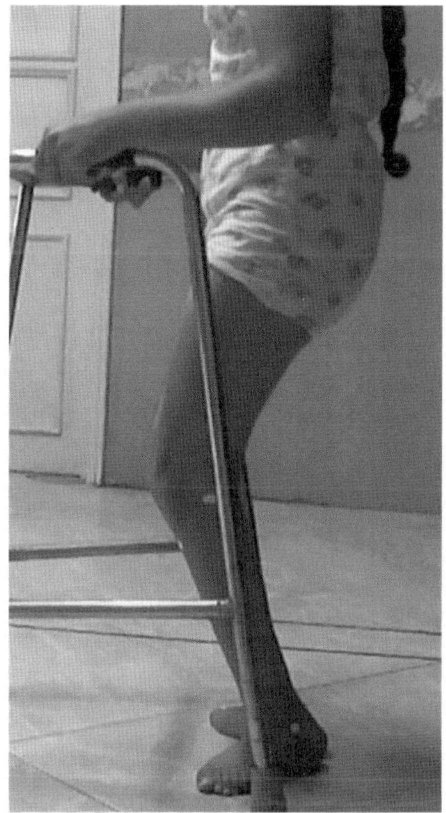

Fig. 14.1 Diplegic CP with crouch gait. Notice the flexed hips and knees

- Dystonic hypertonia shows:
  - An increase in muscle activity when at rest.
  - Increases resistance with movement of the contralateral limb.
  - **Exaggerated with emotional state or posture**.
  - **There are involuntary sustained or intermittent muscle contractions causing twisting and repetitive movements, abnormal postures, or both**.

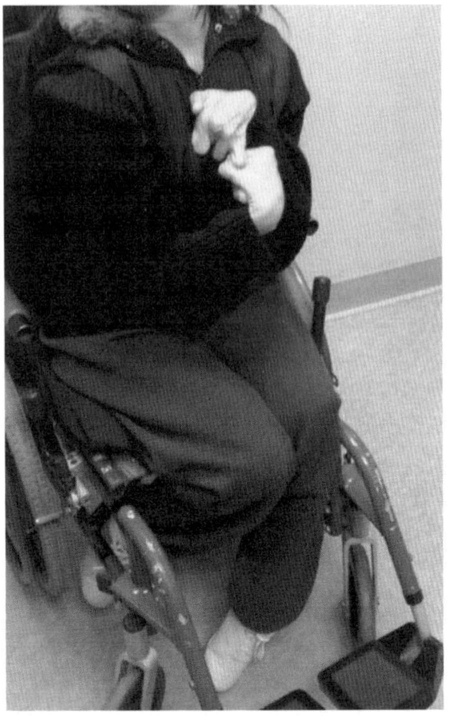

Fig. 14.2 Quadriplegic Cerebral palsy. A 26-year-old female with quadriplegic cerebral palsy. Notice the involvement of four extremities

- A tendency to return to a fixed posture.
- Higher incidence of developing early contractures.

Rigidity:

- Rigid hypertonia may be encountered in post encephalitic Cerebral Palsy.
- Rigidity is defined as hypertonia in which all of the following are true:
  - The resistance to externally imposed joint movement is present at very low speeds of movement, does not depend on imposed speed, and does not exhibit a speed or angle threshold.

- Simultaneous co-contraction of agonists and antagonists may occur, and this is reflected in an immediate resistance to a reversal of the direction of movement about a joint.
- The limb does not tend to return toward a particular fixed posture or extreme joint angle.
- Voluntary activity in distant muscle groups does not lead to involuntary movements about the rigid joints, although rigidity may worsen.

Pathophysiology of Cerebral Palsy

The neurological lesion may produce different tone abnormalities (spastic, dystonic, or mixed):

- In pure **spasticity**, only the corticospinal system is damaged.
- In pure **dystonia**, only the basal ganglia and/or its connecting pathways are involved.
- In **a mixed pattern**, both systems are injured.

Gait in Cerebral Palsy:

Gait deviations in Cerebral Palsy are due to:

- ***Primary anomalies***: are due to the damage to the central nervous system. These are:
  - Deficiency of selective muscle control (this increases distally down the limb, i.e., proximal control is better).
  - Dependence on primitive reflex patterns for ambulation.
  - Abnormal muscle tone.
  - Relative imbalance between muscle agonists and antagonists.
  - Deficient equilibrium reactions.
- ***Secondary anomalies***: are due to abnormal bone/muscle growth.
  - Progressive skeletal deformities:
    - □ Progressive hip subluxation.
    - □ Torsional deformities of long bones.
    - □ Foot deformities.

- Soft tissue contractures (musculotendinous units and capsular structures):
  - Muscle contractures.
  - Joint contractures.

- ***Tertiary abnormalities***:
  - Are the compensations that the patient uses to circumvent the primary and secondary abnormalities of gait (the coping responses).
  - Coping responses depend on selective control. Thus, are usually provided by proximal muscles.

Examples:

- Co-spasticity of the rectus femoris and hamstrings (primary abnormality) will lead to stiff knee gait and difficulty with toe clearance. The child will compensate with hip circumduction to clear the foot (coping response).
- Spastic equinus deformity (primary anomaly) will lead to knee hyperextension during midstance phase of gait cycle to be able to rest the whole foot on the ground (coping response).

The three anomalies interact to produce a specific gait pattern for a Cerebral Palsy child. The primary and secondary abnormalities require operative or orthotic correction. Whereas the coping responses will disappear spontaneously once they are no longer necessary.

Assessment of a child with Cerebral Palsy:

- Medical history:
  - Birth history.
  - Developmental milestones.
  - Medical problems.
  - Surgical history.
  - Current physical therapy treatment.
  - Current medication.

- **Detailed physical examination**:

1. ***Strength*** (the 5-point Kendall scale) and ***selective motor control*** of isolated muscle groups; a scale of 3 grades that assess ability to isolate and control movements on request.
2. Assessment of the ***Degree and type of muscle tone***: Important for evaluation of the effectiveness of the therapeutic interventions, to guide treatment decisions, and to measure progress in patients with spasticity.

   - **Modified Ashworth Scale (MAS)**

     - Grade 0 = no increase in muscle tone.
     - Grade 1 = slight increase in muscle tone, manifested by a catch and release or by minimal resistance at the end of the range of motion when the affected part is moved in flexion or extension.
     - Grade 1+ = mild increase in muscle tone, manifested by a catch, followed by minimal resistance throughout the remaining (less than half) range of motion (ROM).
     - Grade 2 = moderate increase in muscle tone through most of the ROM, but affected part easily moved.
     - Grade 3 = marked increase in muscle tone, passive movement difficult.
     - Grade 4 = obvious limitation in range of motion, the affected part is fixed in flexion or extension.

   - **Modified Tardieu Scale**:

     - Defines the moment of "catch," seen in the range of motion of a particular joint angle at a fast passive stretch.

3. ***Degree of static muscle and joint contracture***:

   - Variation in ROM measurements between observers is common.
   - These errors are most likely the result of how much stretch is applied before recording the value for the range of movement.
   - Differentiation between static (due to joint contracture) and dynamic (due to muscle spasm) deformity may be difficult in the non-anesthetized patient.
   - Dynamic contracture disappears under general anesthesia. Dynamic contracture needs tone lowering procedure but static contracture needs tendon lengthening.

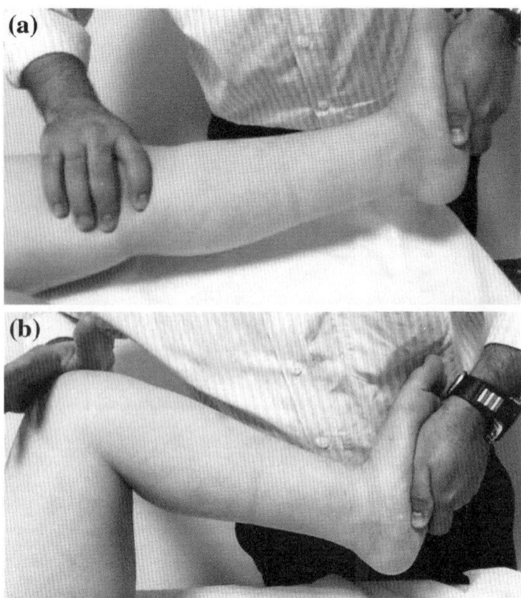

Fig. 14.3 Silfverskiold test. Assessment of ankle dorsiflexion with the knee extended (**a**) and with the knee flexed 90° (**b**). In cases of isolated gastrocnemius contracture, there will be equinus contracture with knee extended and when the knee is flexed to 90°, ankle dorsiflexion significantly improves

- Differentiation between contracted bi-articular and mono-articular muscles is important;
  - The **Silfverskiold test** (Fig. 14.3) assesses the difference between gastrocnemius and soleus contracture.
    - Increase in the amount of ankle dorsiflexion by knee flexion indicates gastrocnemius contracture (bi-articular).If dorsiflexion is the same whether the knee is extended or flexed, it indicates soleus muscle contracture.
  - The **Duncan-Ely test** (Fig. 14.4) differentiates between contracture of the monoarticular vasti and the biarticular rectus femoris.
    - Hip flexion with knee flexion indicates contracture of the rectus muscle.

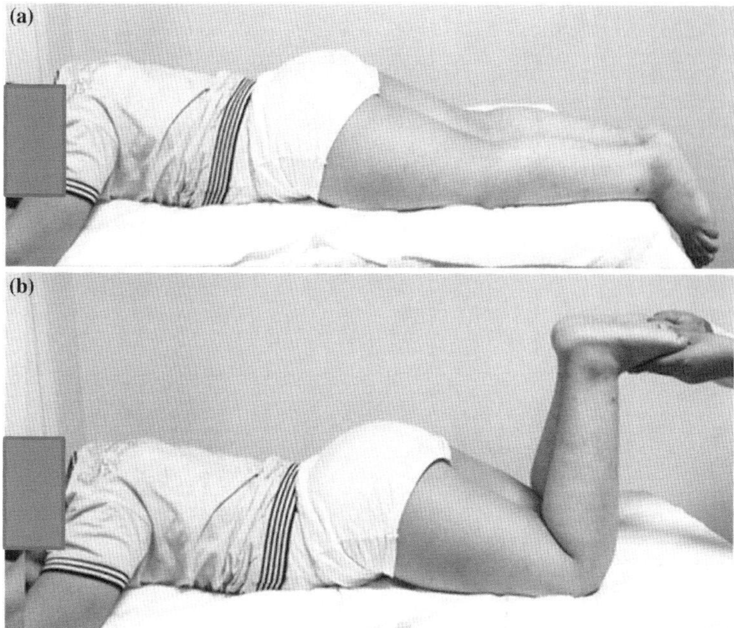

Fig. 14.4 The Duncan-Ely test. **a** Passively flexing the knee while the patient lies prone position. **b** Hip flexion (hip lifting from table) indicated tight Rectus muscle

- Hip:
  - Flexor tightness (i.e., Iliopsoas muscle) by **Thomas test (see hip chapter)** (Fig. 6.4/**hip**).
  - Adductor tightness by Abduction in flexion and extension (to isolate tightness of the biarticular gracilis).
- Knee: it is important to differentiate between knee joint contracture and hamstring tightness;

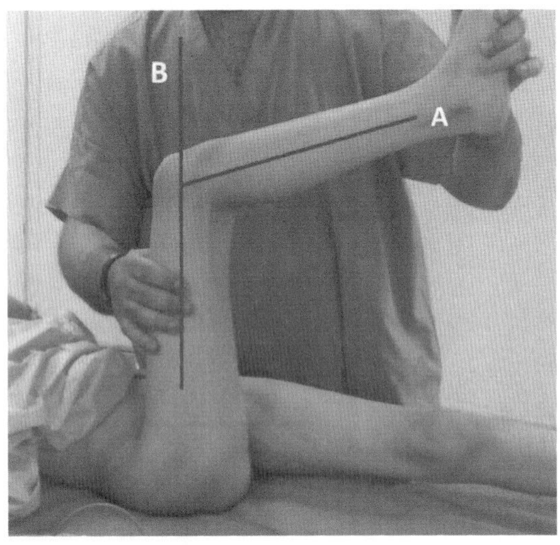

Fig. 14.5 Popliteal angle. For assessment of hamstring tightness. The examiner flex the hip and try to extend the knee maximally. The angle between the tibia and vertical is the popliteal angle

- Joint contracture: lack of full knee extension with the hip extended (to relax the hamstrings) and the ankle in equinus (to relax the gastrocnemius).
- Hamstring contracture: limited knee extension with the hip flexed to 90° (the popliteal angle) (Fig. 14.5).

■ Torsional and other bone deformities: femoral anteversion, tibial torsion, patella alta, and limb length (Fig. 14.6).

- Limb length inequality in Cerebral Palsy can be caused by:

  - Scoliosis.
  - Hip subluxation.
  - Pelvic obliquity caused by unilateral contracture of the hip adductors or abductors.
  - Unilateral knee flexion contracture.

■ Fixed and mobile foot deformities (Fig. 14.7).
■ Balance, equilibrium responses, and standing posture.

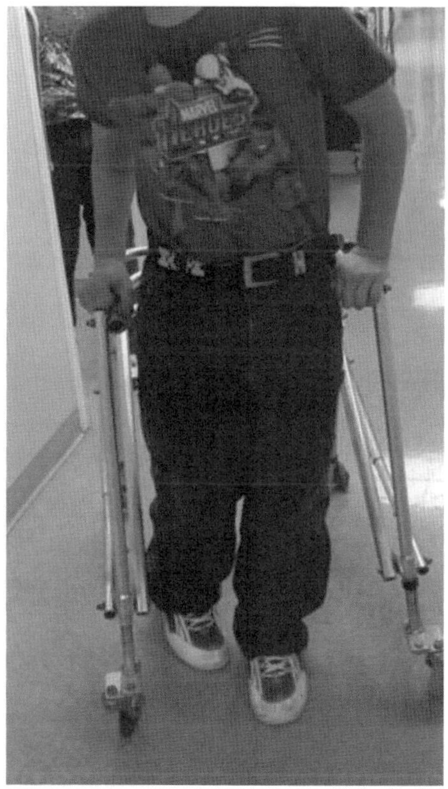

Fig. 14.6 Femoral anteversion. A 14 year old boy with diplegic cerebral palsy. The right foot in turned inward as a result of excess femoral anteversion which is common in cerebral palsy patients

4. Functional assessment:

   - Functional level of children with Cerebral Palsy with the Gross Motor Function Classification System (GMFCS) (Fig. 14.8):

     - ***Level I***: Walks without limitations.
     - ***Level II***: Walks with limitations.
     - ***Level III***: Walks using a hand-held mobility device (walker or crutches).

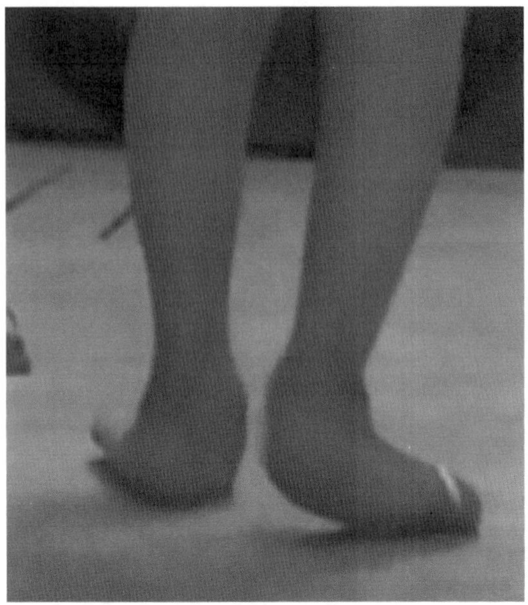

Fig. 14.7 Bilateral valgus feet deformity in 8-year-old girl

- *Level IV*: Self-mobility with limitations; may use powered mobility.
- *Level V*: Transported in a manual wheelchair.

- Functional assessment questionnaire (FAQ) of the Pediatric Orthopaedic Society of North America.
- Pediatric outcomes data collection instruments (PODCI).
- The functional mobility scale (FMS).

5. Electrophysiological evaluation of spasticity: Detailed electromyography motor-control analysis can alter surgical planning (i.e., H/M ratio).
6. Imaging studies.

   - Plain X-Rays (i.e., for hip joints).
   - Computed tomography (CT) with reconstruction (i.e., for dislocated hip joints).

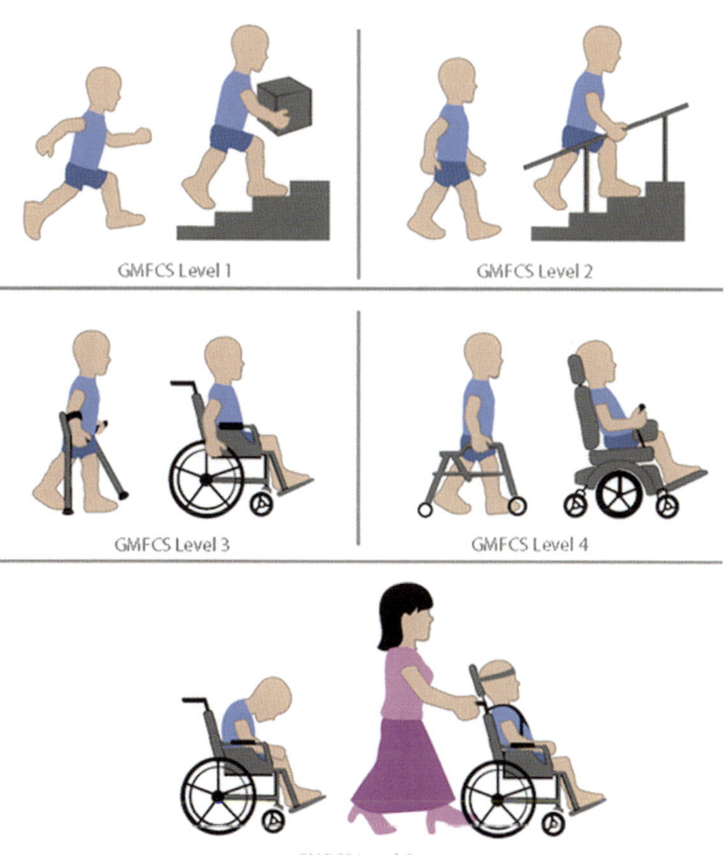

Fig. 14.8 GMFCS

- Magnetic Resonance Imaging (MRI) (e.g., for the brain to confirm the diagnosis of Cerebral Palsy).

7. Observational gait analysis.
8. Computerized gait analysis including dynamic electromyography.
9. Assessment of patient and family goals.

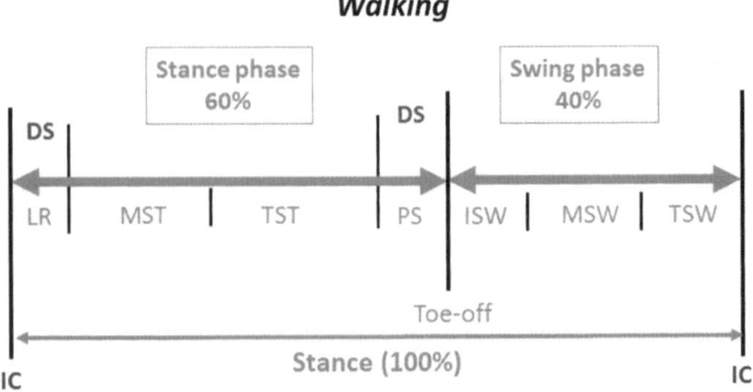

Fig. 14.9 Normal walking (gait cycle). 60 % of the gait cycle is the stance phase (the foot or part of it is on the ground) and 40 % is swing phase (the foot is off ground). DS (Double stance); LR (Loading response); MST (mid stance); TST (terminal stance); PS (pre swing); ISW (initial swing); MSW (mid swing); TSW (terminal swing); IC (initial contact)

Normal gait:

- **Normal walking (**Fig. 14.9**) is defined** as a highly controlled, coordinated, and repetitive series of limb movements whose function is to advance the body safely from one place to another with a minimum expenditure of energy.
- **The prerequisites** of normal gait, in order of priority, are:

  1. Stability of the foot, the ankle, and the entire lower limb in stance phase.
  2. Clearance of the ground by the foot in swing phase.
  3. Proper prepositioning of the foot in terminal swing.
  4. Adequate step length.
  5. Maximization of energy conservation.

- **Important definitions**:

  - ***Gait cycle*** is defined as the movement of a single limb from heel-strike to heel-strike again. It divides into two phases: stance (60 % of the cycle) and swing (40 % of the cycle) (Fig. 14.10).
  - ***Step length*** indicates the distance from a specific stance-phase event of one foot to the same event of the other foot.

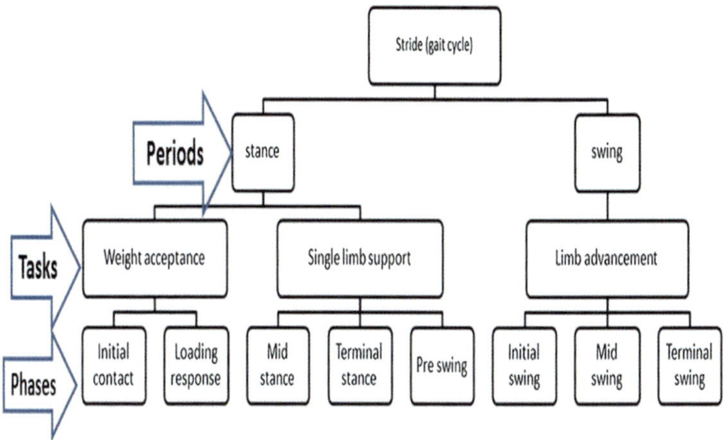

Fig. 14.10 Gait cycle. The stance phase has two tasks (weight acceptance and limb support) while swing phase has the task of limb advancement

- ***Stride length*** (***cycle length***) is the distance from the initial contact of one foot to the following initial contact of the same foot.
- ***Velocity*** refers to the average horizontal speed of the body along the plane of progression, measured over one stride or more.
- ***Cadence*** is the number of steps per unit of time, represented as steps per minute.

- **Ankle rockers** (Table 14.1)
- **Components of gait analysis**:

  - **Kinematics**: describes the movement of the body regardless of the forces that caused them (actual movement happening). Hip, knee, and ankle joint kinematics in normal gait can be seen in (Fig. 14.11).
  - **Kinetics**: describes the mechanism that caused movements. These are:

    - The internal joint moments
    - The ground reaction force

TABLE 14.1 SHOWS ANKLE ROCKERS WITH THE MAIN RESPONSIBLE MUSCLES

	First rocker	Second rocker	Third rocker
Event	From initial contact till foot flat	Foot remains flat and tibia advances forward to advance the whole body. Quadriceps contracts initially to slow down tibial advancement	It is the push off required for body advancement
Muscles involved	Eccentric contraction of ankle dorsiflexors	Eccentric contraction (lengthening) of plantar flexors. Plantar flexors take over the quadriceps action by bringing the ground reaction force anterior to the knee i.e. leads to passive knee extension without much quadriceps power	Concentric (shortening) contraction of triceps-surae

- **Dynamic polyelectromyographic data**: these are the electrical signals generated by muscle actions that are detected by surface electrodes during gait cycle.
- **Oxygen consumption.**
- **Observational video gait analysis.**

■ Although not a substitute for clinical judgment and experience, instrumented gait analysis (IGA) is extremely valuable as it allows:

- Increases understanding of the gait patterns.
- Suggest possible treatment options.
- Measures treatment outcomes.

Functional gait patterns in ambulatory Cerebral Palsy:

■ The most common gait abnormalities occur in the sagittal plane.

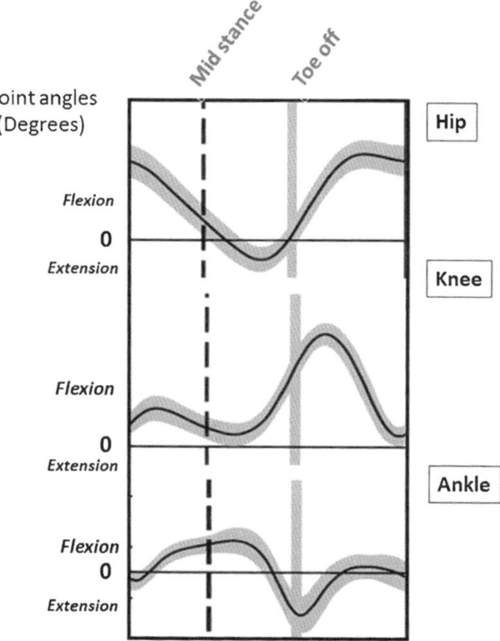

Fig. 14.11 Kinematics of the sagittal movement (flexion/extension) of the hip, knee, and ankle in normal gait cycle. The *black curve* represents mean value while the gray shadow represent two standard deviations

- In Cerebral Palsy the key muscle groups whose spasticity affect the pattern of gait are:

  1. Hip flexors (mainly iliopsoas)
  2. Knee flexors (hamstrings)
  3. Ankle plantar flexors (gastrosoleus)

1. **True equinus**:

   - The ankle is in equinus; forefoot initial contact persisting throughout stance (lost first rocker).
   - This pattern is seen in younger diplegic children as soon as they begin to walk.
   - ***Treatment***:

     - Focal spasticity management and hinged ankle foot orthosis (AFO).

- Surgical management (orthopedic/neurosurgical referral):
  - Gastrocnemius recession with or without selective tibial neurotomy, if persists to the age of 7–8 years or there is evidence of contracture.
  - Selective dorsal rhizotomy (SDR): if spasticity is regional and other criteria are met (see later).

2. **Crouch gait**:

- The knee and hip are excessively flexed (Fig. 14.1).

Treatment:

- Orthopedic referral:
  - **One stage surgery** (**SEMLS**: **Single Event Multi Level Surgery**)
    - Spasticity management.
    - Correction of fixed knee contracture by supracondylar extension osteotomy.
    - Lengthening of muscle contractures.
    - Correction of lever-arm dysfunction (rotational mal alignment).
    - Extensor mechanism advancement (tibial tubercle advancement).
    - Possible distal rectus transfer.
    - Ground reaction AFO.

3. **Stiff knee gait**:

- This pattern is due to spasticity and abnormal activity of the **rectus femoris** which leads to restricted knee flexion throughout the swing phase.
- This makes foot clearance and the task of limb advancement difficult, and can result in tripping.

Treatment:

Orthopedic referral.

- Early:
  - Focal spasticity management targeting the rectus femoris.

- Late:
  - Distal rectus transfer.

Rotational malalignment and mechanical axis deviations in Cerebral Palsy:

- **Excess Femoral anteversion**:
  - **Compensated** by hip internal rotation
  - **Consequences**:
    - internal foot progression angle (Fig. 14.6)
    - abnormal patellofemoral mechanics
    - anterior pelvic tilt to maintain coverage of the femoral head
    - hip abductor weakness
  - **Treatment**:
    - Orthopedic referral:
    - Femoral derotational osteotomy
      - better delayed until the age of 9 years due to high incidence of recurrence
      - Can operate earlier in severe cases. Family counseling should be done about recurrence rate.
      - Done as part of SEMLS
- **Abnormal tibial torsion**:
  - Tibial position usually follows foot position (internal tibial torsion with equinovarus and external tibial torsion with equinovalgus position).
  - The position of the tibia is commonly external more than internal.
  - Torsion of the tibia is less tolerated than femoral rotation (no compensation).
  - Correction should be considered even if torsion is relatively minimal ($\geq$15°).
  - **Treatment**:
    - Orthopedic referral:

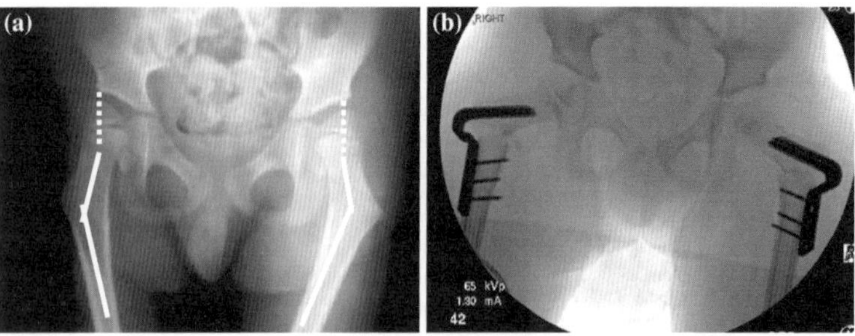

Fig. 14.12 Hip dysplasia. A 7-year-old boy with diplegic cerebral and bilateral hip dysplasia. **a** Notice the increased neck shaft angle (*lines*), shallow acetabulum and subluxation of the femoral head (increased part of the head of femur lateral to the edge of acetabulum (*dotted line*). **b** Bilateral varus osteotomy was done to correct the above deformity

- Better delayed after age of 10 years.
- Supramalleolar osteotomy.

Hip Subluxation/dislocation:

Etiology:

- Muscle imbalance
  - Weak hip **abd**uctors and spastic hip **add**uctors.
  - The femoral head starts to subluxate from the acetabulum and slowly progress to complete dislocation (Fig. 14.12).

Clinical picture:

- Usually the condition is asymptomatic in the beginning,
- The parents may complain from decrease abduction of the hips (difficulty during cleaning the child perineum)
- For advanced dislocation of the hips, the child may start complaining of hip pain (grimace during movement of the leg if he/she is non verbal)

Treatment:

- Early identification of hip subluxation by regular monitoring especially in patients with diplegic and quadriplegic Cerebral palsy.

- Radiographs should be taken for the pelvis yearly until the age of 4–5 years of life then it can be every other year until skeletal maturity.
- If there is subluxation or dislocation, orthopedic referral (Fig. 14.12).

Decision-making in ambulatory cerebral palsy

- Management principles:
  - Spasticity reduction.
  - Correction of contractures.
  - Preservation of power generators.
  - Correction of lever-arm dysfunction.

1. The management of children with cerebral palsy ideally involves a team of professionals, including:
   - Physical therapists.
   - Occupational therapists.
   - Physiatrists.
   - Developmental pediatricians.
   - A neurologist/neurosurgeon.
   - An orthopedic surgeon.
     - The pediatric orthopedic surgeon manages contractures and skeletal malalignment, while the neurologist/neurosurgeon is concerned with the management of spasticity.
2. **Spasticity management:**
   - Spasticity management is essential before and after orthopedic surgery to ensure best results:
     (a) **Relieve pain or discomfort related to stiffness/spasms**.
     (b) Allow the child to have greater range of motion.
     (c) Facilitate and increase the efficiency of muscle strengthening programs.
     (d) Better potential for the development and use of voluntary muscle activity during gait.
   - There is no worldwide acceptance for a specific protocol for treatment of spasticity.
   - **Modalities**:

(1) Physical therapy.
(2) Passive stretch:

- Needs to be at least 6 h daily to effectively prevent contractures.
- Emphasis should be done regarding the importance of parent's stretching of the child's joint at home and not mere dependence on the stretching exercises during therapy session.

(3) Night splinting.
(4) Systemic pharmacological agents, for generalized spasticity (baclofen, dantrolene, clonazepam, diazepam, and tizanidine).
(5) **Intramuscular chemodenervation with BTX-A** :

- **Mechanism of action**: Block acetyl choline release at the synaptic cleft of the myoneural junction.
- **Indications**:
  - Focal spasticity due to muscle spasticity
  - Dynamic shortening
  - Good residual muscle power
- **Contraindications**:
  - Fixed contractures
  - Autoantibodies
  - Parents are hesitant or does not fully understand risk/benefits is considered a relative contraindication
- **Dosing**:
  - For Botulinum toxin- A (BOTOX®, Allergan)
    - 3–6 units/muscle/Kg BW
    - Total maximum dose per visit: 400 Units
    - Maximum volume per site: 0.5–1.0 ml
    - Single or double sites for injection according to muscle size
    - Reinjection can be done after 3 months
    - Onset of effect 24–72 h, peak at 1–4 weeks
    - Duration of clinical benefit 3–6 months

(6) **Neurosurgical procedures**:

- **Neuromodulation:**

1. **Intrathecal Baclofen (ITB):**

Indications:

a. Severe regional spasticity.
b. Child weight ≥25 kg m.
c. Good response to test dose of ITB.

2. **Deep Brain Stimulation (DBS):** indicated in mixed Cerebral Palsy with predominance of dystonia and tremors.

- **Neuroablative procedures**

1. **Selective Peripheral Neurotomy (SPN):**

- Indications:

a. Severe focal spasticity of upper and lower limbs in ambulant or severely disabled child.
b. Multifocal spasticity.
c. H/M ratio in the nerve conduction (NC) study is more than 0.5.
d. Preoperative nerve block test showing satisfactory relaxation with positive impact on function.

2. **Selective Dorsal Rhizotomy (SDR):**

- Indications:

a. Severe regional spasticity
b. Ambulant or severely disabled child
c. Age from 3- to 10-year old

- Contraindications: Dystonic Cerebral Palsy

3. **Dorsal Root Entry Zone lesioning (DREZ):** in cases of severely painful spasticity in severely disabled and for hyperactive bladder

4. **Combined Ventral and Dorsal Rhizotomy (CVDR):**

- Indications:

a. Severe mixed spastic dystonia.
b. Failed oral medications.
c. DBS or ITB are inaccessible.

(7) Orthopedic procedures.

- Musculotendinous lengthening.
- Reconstruction procedures.

REFERENCES

1. Sanger TD, Delgado MR, Gaebler-Spira D, Hallett M, Mink JW. Task force on childhood motor disorders. Classification and definition of disorders causing hypertonia in childhood. Pediatrics. 2003;111(1):89–97.
2. Sanger TD, Chen D, Delgado MR, Gaebler-Spira D, Hallett M, Mink JW. Taskforce on childhood motor disorders. Definition and classification of negative motor signs in childhood. Pediatrics. 2006;118(5):2159–67.
3. Sanger TD. Toward a definition of childhood dystonia. Curr Opin Pediatr. 2004;16(6):623–7.
4. Hoon AH Jr, Nagae LM, Lin DD, Keller J, Bastian A, Campbell ML, Levey E, Mori S, Johnston MV. Sensory and motor deficits in children with cerebral palsy born preterm correlate with diffusion tensor imaging abnormalities in thalamocortical pathways. Dev Med Child Neurol. 2009;51(9):697–704.
5. Deon LL, Gaebler-Spira D. Assessment and treatment of movement disorders in children with cerebral palsy. Orthop Clin North Am. 2010;41(4):507–17.
6. Steinbok P. Neurosurgical management of hypertonia in children. Neurosurg Q. 2002;12(1):63–78.
7. Chang FM, Rhodes JT, Flynn KM, Carollo JJ. The role of gait analysis in treating gait abnormalities in cerebral palsy. Orthop Clin North Am. 2010;41(4):489–506.
8. Rosenbaum P, Paneth N, Leviton A, Goldstein M, Bax M, Damiano D, Dan B, Jacobsson B. A report: the definition and classification of cerebral palsy April 2006. Dev Med Child Neurol Suppl. 2007;109:8–14.
9. Palisano R, Rosenbaum P, Walter S, Russell D, Wood E, Galuppi B. Development and reliability of a system to classify gross motor function in children with cerebral palsy. Dev Med Child Neurol. 1997;39(4):214–23.
10. Novacheck TF, Trost JP, Sohrweide S. Examination of the child with cerebral palsy. Orthop Clin North Am. 2010;41(4):469–88.
11. Wren TA, Do KP, Hara R, Dorey FJ, Kay RM, Otsuka NY. Gillette Gait Index as a gait analysis summary measure: comparison with qualitative visual assessments of overall gait. J Pediatr Orthop. 2007;27(7):765–8.
12. Rodda JM, Graham HK, Carson L, Galea MP, Wolfe R. Sagittal gait patterns in spastic diplegia. J Bone Joint Surg Br. 2004;86(2):251–8.
13. Sutherland DH, Davids JR. Common gait abnormalities of the knee in cerebral palsy. Clin Orthop Relat Res. 1993;288:139–47.
14. Aiona MD, Sussman MD. Treatment of spastic diplegia in patients with cerebral palsy: part II. J Pediatr Orthop B. 2004;13(3):S13–38.
15. Ward AB. A summary of spasticity management–a treatment algorithm. Eur J Neurol. 2002;9(suppl 1):48–52; discussion 53–61.
16. Lazorthes Y, Sol JC, Sallerin B, Verdié JC. The surgical management of spasticity. Eur J Neurol. 2002;9(suppl 1):35–41; dicussion 53–61.
17. Albright AL, Tyler-Kabara EC. Combined ventral and dorsal rhizotomies for dystonic and spastic extremities. Report of six cases. J Neurosurg. 2007;107(suppl 4):324–7.
18. Sindou M, Keravel Y. Microsurgical procedures in the peripheral nerves and the dorsal root entry zone for the treatment of spasticity. Scand J Rehabil Med Suppl. 1988;17:139–43.
19. Thomason P, Baker R, Dodd K, Taylor N, Selber P, Wolfe R, Graham HK. Single-event multilevel surgery in children with spastic diplegia: a pilot randomized controlled trial. J Bone Joint Surg Am. 2011;93(5):451–60.

Chapter 15
Non Accidental Trauma

Amr Abdelgawad and Osama Naga

Definition:

- Non accidental trauma (NAT) is an injury that was induced to the child intentionally or as a result of an obvious neglect.
- The old name was 'child abuse'.

Incidence:

- 1–1.5 % of children are abused per year.
- 70,000–2,000,000 children are abused annually in US.
- More than 1,000 deaths annually in the United States are caused by child abuse.
- It occurs most frequently in infants and children under 3 years of age.

Risk factors:

- Young children (less than 3 years of age).
- First born children.
- Premature infants.
- Disabled children.
- Stepchildren.
- Single parent families.
- Children for parents who were abused when they were children.

Clinical presentation:

- Inappropriate clinical history:
  - Discrepancy of the history between guardians and/or children.
  - Change of the story given by the same person to different providers.

A. Abdelgawad and O. Naga (eds.), *Pediatric Orthopedics*,
DOI: 10.1007/978-1-4614-7126-4_15,

  - The mechanism of injury does not explain the resultant trauma.

- Delay in seeking medical attention.
- Caregivers: can be hostile or indifferent.
- Non-skeletal manifestations of NAT:
  - Soft tissue injuries:
    - Bruising (belt marks, finger marks).
    - Burns:
      - Gluteal burns (immersion injuries from putting the child in hot water).
  - Intra-abdominal injuries:
    - Result from "kicking" the child in his abdomen.
  - Intracranial injuries:
    - Hitting the child head against the wall.

Skeletal manifestation of Non Accidental Trauma:

- Fractures with high suspicion for NAT:
  - Corner fractures (metaphyseal fractures) (Fig. 15.1).
  - Rib fracture.
  - Distal humeral physeal fractures.
  - Femur fracture in less than 1-year-old child (Fig. 15.2).
  - Humeral shaft fracture in less than 3-year-old child (Fig. 15.1).
  - Fractures of different stages of healing:
    - Periosteal reaction.
    - Callus formation.
  - Scapular fractures.
  - Fractures of the outer end of the clavicles.
  - Finger fracture in non-ambulant children.
  - Bilateral fractures.
  - Complex skull fractures.

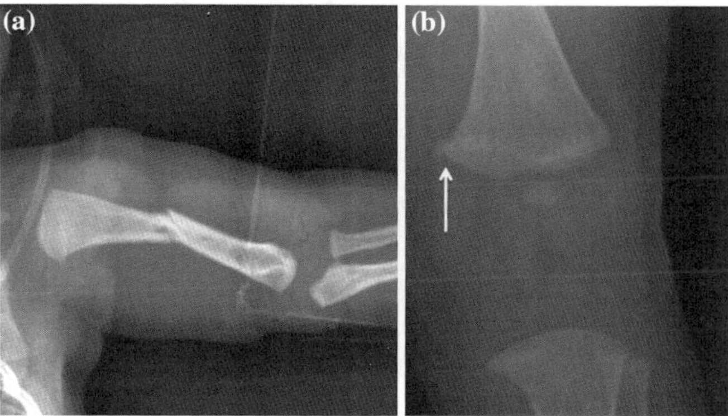

Fig. 15.1 A 5-month-old boy is brought to the emergency department because of swelling and deformity of *left arm*. **a** Radiograph shows mid shaft humeral fracture. **b** Bone survey was done which showed metaphyseal corner fracture in the *left distal femur* (*arrow*)

Pattern of fracture and its association with child abuse:

- Spiral fracture (Fig. 15.2):
  - Spiral fracture can occur in both accidental and NAT.
  - **Spiral fracture is more common in accidental injuries than in non accentual injuries.**
  - Only about one-third of the cases non accidental injuries are spiral fractures.
- Transverse fracture:
  - Transverse fractures are common in both accidental and non accidental trauma

Metaphyseal fractures [Corner Fracture]

- Commonly affects the distal femur or the proximal tibia (Fig. 15.1).
- Very specific fracture for NAT.
- Metaphyseal fractures can be undetectable clinically and show only in bone survey.
- **Differential diagnosis for corner fractures:**

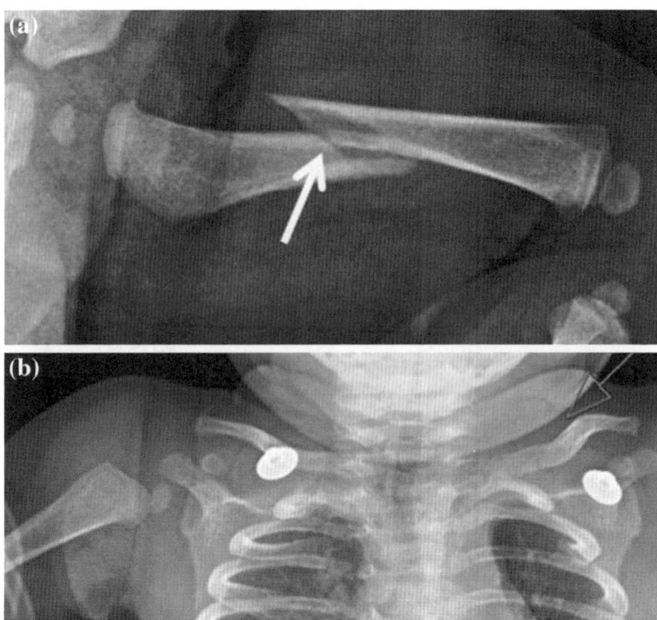

Fig. 15.2 A 3-month-old boy was brought to the emergency department because of swelling and deformity of *left thigh*. **a** Radiograph shows mid shaft femoral spiral fracture (*arrow*). **b** Bone survey was done which showed callus formation of the *left clavicle* indicating healed fracture (*arrow*)

- Spurs or small peaks adjacent to growth plate.
- Osteomyelitis.

Periosteal bone injuries

- **Mechanism:**
  - Periosteal reaction is a sign of fracture repair (Fig. 15.3).
  - Less commonly, can occur without fractures in cases of:
    - □ Rough gripping of limb;
    - □ Shaking: acceleration and deceleration applied to unsupported limb.

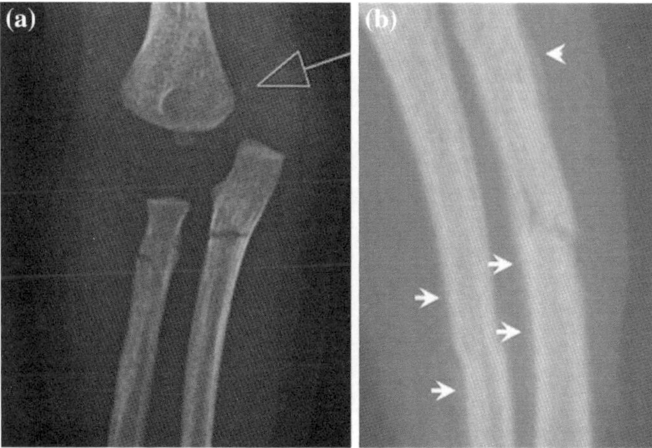

Fig. 15.3 A 2-year-old boy with bilateral upper extremity pain, deformity and swelling. **a** *Right elbow* shows trans-physeal fracture of the distal humerus with acute fracture proximal ulna and radius (no callus or periosteal reaction). **b** Radiograph of *left forearm* shows periosteal reaction around the radius and ulna indicating healing fracture (few weeks old fracture)

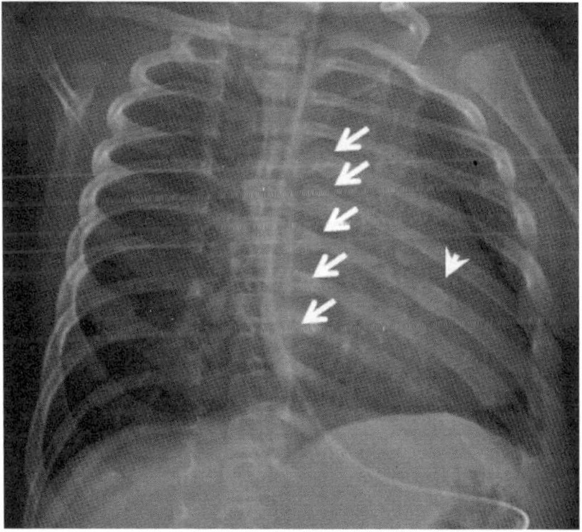

Fig. 15.4 Bone survey done for suspected child abuse showing callus formation posteriorly in ribs 5–9 on the *left side* (*arrows*). Callus formation is seen also on the *left seventh* more laterally (*arrow head*)

- **Differential diagnosis of Periosteal reaction:**
  - Periosteal bone formation may be seen as a **normal variant in infants from 6 weeks to 6 months**.
  - Infection.

Rib Fracture (Fig. 15.4)

- Very specific for child abuse.
- **Mechanism:**
  - Squeezing injury of the chest.
- Differential diagnosis of rib fractures due to NAT:
  - Very high energy injuries (motor vehicle collision).
  - Osteogenesis imerfecta.

Humeral fractures

- **Fractures common with NAT:**
  - **Diaphyseal fractures** in children less than 3-year old.
  - **Transphyseal fractures**
    - □ Very specific for NAT (Figs. 15.3 and 15.5).
    - □ Because the epiphysis is still cartilaginous and cannot be seen in the radiograph, the lesion is sometimes confused with elbow dislocation.
- **Fractures common in accidental trauma:**
  - Supracondylar fracture of the humerus:
    - □ Occur as a result of falling on outstretched hand.
    - □ Very common injury in children and has low association with NAT.

Differential Diagnosis of NAT

- Accidental trauma.
- Osteogenesis Imerfecta.
- Metabolic Bone Disease (rickets, etc.).
- Birth trauma.
- Physiologic periostitis.

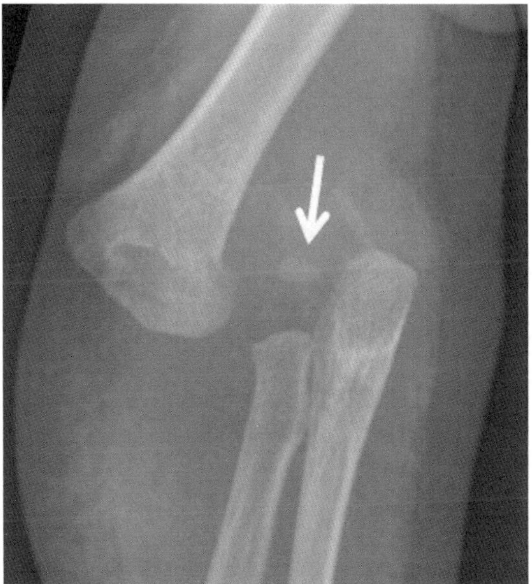

Fig. 15.5 A 2-year-old girl is brought to emergency room because of pain, swelling, and deformity of the right elbow. Radiograph shows transphyseal fracture of the distal humerus. This is not dislocation of the elbow joint, the fracture line cannot be seen because it occurred through the physis of the distal humerus which is not ossified at this age. Notice the capitellum (part of the distal humerus) (*arrow*) aligned with proximal radius indicating the fracture is through the physis of the distal humerus proximal to capitellum

Management of suspected NAT

- **Careful and detailed history.**
  - **History is the most important aspect to suspect NAT.**
  - Ask about the mechanism of injury, where were the caregivers at the time of accident.
  - The physician must have professional nonjudgmental approach in initial encounter and workup.
  - Explain workup to parents as standard approach to specific ages/injury patterns (see inpatient Chap. 12 for management of inpatient wiht suspected NAT).

- Early involvement of child protection team if available.
- Early contact of child's primary care physician.
- **Radiology**

  - **X-ray**

    - Skeletal survey for children with suspicion of NAT.
    - "Babygram" (one radiograph of the whole child) is not sufficient as it does not provide necessary detail of the skeletal structures to identify fractures.
    - Skeletal survey

      - AP/LAT skull, AP/LAT axial skeleton and trunk, AP bilateral arms, forearms, hands, thighs, legs, feet.
      - Repeat skeletal survey at 1 week can be done if there is high suspicious for NAT and the primary survey in negative.

    - **Bone Scan**

      - Usually reserved for highly suspicious cases with negative skeletal survey.
      - Can detect rib fractures and vertebral fractures.

Legal aspect of NAT

- All states require reporting of suspected cases of abuse by medical professionals.
- Need only reasonable suspicion to report suspected abuse.
- Law gives immunity to providers from civil or criminal liability for reporting in good faith.

HIGH YIELD FACTS

- Isolated diaphyseal fractures are common in NAT and accidental trauma.
- Spiral fractures are common in NAT and accidental trauma.
- Fractures with very high suspicious for NAT:

- Humerus diaphyseal fractures in children less than 3 years of age.
- Femur in children less than one year old.
- Posterior rib fractures.
- Corner fractures.
- Transphyseal humeral fractures.

■ Blue sclera may be normal variants until 4 years of age.

CLINICAL SCENARIOS

Case number one: 6-years old with quadriplegic cerebral palsy and mental delay is brought to the clinic with his mother. She reports that since yesterday after coming from the school the child is complaining of pain when she moves or touch his left lower extremity. No local signs of inflammation. No fever	Get radiographs of the pelvis, left femur, and left leg If the radiographs shows spiral fracture, have a high suspicious that this is a case of NAT by his care giver at school Report to child protective service (CPS)
18-month-old girl brought to the emergency room by her 16-year-old mother who lives with her boy friend. She noticed the child had been fussy for the last few days and she is not able walk. On exam, you noticed the swollen right thigh	Get radiographs of the femur If radiograph showed femoral fracture: • Get bone survey • Admit the child • Inform CPS • Orthopedic consult

REFERENCES

Kocher MS, Kasser JR. Orthopaedic aspects of child abuse. J Am Acad Orthop Surg. 2000;8:10–20.

King J, Diefendorf D, Apthorp J, Negrete VF, Carlson M. Analysis of 429 fractures in 189 battered children. J Pediatr Orthop. 1988;8:585–9.

Carty HM. Fractures caused by child abuse. J Bone Joint Surg Br. 1993;75(6):849–57.

Mulpuri K, Slobogean BL, Tredwell SJ. The epidemiology of nonaccidental trauma in children. Clin Orthop Relat Res. 2011;469(3):759–67.

Jayakumar P, Barry M, Ramachandran M. Orthopaedic aspects of paediatric non-accidental injury. J Bone Joint Surg Br. 2010;92(2):189–95.

Chapter 16
Orthopedic Trauma

Amr Abdelgawad and Enes Kanlic

FRACTURES

Definition:

- Failure of the bone structure.

Types of bone fracture in children:

- **Complete fracture:**
  - Fracture with **displacement** of the bone ends (Fig. 16.1).
- **Green stick fracture:**
  - Fracture with **angulation** without displacement (Fig. 16.2).
- **Torus fracture** (buckle fracture):
  - Failure of one side of bone cortex, the opposite cortex is still intact (no angulation or displacement) (Fig. 16.3).
- **Plastic deformation:**
  - The bone is bent throughout its length.
  - Occurs because of the elasticity of the bone in children, so the bone can be bent along its entire length without being fracture at a certain spot.
  - Common to occur in the ulna and fibula (Fig. 16.4).
- **Fracture through the growth plate** (Salter-Harris injury)
  - The failure of the bone structure happens through the growth plate (see later).

A. Abdelgawad and O. Naga (eds.), *Pediatric Orthopedics*,
DOI: 10.1007/978-1-4614-7126-4_16,

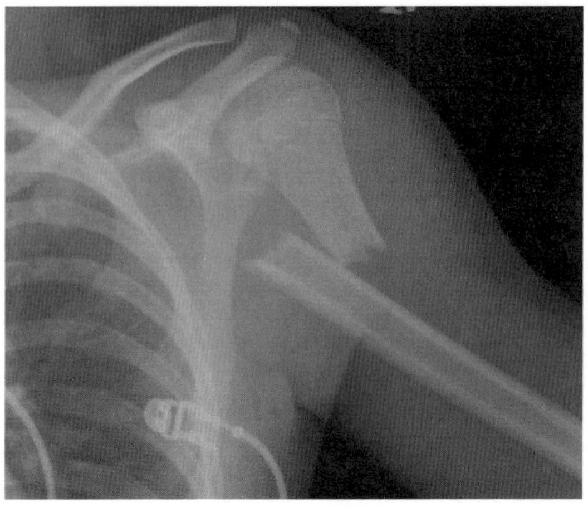

Fig. 16.1 Complete fracture of the proximal humerus. Notice the displacement of the fracture ends

General management of fractures:

History:

- Inquire about the mechanism of injury and time between injury and seeking medical treatment (for possible child abuse).
- Inquire about loss of consciousness or abdominal trauma.

Clinical presentation:

- **Pain** and **swelling** at the affected side.
- **Deformity** of the affected limb (if there is displacement or angulation).

Radiograph:

- Will show the fracture as interruption in the cortex. (see Figs. 16.1, 16.2, and 16.3).
- Fractures have to be differentiated from normal physeal cartilage:
  - The physeal cartilage has specific anatomic sites (proximal and distal ends of the bones).

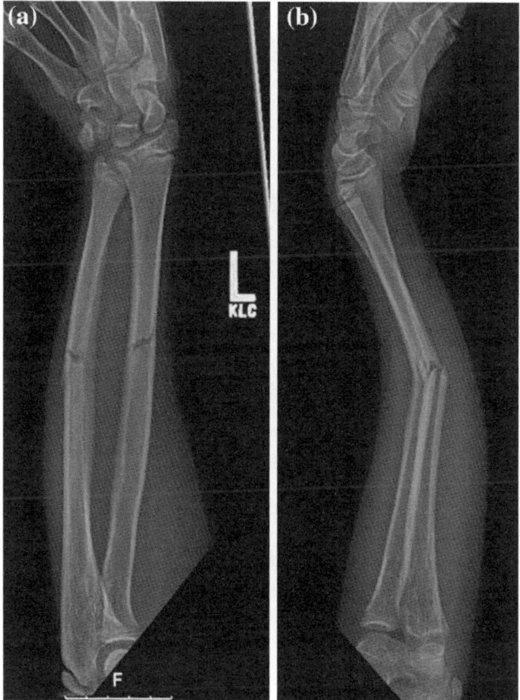

Fig. 16.2 Greenstick fracture. Fracture of the radius and ulna. Notice the angulation of the fracture in the lateral view (**b**) with no displacement of the fracture ends in both the anteroposterior (**a**) and lateral views (**b**)

- The growth plate has a smooth outline

- The radiograph should show the following:
  - **The joint below and the joint above the affected area.**
  - Two perpendicular view are needed to assess the fracture (a fracture which appear aligned in one view may be quite displaced in the other view)

Other imaging studies:

CT:

- Rarely needed in orthopedic trauma.

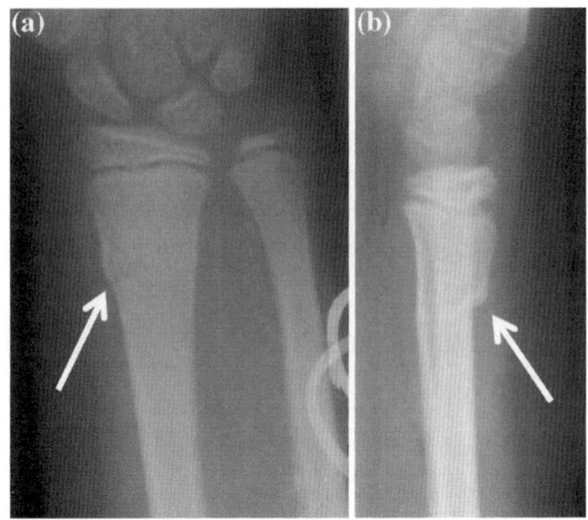

Fig. 16.3 Anteroposterior (**a**) and lateral (**b**) view of the distal radius and ulna showing distal radial torus fracture (*arrow*). Please notice in the lateral view the volar cortex of the radius is intact and there is compression fracture in the dorsal cortex

- Sometimes needed to assess intra-articular fractures or complex fracture patterns.

MRI:

- Can show ligamentous injury (knee injury) or stress fractures.

Bone scan:

- Rarely used, in cases of suspected stress fracture (MRI is more commonly used nowadays for this indication).

Treatment:

- Adequate control of the pain.
- Splinting the fracture.
- ***Neurovascular assessment before and after application of the splint.***
- According to the pattern of fracture:

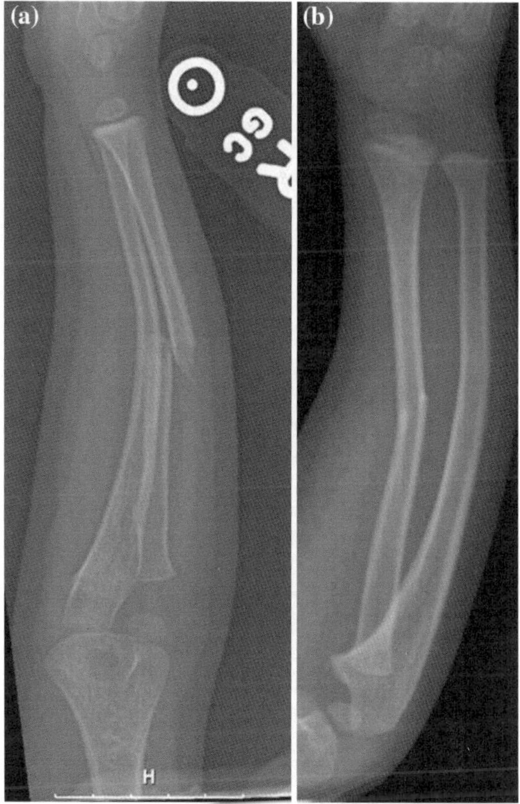

Fig. 16.4 Plastic deformation of the ulna. A 4-year-old boy fell down while jumping on the couch on outstretched hand with immediate development of pain and deformity of the forearm. Radiographs [AP (**a**) and LAT (**b**) of the forearm] shows fracture mid shaft radius and plastic deformation of the ulna)

- If the fracture is displaced or angulated, urgent orthopedic consultation.
- If the fracture in non displaced, splint for comfort and orthopedic referral.
- Buckle (torus) fractures can be totally managed by the pediatrician (without need for orthopedic referral).

Open fractures:

Definition:

- Fractures with connection between the fracture hematoma and the external environment.
- The connection in most cases is through interruption of the skin integrity (wound), in some pelvic fractures, the connection can be through break in the mucosa of the rectum or the vagina.

Clinical picture:

- Usually associated with higher energy injuries.
- Same as regular fracture (pain, swelling, and deformity) with the addition of wound in the vicinity of the fracture.
- The wound, even if very small, will keep oozing blood for long time (because it is connected with the fracture hematoma).

Classification of open fractures:

- Type 1:
  - Puncture wound, less than 1 cm.
  - Usually caused by the displaced sharp bone ends penetrating the skin (from within) (Fig. 16.5).
  - Carries minimal risk on infection.
- Type 2
  - The wound is between 1 and 10 cm.
  - No exposed bone that can be seen from the wound or marked stripping of periosteum (Fig. 16.6).
- Type 3:
  - Further classified to A, B, and C.
    - Type 3A:
      - Wound is larger than 10 cm or with exposed bone ends.
      - Wounds can be closed primarily (no need for flap reconstruction) (Fig. 16.7)

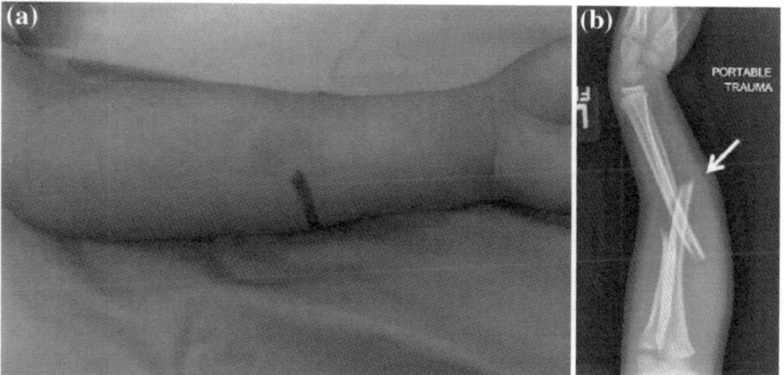

Fig. 16.5 Open fracture type 1. (**a**) A 9-year-old boy who fell down from the swing. Patient had fracture of the forearm with small "7 mm' wound that had continuous blood oozing. Radiographs shows displaced fracture of the radius and ulna. The proximal end of the ulna (*arrow*) had caused the wound in the skin

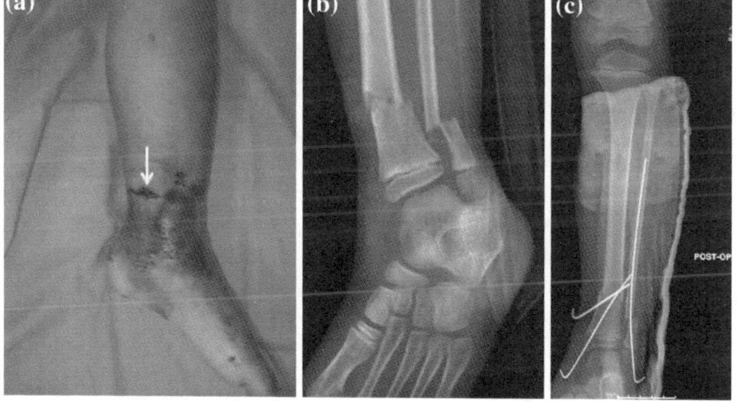

Fig. 16.6 Type 2 open fracture. A 9-year-old boy hit by a car. (**a**) Notice the wound on the medial side of the leg (*arrow*) and the road rash. The wound is about 2 cm with continuous oozing of blood. (**b**) Radiograph shows fracture of the distal tibia and fibula. Patient was taken to operating room where debridement was done followed by the fixation with K-wire

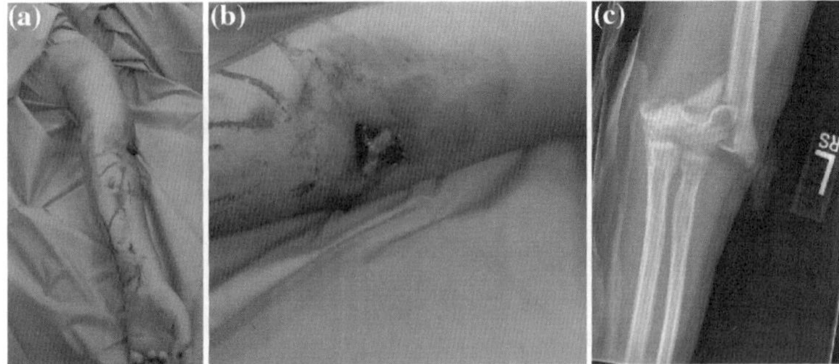

Fig. 16.7 Type 3A open fracture. A 12-year-old girl fell down while running. She had an open 3A distal humeral fracture. Notice the exposed bone from the wound

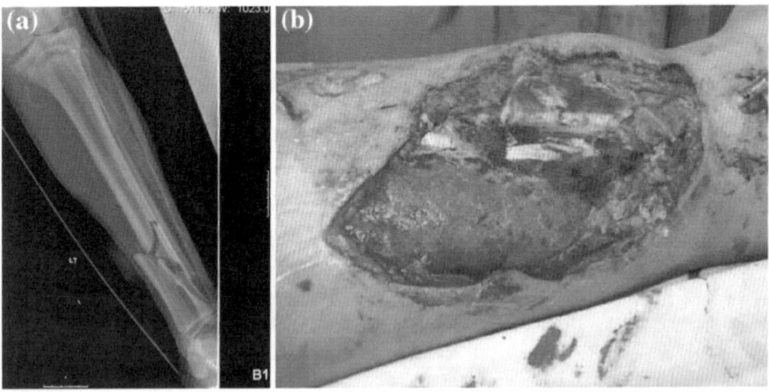

Fig. 16.8 Open fracture type 3B. A 13-year-old in an all-terrain vehicle (ATV) roll-over accident. Patient had open 3B fracture tibia. Notice the extent of tissue loss and exposed tibia. The patient needed application of negative pressure wound dressing and skin graft to cover the defect

- Type 3B:
  - Wound cannot be closed without flap or other forms of plastic reconstruction (Fig. 16.8).
- Type 3C:
  - Open fractures with neurovascular lesions that requires repair.

Complications of open fractures:

- **Infection:** open fracture becomes contaminated at the time of trauma. There is higher incidence of infection if internal hard ware is used to fix these fractures.
- **Delayed union and non union:** at the time of injury, the fracture hematoma (which is the first stage of healing) is disturbed and lost outside the body, this causes delay in healing. Also there is higher incidence of stripping of the periosteum which also can cause delayed union/non union.

Treatment of open fractures:

- The open fractures are contaminated with bacteria from external environment, **antibiotics should be given.**
    - Antibiotic for open fracture should be given **as soon as possible**. This has been found to decrease the risk of infection.
    - The type of antibiotic depends on the classification of the open fracture, which in turn reflects its degree of contamination:
        - For types I and II open fractures: first-generation cephalosporin (cefazolin 50 mg/kg/d on three divided doses).
        - For type III fractures: aminoglycoside should be added to the first-generation cephalosporin (gentamicin 5 mg/kg/d on three divided doses.
        - Penicillin (100,000–400,000 units/kg/d on four divided doses) is added for gross contamination, farm injuries, and deep wounds to guard against anaerobes.
        - The duration of antibiotic administration is 48 h, this should be repeated with any additional orthopedic intervention (e.g., debridement, fixation, or coverage).
- Urgent orthopedic consult for surgical debridement and evaluation.

Complications of fractures in children:

- **Neurovascular injury:**
    - The injury can occur either by the trauma itself or the sharp ends of the fractured bone.

- There are certain fractures which are more prone to neurovascular injury like pelvic fractures, supracondylar fracture of the humerus, and distal femur fracture (Fig 12.1 Chap. 12).
- Careful assessment of the neurovascular bundle should be carried out in all fractures.

- **Growth disturbance:**

  - Fractures through the growth plate can affect the future growth of the bone.
  - If the growth disturbance is through the whole growth plate (complete), it will result in a short bone (and possible limb length discrepancy).
  - If the growth disturbance is partial (only part of the growth plate is affected), the bone will grow in deformed position (Fig. 16.9).

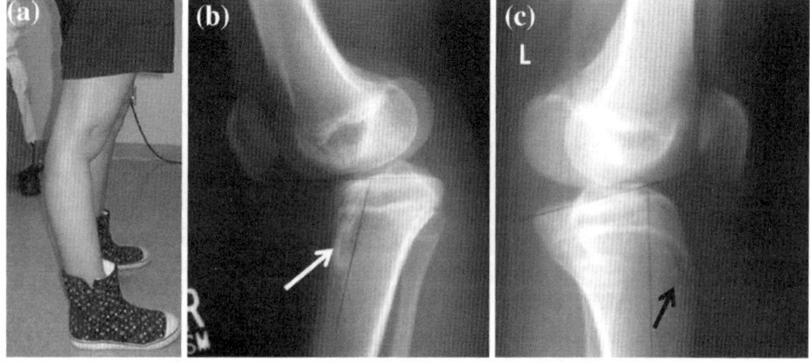

Fig. 16.9 A 13-year-old girl with history of trauma to the right lower extremity 2 years earlier. (**a**) The patient started to notice gradual deformity of the right knee (hyperextension of the knee or knee recurvatum). Radiographs of both knees show the closure of the anterior part of the physis of the proximal tibia in the right knee (**b**, *white arrow*) while the growth plate is still open (active) in the left knee (**c**, *black arrow*). This premature closure of the right proximal tibial physis was due to type V physeal injury of the proximal tibial physis that result in partial closure of the anterior part. As the tibia continued to grow from the posterior part only, the deformity developed

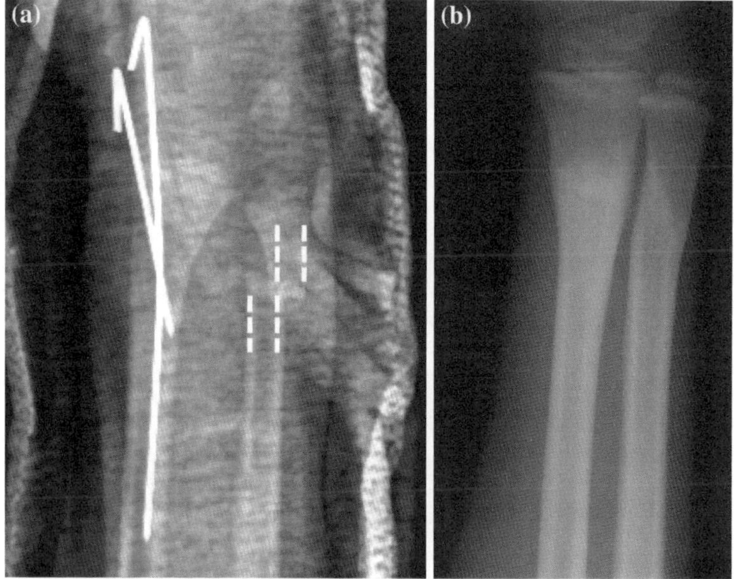

Fig. 16.10 Remodeling. A 9-year-old boy fell on out stretched hand and fractured the distal radius and ulna. The radius was reduced and treated with percutaneous fixation with two wires. The ulna was left without fixation. (**a**) Postoperative radiographs. Notice the displacement of the fracture ends (*dotted lines*). (**b**) Five months later, remodeling of the fractured ulna had occurred and the bone became more aligned

- **Malunion:**
  - Healing of the fracture ends in non anatomical position.
  - In skeletal immature patients, **remodeling** can result in re-aligning of the affected bone (Fig. 16.10).
  - There are certain fractures that are more prone to malunion.
    - Supracondylar fracture of the humerus can heal in varus position resulting in cubitus varus deformity and obvious elbow deformity (Fig. 16.11).

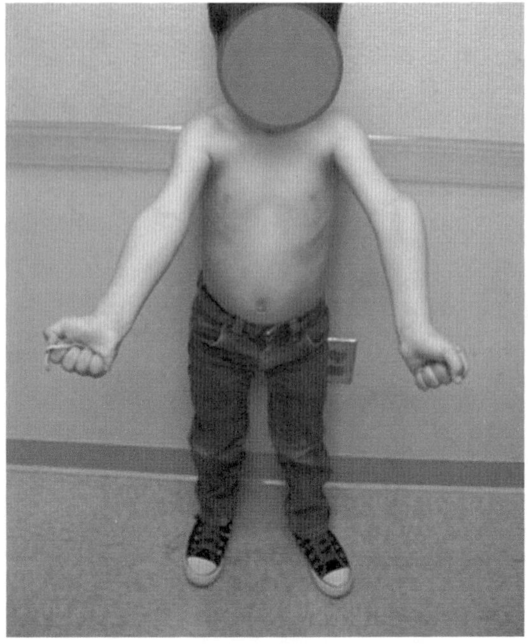

Fig. 16.11 Malunion of the fracture. A 5-year-old boy with supracondylar fracture of the humerus on the left side that had healed in varus, causing cubitus varus deformity

- **Remodeling** power is highest in
  - Very young (the more growth potential the child has, the more remodeling will occur).
  - Near the physis (metaphyseal fractures remodel more than diaphysial fractures).
  - Coronal and sagittal plane. There is very limited remodeling power in the rotational plane.

- **Non union:**
  - The problem of non union is not as common in children as in adults as children have better healing potential and they do not smoke.

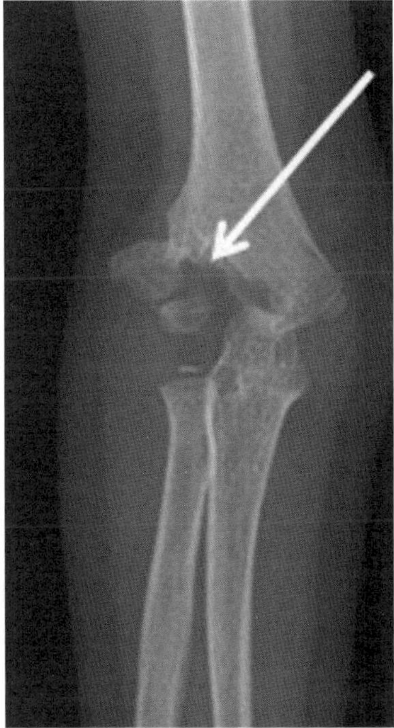

Fig. 16.12 Non union of the fracture. Anteroposterior radiograph of a 5-year-old girl with fracture of the lateral condyle 1 year ago. The fracture was managed non surgically and developed non union (*arrow*)

- There are certain fractures which have high probability of developing non union like **proximal femur fracture and fracture of lateral condyle of humerus** (Fig. 16.12). These fractures usually require surgical intervention.

- **Limb length discrepancy:**
  - Can occur due to:
    - Shortening at the fracture level (overlap of the fracture ends).
    - Growth disturbance due to injury to the growth plate.
  - Management: see limb length discrepancy in Chap. 2

▪ Compartment syndrome:

- **Definition:**
  - An elevation of the interstitial pressure in a closed osteofascial compartment that results in microvascular compromise.
- **Clinical presentation:**
  - Compartment syndrome should be suspected in children involved in accidents with high-energy trauma to the extremities.
  - **Tense non compressible** swelling of the affected compartment (Fig. 16.13).
  - **Increase in the narcotic requirements** to keep the child comfortable is an early sign of increased compartment pressure (remember: children with splinted reduced fracture should have minimal pain).
  - **Severe excruciating pain with passive stretch of the distal joints** is a characteristic feature of compartment syndrome.

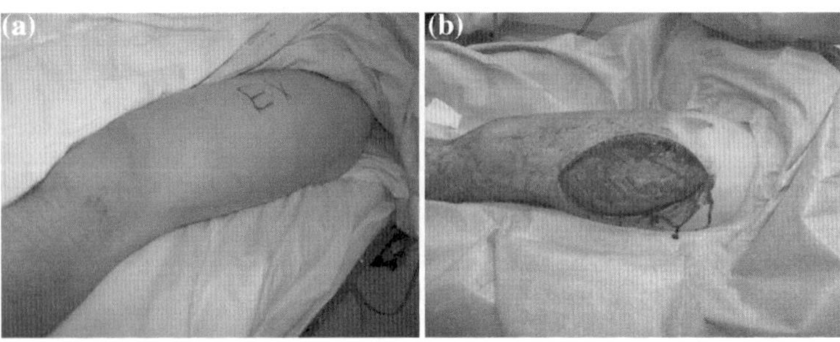

Fig. 16.13 Compartment syndrome of the thigh. A 16-year-old boy who was kicked in his left thigh while playing football. A few hours later, he started to have severe excruciating pain in the thigh. Radiographs were negative for fractures. (**a**) On examination, swollen tense non compressible thigh compartments (notice the swollen thigh). The diagnosis was compartment syndrome for thigh. (**b**) Surgical release of the fascia (fasciotomy) was done emergently. Notice the muscle bulge once the fascia is released (sign of increased tension in the compartment)

- **Paresthesias, pulselessness, and paralysis are late findings**, and the absence of these signs does not rule out this diagnosis.
- **More common with fractures of the leg and forearm**.
- Compartment pressure can be measured using pressure needle. If the compartment pressure is more than 30 mm Hg or the difference between the patient diastolic pressure and the compartment pressure is less than 30 mm Hg, this indicates that patient has compartment syndrome.
- The diagnosis of compartment syndrome is a clinical decision. **No need to measure the compartment pressure in every case.** Measuring the pressure is used in cases of:
    - The examiner is not sure about the diagnosis.
    - The patients is not responsive (either from head injury or from medications), the pain level becomes a non reliable parameter for assessment of the development of compartment syndrome.

- **Management:**
    - Once compartment syndrome is suspected, **cast and splints should be removed or split immediately** (this should include splitting the padding material underneath the cast as well; failure to completely split the padding layer can cause continuation of compression).
    - The affected extremity should be elevated to **the level of the heart** (elevating the extremity above the level of the heart will **decrease tissue perfusion)**
    - **Urgent orthopedic consult is needed:**
        - Definitive treatment of compartment syndrome consists of wide prompt release of the affected compartments (**fasciotomy**).
        - Delay in diagnosis or treatment for more than 8 hours can seriously affect the prognosis.

SALTER HARRIS INJURIES

- **Definition:**
  - Injuries of the bone that go through the growth plate (physis)
- **Classification:**
  - Type I through type V (Fig. 16.14).
  - Type I:
    - The fracture passes completely through the growth plate.

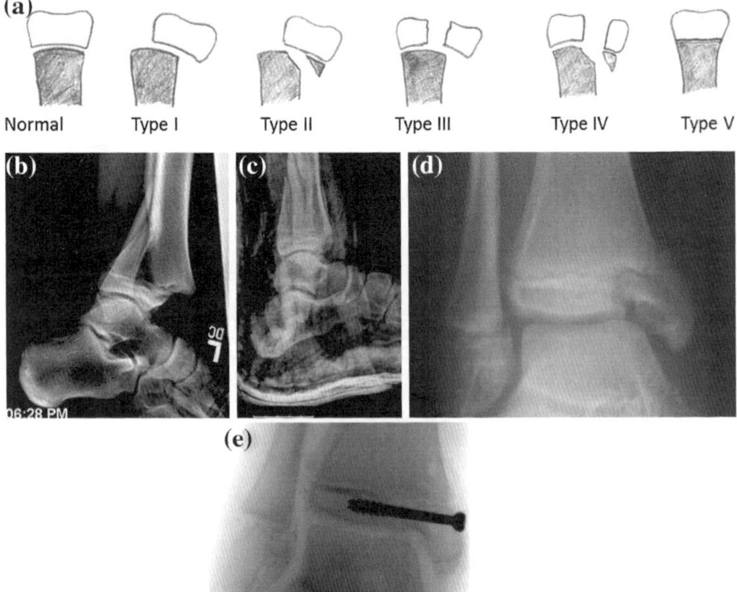

Fig. 16.14 (**a**) Physeal (Salter Harris) injuries classification. Type V is usually a retrospective diagnosis after growth disturbance occurs (see Fig. 16.9). **b**, **c** Type II distal tibial fracture before and after closed reduction. **d**, **e** Type IV distal tibial fracture before and after open reduction and internal fixation

- Type II:
  - □ The fracture passes through the growth plate and part of the metaphysis.
  - □ **Most common type.**
- Type III:
  - □ The fracture separates part of the epiphysis.
- Type IV:
  - □ The fracture separates part of the epiphysis and part of the metaphysis.
- Type V
  - □ Compression injury of the growth plate.
  - □ In most cases, it is a **retrospective diagnosis** (few months after injury to the growth plate, the child develop growth disturbance due to type V injury to the growth plate (Fig. 16.9).

■ **Complication of Salter Harris injuries**:

- These fractures can cause injury to the growth plate and possible **growth disturbance.**
- Effect of growth disturbance:
  - □ If the growth disturbance is through the whole growth plate (complete), it will result in a short bone (and possible limb length discrepancy).
  - □ If the growth disturbance is partial (only part of the growth plate is affected), the bone will grow in deformed position (Fig. 16.9).
- The growth disturbance is more common in:
  - □ Certain fracture pattern: **types III and IV** more commonly lead to growth disturbance than type I and II.
  - □ Certain growth plates are more prone to develop growth disturbance with Salter-Harries injuries (e.g., **distal femur and proximal tibia growth plates**).

- **Management of Salter Harris injuries**:
  - **Urgent Orthopedic referral**, physeal injuries **heal faster** than other fractures because they occur through rapidly dividing cells. They have to be reduced as soon as possible.
  - The reduction should be gentle (repeated reduction attempts will cause more damage to the dividing cells which can cause growth disturbance).
  - Affected children should be followed after the healing for about 1 year to assess possible growth disturbance.
  - Type III and type IV fracture if they are displaced, need open reduction and internal fixation to obtain anatomical reduction and decrease the incidence of growth disturbance.

COMMON FRACTURES IN PEDIATRIC PATIENTS

Clavicle fracture:

- **Overview**
  - Common fracture in pediatric patients due to clavicle's superficial location.
- **Clinical presentation:**
  - Pain over the clavicle after falling on the outstretched hand.
  - Deformity and swelling over clavicle.
- **Radiographs:**
  - Will show the fracture of the clavicle with possible deformity (angulation and/or displacement) (Fig. 16.15).

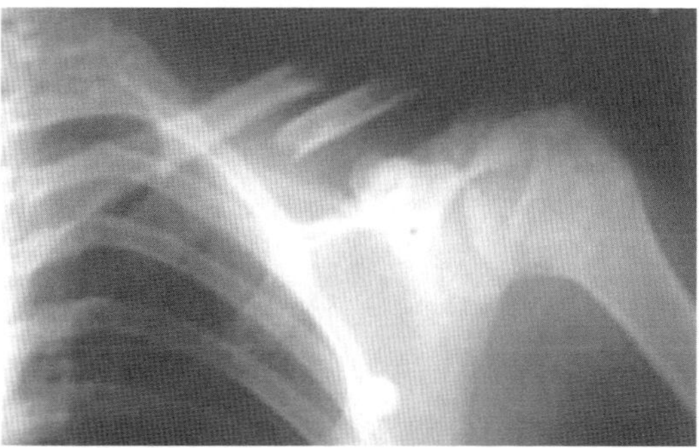

Fig. 16.15 Radiograph of a 12-year-old boy, who fell down and had pain over the clavicle. The radiograph shows a mid-shaft clavicle fracture

- **Management:**
  - Arm sling for comfort.
    - The child can take it off when he/she feels more comfortable.
    - No need for the "figure of 8" sling.
  - Fracture clavicle will heal with obvious bump (bony callus), so you should warn the parents about that in advance (Fig. 16.16).
  - The primary care physician can manage most cases of fracture clavicle with no need for referral to orthopedic surgeon.
    - Indication for referral:
      - Open fracture
      - Fractures associated with neurovascular injuries
      - Fracture ends tenting the skin (Fig. 16.17).
      - Markedly displaced or shortened fractures (more than 2 cm).
      - Adolescent patients, it is better to refer adolescent patients to orthopedic surgeons as they may develop pain with malunion of the clavicle (relative indication for surgery).

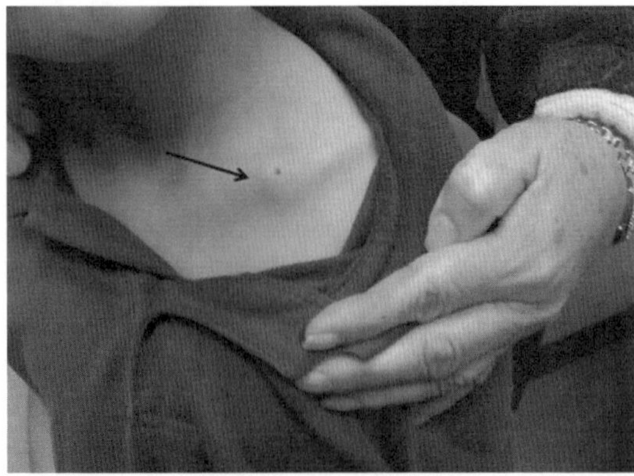

Fig. 16.16 A picture of a 9-year-old boy with healed fracture clavicle. The callus had formed a bony swelling that can be easily seen and felt (*arrow*)

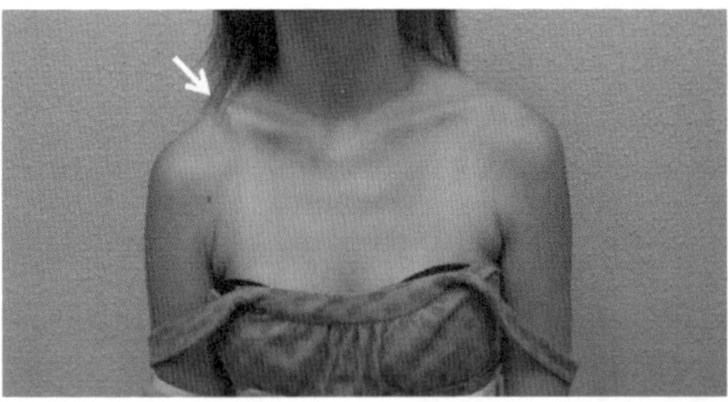

Fig. 16.17 A 16-year-old girl with a fractured right clavicle that is tenting the skin. This patient needed surgical intervention to prevent soft tissue complications

PROXIMAL HUMERAL FRACTURE

Clinical presentation:

- Pain and swelling of the proximal arm.

Management:

- 80 % of the growth of the humerus comes from the proximal end, so there is high remodeling power in this area. Most of the fractures can be managed non operatively especially in young children.
- Sometimes, this fracture can be associated with simple bone cyst of the proximal humerus (pathological fracture) (Fig. 16.18) (The proximal humerus is the commonest site to have simple bone cyst).
- Most cases do not need reduction or surgery.

  - Minimally displaced fractures: sling for comfort.
  - Displaced fractures (especially in adolescent): orthopedic referral for possible intervention.
  - Salter Harris injuries of the proximal humerus or those associated with simple bone cyst: orthopedic referral (Fig. 16.19).

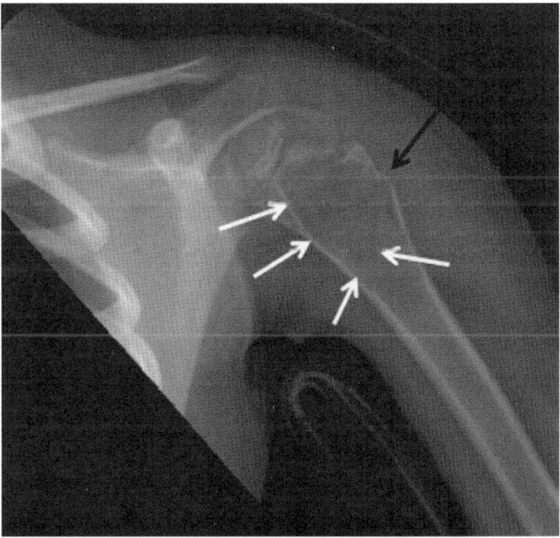

Fig. 16.18 Radiograph of a 6-year-old boy who had sudden left shoulder pain while playing. The radiograph shows proximal humeral fracture (*black arrow*). Notice the simple bone cyst that affected the proximal humerus (*white arrows*)

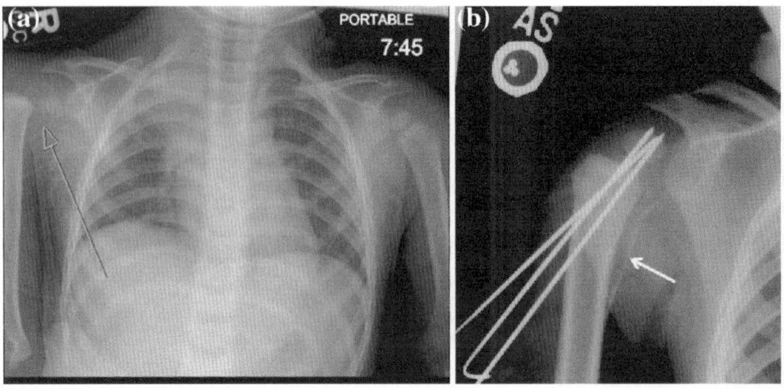

Fig. 16.19 (**a**) Chest radiographs of a 2-year-old boy involved in a motor vehicle collision. The patient had physeal injury of the right proximal humerus (type 1 Salter-Harris injury of the proximal humerus, *arrow*). Note the difference in position of the proximal humeral epiphysis to the shaft between right and left side. Closed reduction was done and fixation by K wires. (**b**) Radiographs taken after 2 weeks show the periosteal new bone formation indicating the healing process (*arrow*)

HUMERAL SHAFT FRACTURE

Clinical presentation:

- Pain, swelling, and deformity of the arm. Radiographs will show the fracture (Fig. 16.20).
- Radial nerve palsy (about 10 % of cases of humeral fracture).
  - The child will have **wrist drop.**
  - The vast majority of these palsy are neurapraxia (see later) and will recover spontaneously.

Treatment:

- **Orthopedic referral** is needed to assess these patients and treat them.

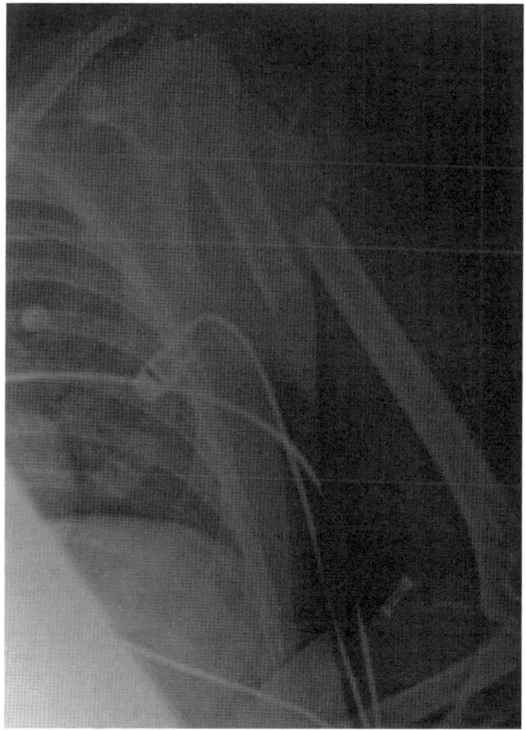

Fig. 16.20 Transverse fracture of the shaft of the humerus in an 11-year-old boy who had ATV accident

- Humerus shaft can tolerate relatively big deformity with minimal functional deficit.
- Most of humeral shaft fractures can be managed non operatively in braces.

ELBOW FRACTURES

- **Elbow fractures are common in children.**
- They may be associated with various complications and long-term sequels.

- The most common elbow fractures are:
  - **Supracondylar fracture of the humerus (most common elbow fracture).**
  - **Lateral condyle fracture**.
  - Medial epicondyle fracture.
  - Olecranon fracture.
  - Radial head fracture.

SUPRACONDYLAR FRACTURE OF THE HUMERUS

Definition:

- Transverse fracture of the distal part of the humerus proximal to the articular surface.

Incidence:

- 60–70 % of elbow fractures.
- **Can be associated with many complications.**
- More common in boys, between 5–7 years old.

Clinical picture:

- Pain, swelling, and deformity of the affected elbow.
- With marked displacement of the fracture ends, bruises of the anterior elbow will occur (the proximal fragment button through the brachialis muscle) (Fig. 16.21).
- **Evaluation of the neurovascular structures** distal to the fracture site is very important in cases of supracondylar fracture of the humerus because of the frequent injury to these structures.
  - Assess radial and ulnar pulses. If absent, urgent orthopedic consult.
  - Assess nerve function:

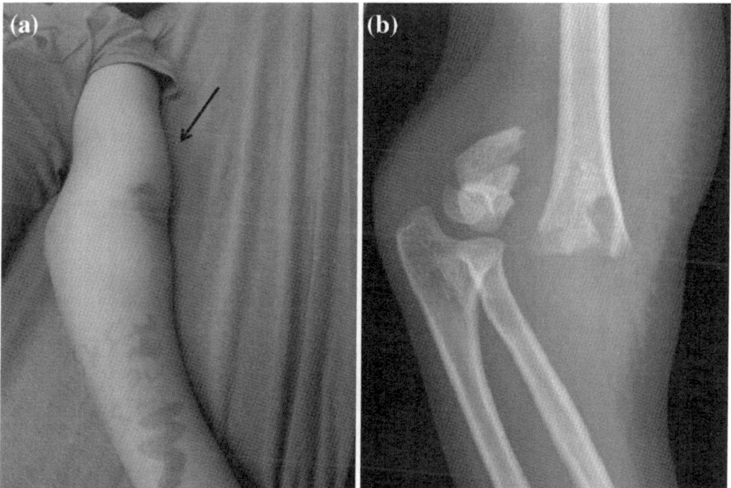

Fig. 16.21 Bruising of the anterior elbow with displacement of the fracture in a 7-year-old girl who fell down and has obvious deformity of the left elbow. Cubital fossa shows bruising (**a**). Radiograph (**b**) shows type III supracondylar fracture of the humerus with marked displacement of the fracture ends. The proximal fragment had 'buttoned through' the brachialis muscle causing this bruising

- □ Commonest nerve to be affected: anterior interosseus nerve (this is assessed by asking the patient to do OK sign) (Fig. 16.22).
- □ Radial, ulnar, or median nerve palsy may also be present (see assessment of nerve function later).

Radiograph:

- Will show the fracture line which pass across the supracondylar area.
- According to the displacement; the fracture is classified into (see Fig. 16.23, 16.24 and 16.25):
  - Non displaced (type one).
  - angulated (type two).
  - displaced (type three).

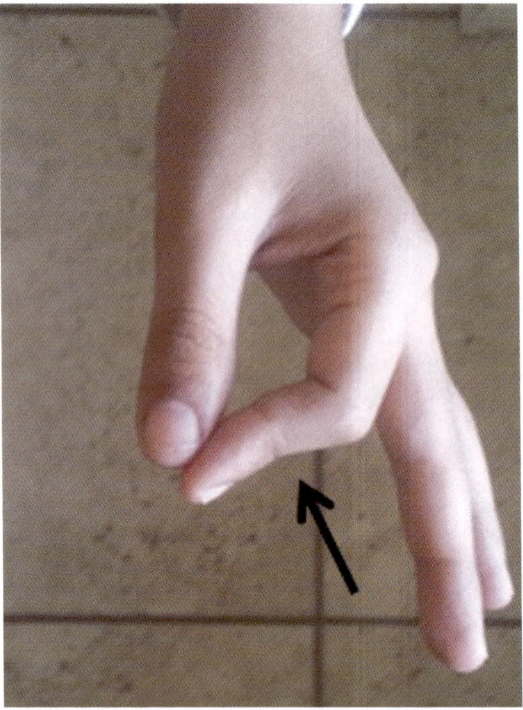

Fig. 16.22 Anterior interosseus nerve injury. When the patient is asked to do 'OK' sign he will not be able to flex the distal interphalangeal (DIP) joint of the index finger and the IP of the thumb to make a circle. The patient will push the pulp of the index and the thumb together; this will lead to extension of the DIP of the index (*arrow*)

- In cases of non displaced fractures '**posterior** fat pad sign' (radio-lucent space behind the olecranon fossa) is an indication of intra articular hematoma which occurs with these fractures (Fig. 16.23).
  - Please note that '**anterior** fat pad' can normally be seen and does NOT signify intra-articular bleeding.

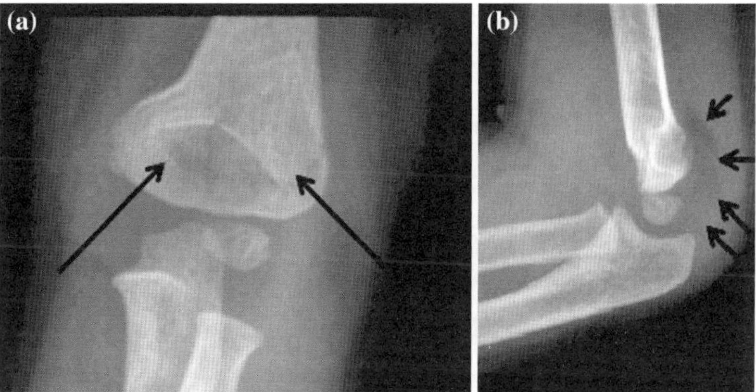

Fig. 16.23 Non displaced fracture supracondylar humerus. Radiographs of a 4-year-old girl who fell down on outstretched hand (FOOSH) and had immediate left elbow pain and swelling. Radiographs show a non displaced fracture of the supracondylar humerus (**a**) and posterior fat pad sign (**b**) (*arrows*)

Treatment:

- Orthopedic referral for possible surgical intervention.
  - Displaced supracondylar humerus fracture (stage 2 and 3), the treatment is closed reduction and percutaneous pinning (Fig. 16.24, 16.25).
- **If there is absent distal pulses or possible compartment syndrome**, urgent orthopedic consult.

COMPLICATIONS OF SUPRACONDYLAR FRACTURE HUMERUS

- **Neurovascular injury:**
  - Most common nerve to be injured is "anterior interosseus nerve".

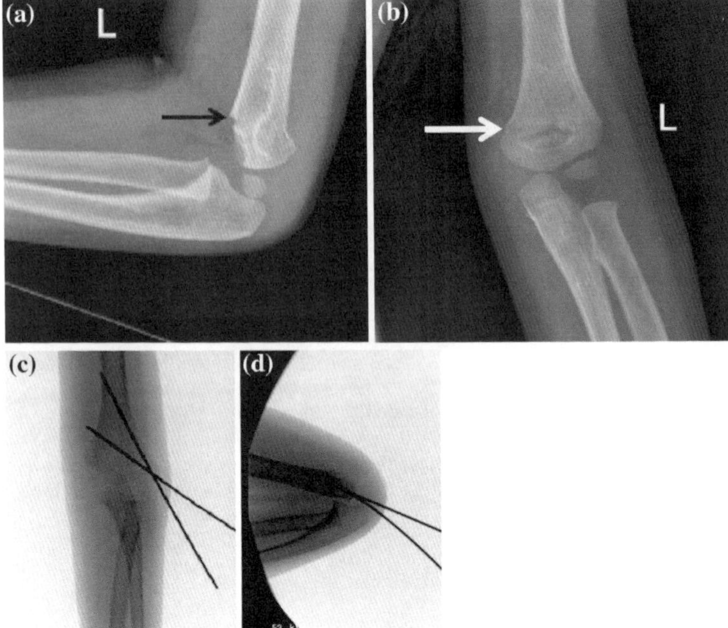

Fig. 16.24 Type 2 supracondylar fracture of the humerus. A 4-year-old boy with left supracondylar fracture of the humerus type 2 (notice the angulation of the fracture end in the lateral view (**a**) with no displacement of the fracture in the anteroposterior view (**b**) (*arrows*). The treatment was closed reduction and percutaneous fixation of the humerus by K wires (**c**, **d**)

- When the patient is asked to do "OK" sign, the child with extend the IP of the thumb and DIP of the index rather than flexing them (Fig. 16.22)
- Vascular injury.
  - Can be due to either spasm of the artery or injury to the vessel wall.
  - Urgent reduction should be done with reassessment of the pulses after reduction (spasm of the artery should improve with reduction of the fracture ends).

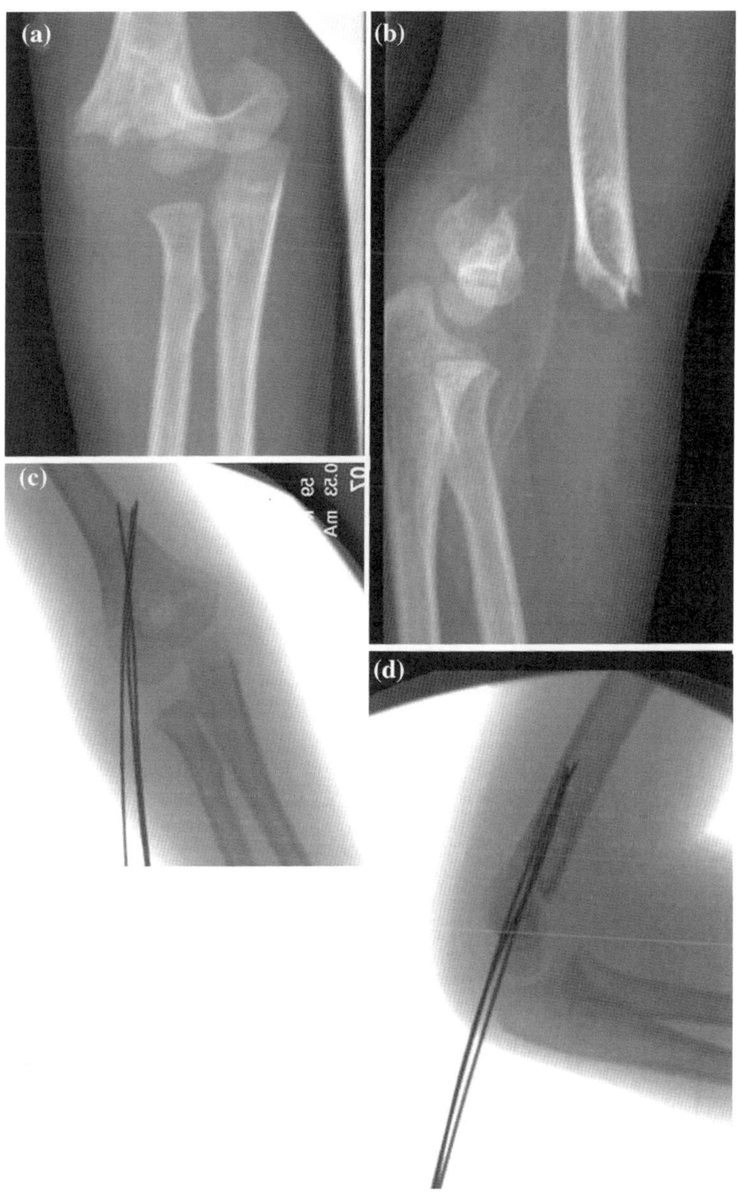
(a)
(b)
(c)
(d)

◀ **Fig. 16.25** Type 3 supracondylar fracture of the humerus (**a**, **b**). A 6-year-old boy with right supracondylar fracture of the humerus type 3 (notice the displacement of the fracture end). The treatment was treated by closed reduction and percutaneous fixation of the humerus by K wires (**c**, **d**)

- **Malunion:**
  - There is usually collapse in the medial side of the fracture with development of **cubitus varus (**see Fig. 16.11**).**
  - There is very minimal remodeling for this deformity.
  - The parents do not like appearance of their kids with this deformity; however, **the functional deficit is usually minimal**.
  - The treatment is osteotomy to correct the deformity if the family desires.
- **Compartment syndrome and Volkmann contracture**:
  - Displaced supracondylar humerus fracture can lead to marked swelling which may lead to development of compartment syndrome.
  - If the compartment syndrome is not appropriately treated, it will lead to fibrosis of the muscles and contracture (**Volkmann contracture**) (Fig. 16.26):
    - Contracture of the long finger flexors and wrist flexors.
    - The child will have flexed position of the wrist and fingers. The only way to extend the fingers is to flex the wrist to relax the long finger flexors and allow the fingers to extend.

LATERAL CONDYLE FRACTURE

Definition:

- Fracture of the lateral condyle of the humerus (which includes the capitellum, see anatomy of the elbow in Chap.11).

Incidence:

- About 10 % of the fractures of the elbow.

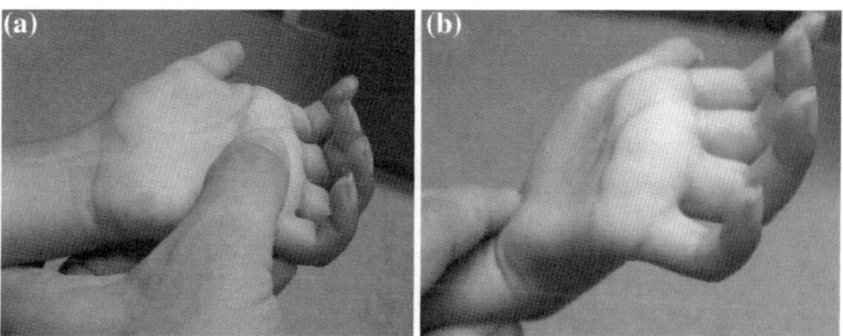

Fig. 16.26 Volkmann contracture. A 5-year-old boy with supracondylar fracture of the humerus and compartment syndrome that was not treated. Patient developed fibrosis and contracture of the finger flexors (Volkmann contracture). **a** With extension of the wrist, the fingers are flexed (tight fingers flexors). **b** With wrist flexion (the fingers flexors are relaxed), the finger can be partially extended

Clinical presentation:

- Pain, swelling, and deformity of the affected elbow.

Radiographs:

- The fracture line will pass through the lateral condyle and the capitellum (Fig. 16.27).
- Oblique radiographs are sometimes needed to identify the amount of displacement of the fracture.

Management:

Orthopedic referral. These fractures are prone to develop non union.

- If non displaced: splint application and **close follow** up to detect possible displacement.
- If displaced: Surgery for internal fixation.

Complication:

- **Non union** is a common complication with the lateral condyle fracture (Fig. 16.12).
- Non union will result in abnormal growth of the distal humerus:

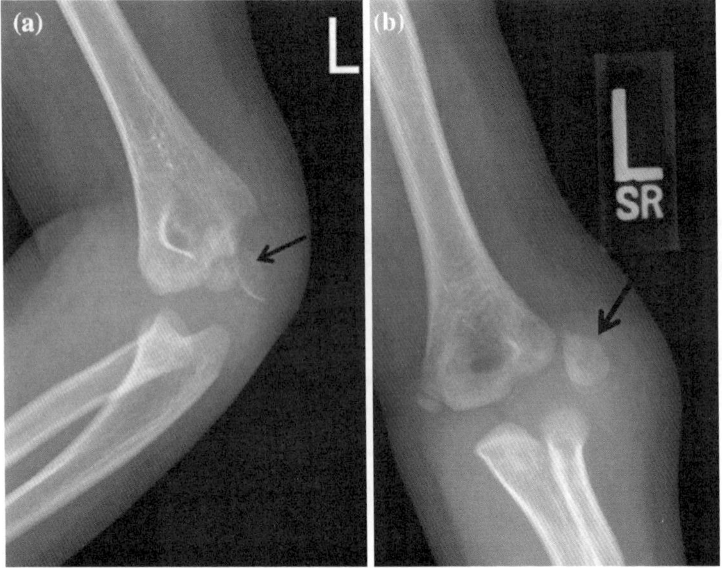

Fig. 16.27 Lateral condyle fracture. A 4-year-old boy fell on outstretched hand and had elbow pain and swelling. The radiographs (**a**, **b**) show a lateral condyle fracture (*arrow*)

- Growth will continue from the medial side only.
- This will result in cubitus valgus deformity (Fig. 16.28).
- Cubitus valgus deformity will cause stretching of the ulnar nerve with possible development of **tardy ulnar nerve palsy**.

MEDIAL EPICONDYLE FRACTURE

Pathology:
Two types of fractures can occur:

- It can occur as a **stress fracture** (repeated stress to the medial epicondyle during throwing activities will cause the fracture with low energy injury) (see Chap.11).

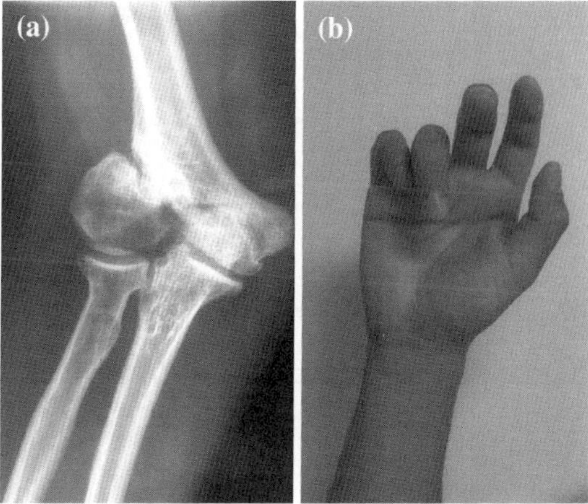

Fig. 16.28 An 18-year-old man with history of right elbow fracture when he was young. **a** Patient has right cubitus valgus as result of non union of the lateral condyle. **b** Cubitus valgus resulted in stretch of ulnar nerve on the medial side of the elbow with development of 'claw hand' deformity (inability to extend the medial two fingers)

- It can also occur as **acute fracture** (Fig. 16.29) due to acute injury to the elbow.
  - Some of the cases of acute fractures can be accompanied by **dislocation of the elbow** (Fig. 16.30).

Management:

- Orthopedic referral.
  - In most cases the fracture can be managed conservatively with no need for surgery
  - Surgery is indicated in cases with fracture-dislocation in which the fractured piece is incarcerated in the joint (Fig. 16.30) or if there is more than 20 mm displacement of the fracture (Fig. 16.29).

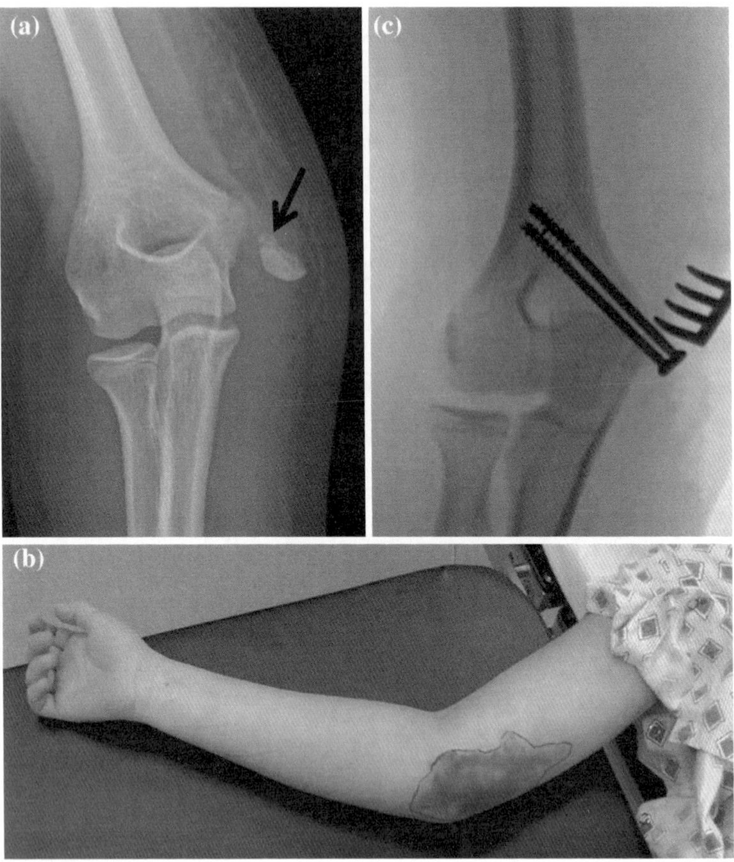

Fig. 16.29 Acute medial epicondyle fracture. A 13-year-old boy who fell while playing basketball. Radiograph shows the fracture displacement *arrow* (**a**). The clinical picture shows the large bruising on the medial aspect of the elbow (**b**). Due to the amount of fracture displacement, surgery was done for open reduction and internal fixation (**c**)

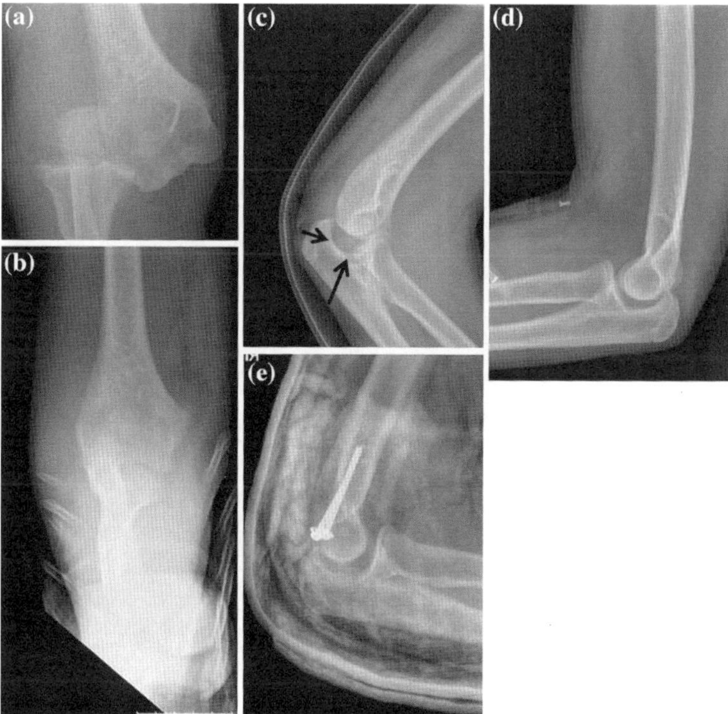

Fig. 16.30 Fracture dislocation of the medial epicondyle. A 12-year-old boy fell on his hand while skating. He dislocated his right elbow (**a**). Closed reduction of the elbow was done. Post reduction radiographs (**b**, **c**) showed incongruence lateral view of the elbow (compare with the normal side (**d**)). The medial epicondyle can be seen in the joint (*arrows*). Surgery was done for removal of the piece from the joint and internal fixation by screws (**e**)

RADIAL NECK FRACTURE

Definition:

- Fracture of the proximal end of the radius (radial neck).

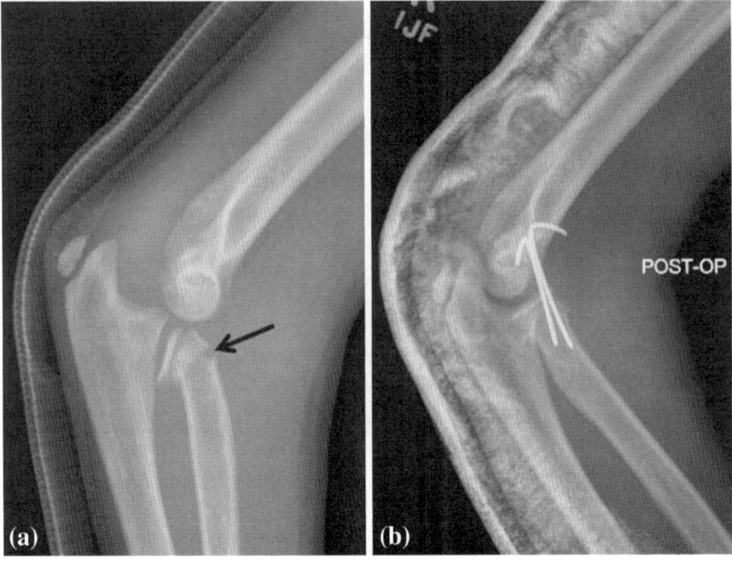

Fig. 16.31 Radial neck fracture. A 14-year-old boy fell down and dislocated the elbow joint and radial neck fracture (**a**). Reduction of dislocation was done and the fracture was fixed percutaneously using K-wires (**b**)

Clinical presentation:

- Pain, swelling, and deformity of the affected elbow.

Radiographs:

- Will show angulation of the radial head in relation to the shaft of the radius (Fig. 16.31).

Management:

- If minimal angulation:
  - Sling for comfort. Encourage early range of motion.
- If angulation is marked:
  - Orthopedic referral:
    - Surgery for reduction of the fracture (Fig. 16.31).

FRACTURE SHAFT OF BOTH BONES OF THE FOREARM

Definition:

Fracture of the shaft (diaphysis) of the radius and ulna.

Incidence:

- More common in boys.
- The cause is usually falling on outstretched hand (FOOSH).

Clinical presentation:

- Pain, swelling, and deformity of the forearm.
- Close observation is needed to ensure that no development of compartment syndrome of affected extremity.

Management:

ORTHOPEDIC REFERRAL

- Adequate reduction is needed to maintain good range of supination-pronation.
- Closed reduction and casting for young children (less than 10-year-old girls or 11-year-old boy).
- For older children or if there is failure to obtain adequate closed reduction, proceed to open surgery (fixation with plates and screws or intra medullary flexible nails) (Fig. 16.32).

FRACTURE OF THE DISTAL RADIUS AND ULNA

Incidence:

- **One of the commonest fractures in the pediatric patients.**
- They occur mostly due to falling on outstretched hand.

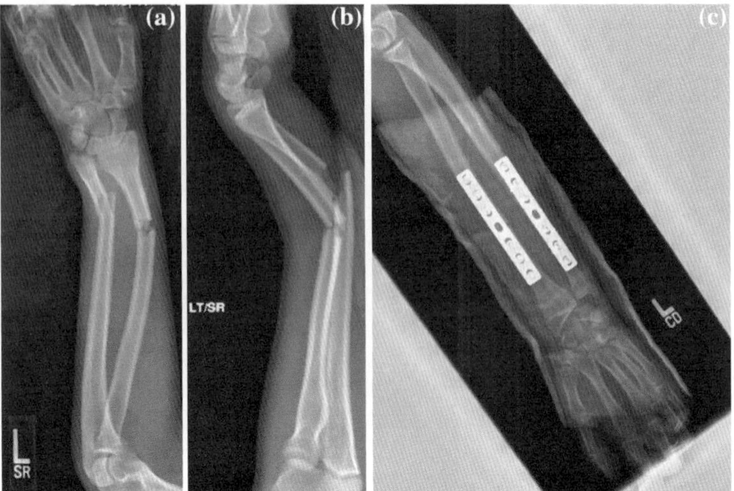

Fig. 16.32 Fractures of both bones of the forearm. A 15-year-old boy who fell on his outstretched hand while skating. Radiographs show the deformity of the forearm and the fracture of the radius and ulna shafts (**a**, **b**). Due to the age of the patient (older than 11-year-old), surgery was done for open reduction internal fixation (ORIF) with plates and screws (**c**)

Clinical presentations:

- Pain, swelling, and deformity of the wrist.

Radiographs:

- Fracture of the distal radius ± ulna.
  - Most of the distal radial fractures are associated with distal ulnar fracture.
- The fracture can be: torus, green stick, or complete displacement (see the introduction of fracture) (Fig. 16.33).
- If the fracture is through the growth plate, it will be considered physeal injury (Salter-Harris) injury (see below).

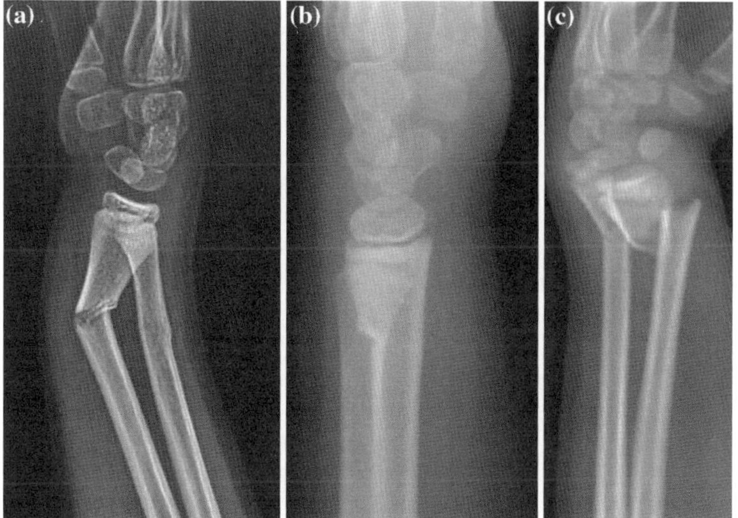

Fig. 16.33 Distal radial fracture. Three types of distal radial fracture ((**a**) greenstick, (**b**) torus, and (**c**) complete fracture)

Treatment:

Torus fracture:

- No need for orthopedic referral. The fracture can be treated by the primary care physicians.
- Splint or brace for comfort for 2–3 weeks.

Angulated or displaced fractures:

- Orthopedic referral.
  - Closed reduction and casting.

DISTAL RADIAL PHYSEAL INJURIES (SLATER-HARRIS INJURY)

Definition:

- Fractures of the distal end of the radius that go through the growth plate.

Radiographs:

- The fracture line will pass through the growth plate of the distal radius.
- In most cases, the fracture will involve part of the metaphysis (type II) (Fig. 16.34).

Management:

- If displaced: urgent orthopedic referral for reduction and casting.

Prognosis:

- Distal radial physis have low incidence of growth disturbance after physeal injury (about 4 %).

GALEAZZI FRACTURE-DISLOCATION

Definition:

- Fracture of the **distal radius** with dislocation of the **distal** radio-ulnar joint (Fig. 16.35).

Clinical presentation:

- Pain, swelling, and deformity of the wrist.
- The ulnar head is usually displaced dorsally.

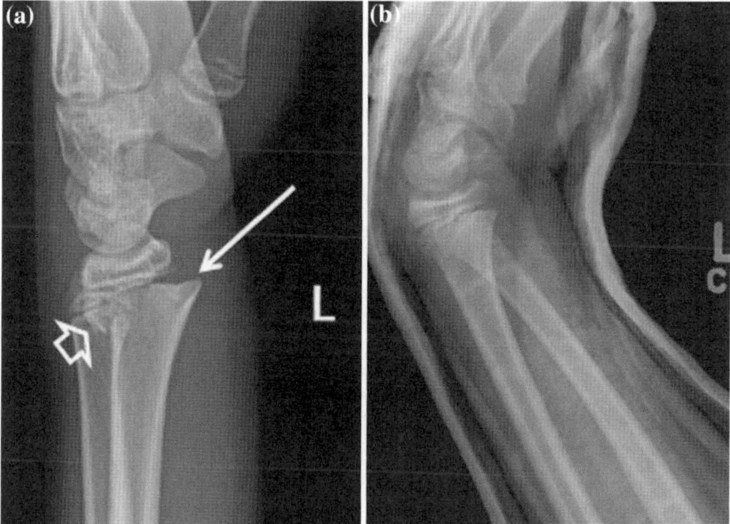

Fig. 16.34 Distal radial Salter-Harris type II fracture. A 12-year-old boy who fell on his outstretched hand had Salter Harris type II fracture distal radius with dorsal displacement and angulation (**arrow**) (**a**). Note the metaphyseal part on the dorsal aspect with the fractured epiphyseal segment (*arrow head*). Closed reduction with casting was done (**b**)

Treatment:

- Orthopedic referral for closed reduction and casting.
- Surgical treatment is rarely indicated in children.

MONTEGGIA FRACTURE DISLOCATION

Definition:

- Fracture of the **proximal ulna** with **dislocation of the radial head** from its articulation in the proximal RUJ (Fig. 16.36).

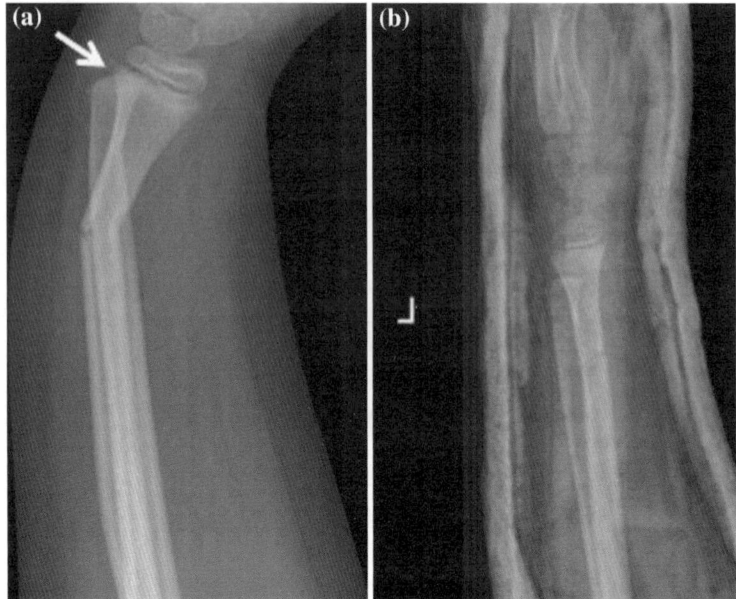

Fig. 16.35 Galeazzi fracture dislocation. A 10-year-old girl, fall down from swing on outstretched hand had fracture of the radius with volar angulation. The ulna is dorsal (posterior) to the radius at the level of the wrist indicating subluxation of the DRUJ (**a**). Closed reduction was obtained with realigning the radius and reducing the ulna to become in line with the radial head (**b**)

Clinical presentation:

- Pain, swelling, and deformity of the proximal forearm.
- Possible posterior interosseus nerve palsy (inability to extend the interphalangeal joint (IP) of the thumb) due to compression by the radial head.

Radiograph:

- The radial head should point to the capitellum in all views.
- If in any view it does not align with the capitellum, this is an indication of radial head dislocation (Fig. 16.36).
- **One of the most commonly missed conditions in the emergency room** (Fig. 16.37).

Treatment:

- **Orthopedic referral**
    - Closed reduction and casting. In most cases, the radial head will reduce with reduction of the ulnar fracture.
    - In cases of old missed Monteggia lesions, open reduction of the radial head is usually needed with possible ulnar osteotomy (16.37).

HAND FRACTURES

See sports injury

Galeazzi and Monteggia fracture dislocation.

- Because the radius and ulna are connected to each other at the proximal (proximal radio-ulnar joint at the elbow) and distal (distal radio-ulnar joint at the wrist) ends; fracture of a single bone with deformity and shortening of the broken bone can result in disruption of the proximal or distal RUJ.
- Two distinct pathologies have been described: Galeazzi and Monteggia.
- The treating physician should be aware of these conditions in order not to miss them and diagnose the injury as simple single bone fracture. As a general rule **"the diagnosis of single shaft radius or ulna fracture should only be given after meticulous assessment of the distal and proximal RUJs."**

LOWER EXTREMITY FRACTURES

Fracture proximal femur:

Definition:

Fractures which involve **the neck of the femur and trochanteric area (** Fig. 16.38).

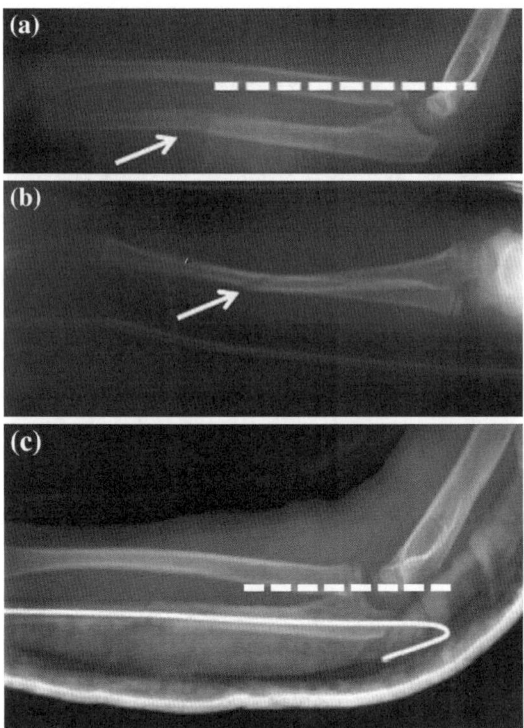

Fig. 16.36 Monteggia fracture dislocation. (**a**, **b**) Patient had fracture ulna (*arrow*). The patient was diagnosed initially as isolated ulnar fracture and long arm cast was applied. Radiographs in the clinic showing the head of the radius is not pointing to the capitellum in the lateral view (*dotted line*). (**c**) Closed reduction was done with percutaneous fixation of the ulna by K wire , the head of radius was closely reduced (radial head in line with the capitellum, *dotted line*)

Clinical presentation:

- History of high energy trauma (e.g., fall from height, motor vehicle collision)
- Pain in the hip region.
- Inability to bear weight on the affected side.
- External rotation deformity of the affected extremity.

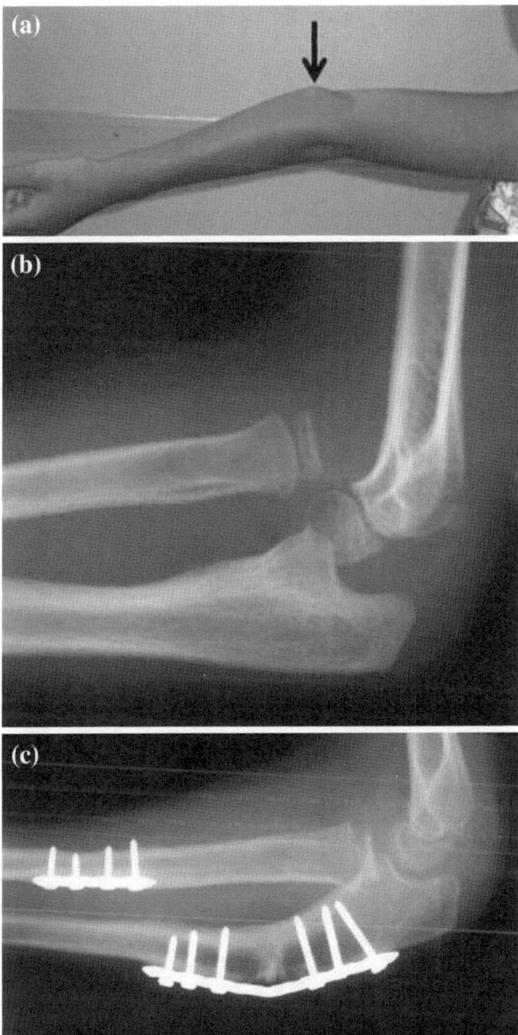

Fig. 16.37 Missed monteggia fracture. A 7-year-old boy with a history of trauma to the left forearm 1 year ago presenting with elbow deformity (**a**). Radiograph shows the radial head anterior subluxation (**b**). The patient was misdiagnosed as isolated ulna fracture and the radial head dislocation was missed. A major reconstruction of the forearm and the elbow [with ulnar and radial osteotomy] was needed to reduce the radial head (**c**)]

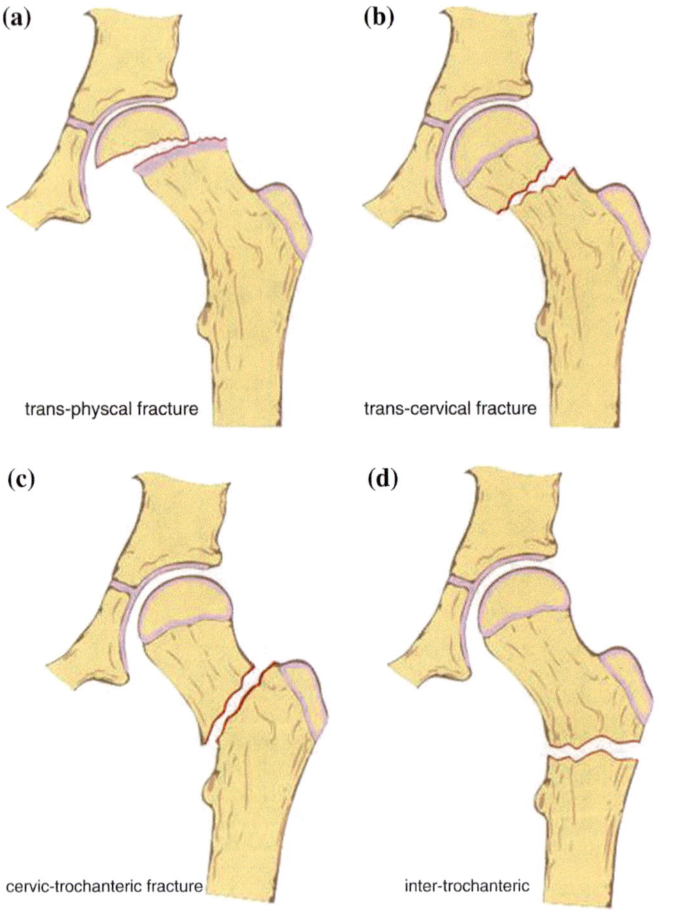

Fig. 16.38 Fracture neck femur. Types of proximal femoral fracture in children

Imaging:

- Radiographs will show the fracture of the proximal femur (Fig. 16.39).
- CT scan to better assess the fracture position.

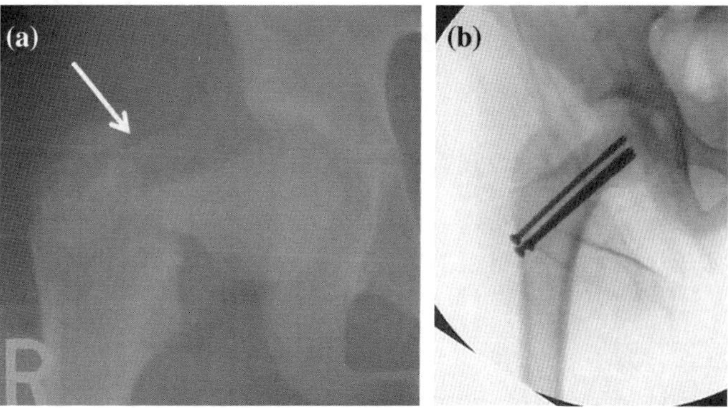

Fig. 16.39 Fracture neck femur. An 8-year-old girl who fell from a tree and had right hip pain. Radiograph showed fracture neck femur (**a**). The fracture was reduced and fixed using three screws (**b**)

Management:

- Because of possible affection of the blood supply, these fractures are considered emergencies and **need urgent orthopedic consultation**.

Complication of fracture neck femur:

- **Avascular necrosis (Osteonecrosis) of the femoral head:**
  - The blood supply to head of the femur will be disrupted by the fracture.
  - The head will become weaker and later collapse. This will cause early arthritis of the joint.
- **Non union of the fracture:**
  - The contact area of the femoral neck is very small with high stresses across the fracture. This makes this fracture prone to non union **(**Fig. 16.40**)**

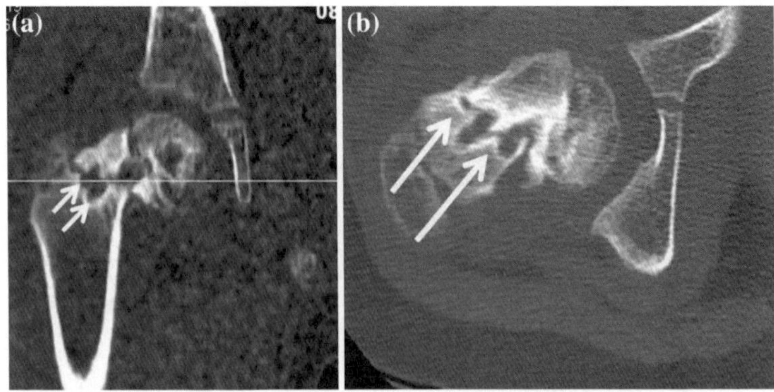

Fig. 16.40 Non union femoral neck. A 6-year-old girl who had femoral neck fracture and treated with internal fixation by screws. Screws started to move in position and had to be taken off. (**a**) Coronal and (**b**) axial **b** CT scan taken after screw removal shows non union of the femoral head and the sites of the previous screws (*arrows*)

FRACTURE SHAFT FEMUR

Mechanism of injury:

- The femur is the thickest bone in the body, considerable amount of energy is needed to break the femur.

Non accidental trauma and femur fracture:

- See Chap.15.

Clinical presentation:

- **Severe pain**, deformity, and swelling of the affected thigh.
- Radiographs will show the fracture.

Management:

- Fracture shaft femur needs orthopedic consultation.
- Treatment will depend on age and severity of the fracture:

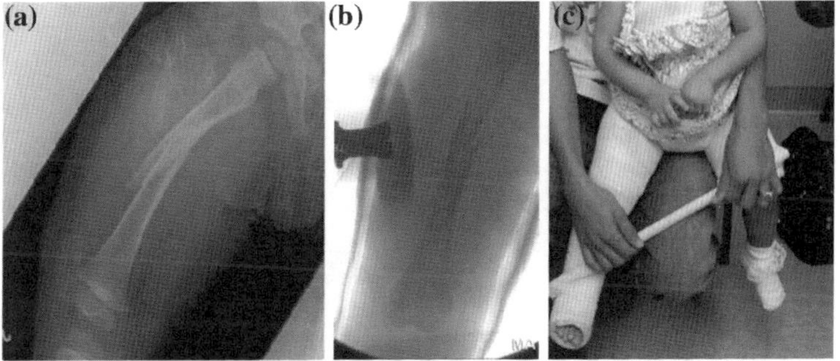

Fig. 16.41 A 4-year-old girl with spiral left femur fracture after falling from monkey bar. Radiograph (**a**) shows the spiral fracture. Closed reduction was done under general anesthesia (**b**) with application of spica cast. (**c**) Follow-up in the clinic with the hip spica applied to the child

- **Fracture at birth**: see Chap.5.
- **Infant and children less the 5- year-old**: casting under anesthesia or sedation (Fig. 16.41).
- Children 6 years and older or with highly comminuted fracture will require internal fixation by either:
  - Intramedullary fixation (flexible or rigid nails) (Fig. 16.42).
  - Plates and screws (Fig. 16.43).

FRACTURE OF THE DISTAL FEMUR PHYSIS (SALTER HARRIS INJURIES)

Clinical presentation:

- Pain, swelling, and deformity of the knee.
- It is critical in these in injuries to assess the pulses (tibialis posterior and pedal pulse) in the affected side and compare with the other side.

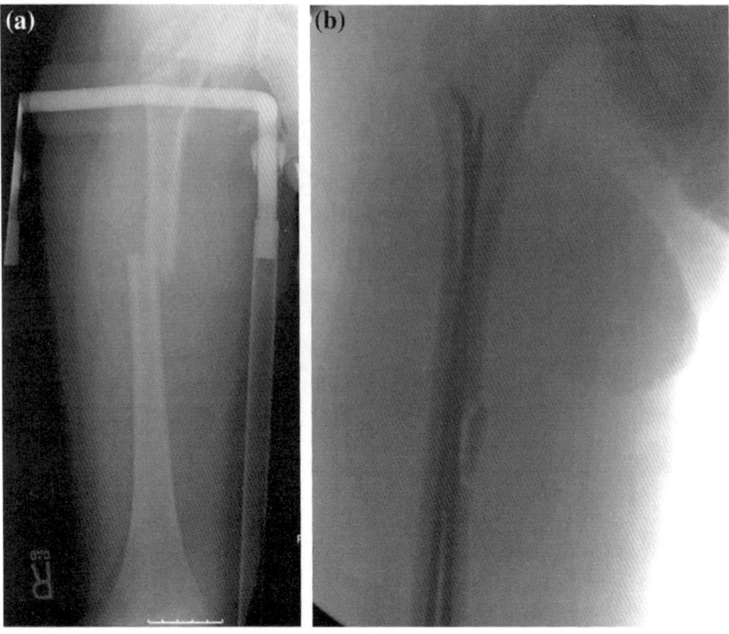

Fig. 16.42 Fracture femur treated by flexible nail. A 10-year-old boy fell down while playing football at school had transverse fracture femur (**a**). The fracture was fixed by flexible intramedullary nail (**b**)

Management:

- Orthopedic referral:
  - Displaced fractures will need reduction and internal fixation.

Complications of distal femoral fractures:

- Have high potential for growth disturbance, must warn the family about that in advance (Fig. 16.44).
- Can be complicated by arterial injury (assess the distal pulses and compare it to the other side) (Fig. 16.45).

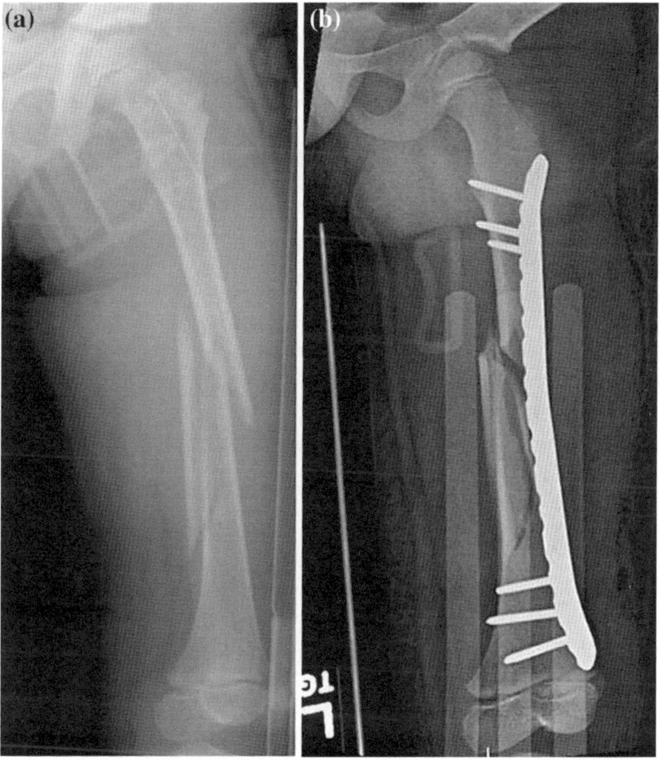

Fig. 16.43 Fracture femur treated by plate and screws. An 8 year-old with motor vehicle collision had left femur fracture [highly comminuted with butterfly segment (**a**)]. Patient was treated with internal fixation by plate and screws (**b**)

PROXIMAL TIBIAL PHYSIS INJURIES (SALTER HARRIS)

Clinical presentation, management, and complications:

- Similar to distal femur physeal injuries (Fig. 16.46).

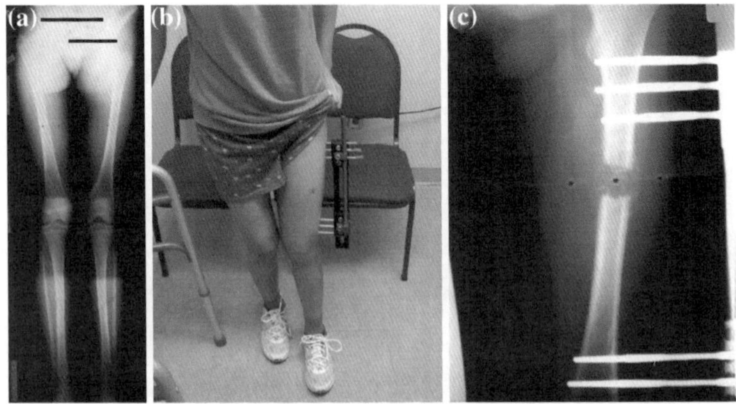

Fig. 16.44 Growth disturbance after distal femur fracture. Radiograph of 13-year-old girl with fracture distal femur few years earlier (**a**) showing 6 cm limb length discrepancy with left side shorter than the right side (lines presenting the upper end of femurs). (**b**) external fixator was applied to length the left femur. (**c**) Radiograph of the left femur showing the distraction lengthening of the left femur

Patellar fracture:

- Pain and swelling of the knee.

Radiographs:

- Will show the fracture (Fig. 16.47).
- Differential diagnosis: Bipartite patella (see Chap.7)

Management:
Orthopedic referral for possible surgical intervention.

TIBIAL SHAFT FRACTURE

Clinical presentation:

- Pain, swelling, and deformity of the affected extremity.

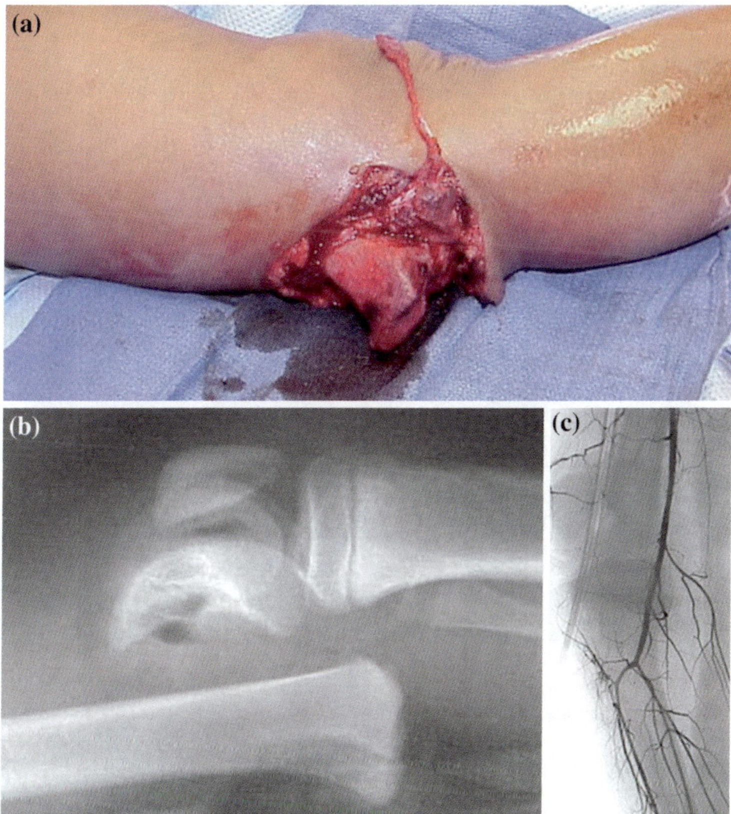

Fig. 16.45 Distal femur physeal fracture. (**a**) 12 years old boy who presented with open fracture distal femur with exposed bone. (**b**) Radiograph showed Salter Harris type I distal femur fracture. (**c**) Because of decrease pulse on the affected side compared to the other side, an arteriogram was performed

- Can be complicated **by compartment syndrome** (pain increases after application of cast).

Treatment:

- Orthopedic referral.
- Treatment is according to age and displacement (Fig. 16.48):

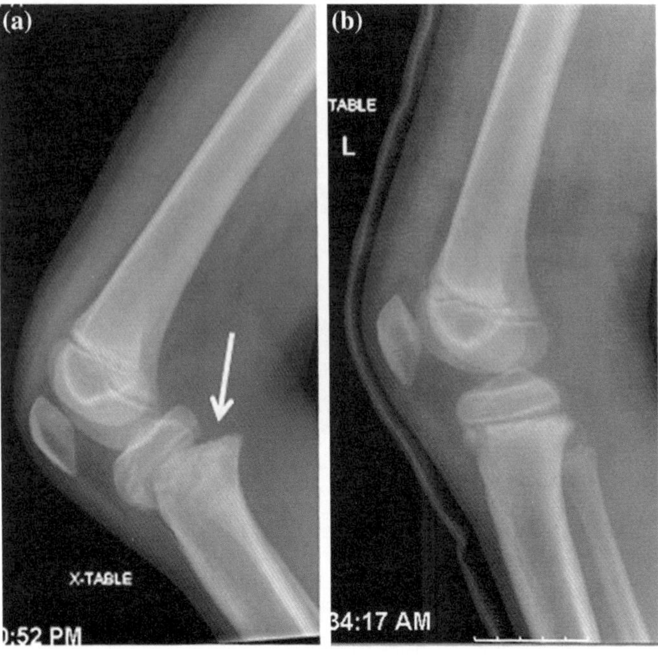

Fig. 16.46 Proximal tibial fracture. A 13-year-old boy with motor vehicle collision, complained of pain and swelling of the left knee. Radiographs showed Salter type 2 of proximal tibial physis (**a**). Closed reduction and application of long leg cast was done (**b**)

- Most cases can be treated by closed reduction and casting.
- Some cases will require internal fixation (flexible nail or plate)

TODDLER FRACTURE

Definition:

- A spiral tibial shaft fracture that occurs in toddler due to twisting trauma.

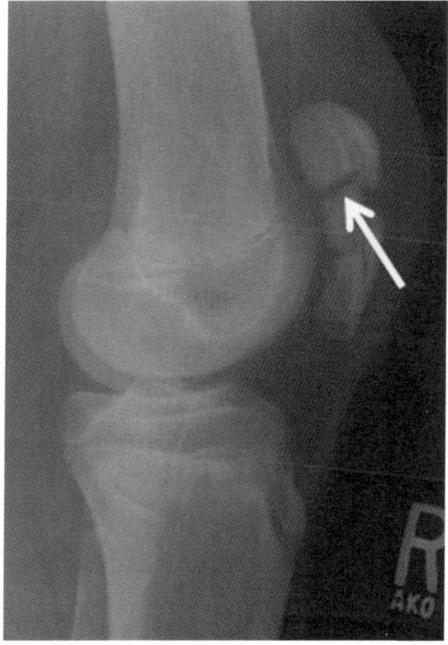

Fig. 16.47 Patella fracture. A 13-year-old boy who fell down and had right patellar fracture (*arrow*)

- **This is a relatively common injury in children less than 4 years old.**

Clinical presentation:

- The parents recall no or minimal trauma in most cases.
- Inability to bear weight on the affected side.
- Minimal swelling and no deformity.
- External rotation of foot will cause pain and discomfort to the child.

Radiographs:

- The radiographs will show spiral fracture of the distal tibia, non displaced (Fig. 16.49).

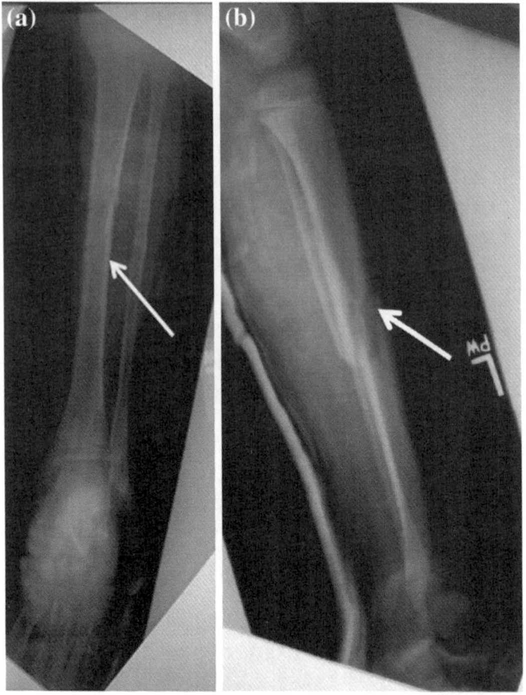

Fig. 16.48 Tibial shaft fracture. A 14-year-old boy fell down while running down the stairs and had left leg pain and swelling. Radiographs (**a**, **b**) show mid shaft tibia fracture (*arrows*). This fracture was managed non surgically with casting

- In some cases, the fracture does not show up in the primary radiograph, but follow up radiograph will show the evidence of healing (periosteal new bone formation and callus at the fracture site).

Management:

- Orthopedic referral (treatment is by above knee cast for 3 weeks).

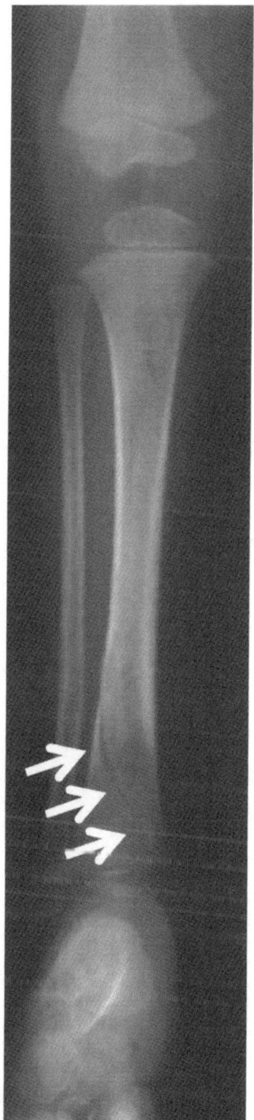

Fig. 16.49 Toddler fracture. A 3-year-old boy presented with his parents because of two days refusal to walk. On exam there was tenderness of the lower leg with pain on external rotation of the tibia. Radiograph shows non displace spiral fracture of the lower end of the tibia (*arrows*)

ANKLE FRACTURE

Mechanism of injury:

- **Twisting** injuries to the ankles.

Pathology

- Fracture of the distal end of the tibial and the fibula.
- Can lead to disruption of the interosseus ligament between the tibia and fibula (syndesmotic injury).

Types of ankle fractures:

- Non physeal injuries (Fig. 16.50):
  - These are treated as adult fractures
    - If non displaced and not associated with syndesmotic injury, non operative treatment by cast immobilization.

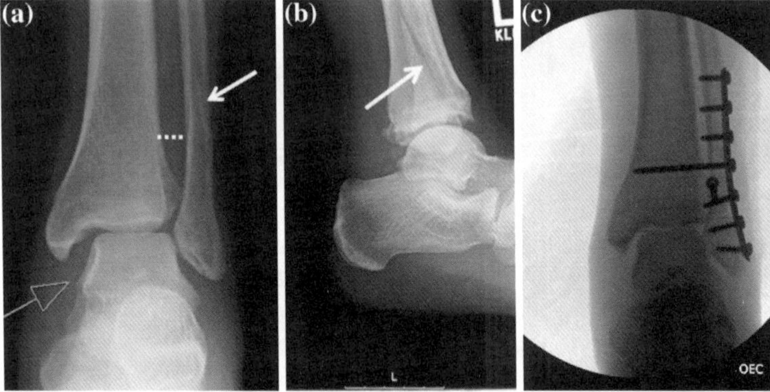

Fig. 16.50 Ankle fracture. A 16-year-old boy had left ankle injury while playing soccer. **a**, **b** Radiographs showed fracture distal fibula (*arrows*) with widening of the distance between tibia and fibula (dotted line) and also widening of the medial joint space (*open arrow*). **c** Surgery was done for fixation of the fracture with plates and screws (notice reduction of the relationship between tibia and fibula and narrowing of the medial joint space

    - If associated with syndesmotic injury (increased distance between tibia and fibula), operative treatment.

- Physeal injuries (Fig. 16.51):
  - Physeal injuries of the distal tibia and fibula can be associated with growth disturbance.
  - Need orthopedic referral.

- Non displaced distal fibular Physeal injury (Salter-Harris type I):
  - **Common injury in children.**
  - Due to twisting injury of the ankle, equivalent to ankle sprain in adults.
  - Tenderness and swelling over the distal fibula.
  - Radiographs:
    - Radiographs can be normal or will show minimal displacement of the distal fibular physis.
    - The diagnosis **depends on the clinical presentation** and not the radiographic picture.
  - Management:
    - Weight bearing as tolerated in a cast or a cam boot.

COMMON FOOT FRACTURES

Calcaneus fracture:

Mechanism of injury:

- Falling from a height.

Clinical presentation:

- Pain, swelling, and deformity of the heel.

Radiographs:

- Calcaneus fractures appear as a compression injury in the calcaneus (Fig. 16.52).

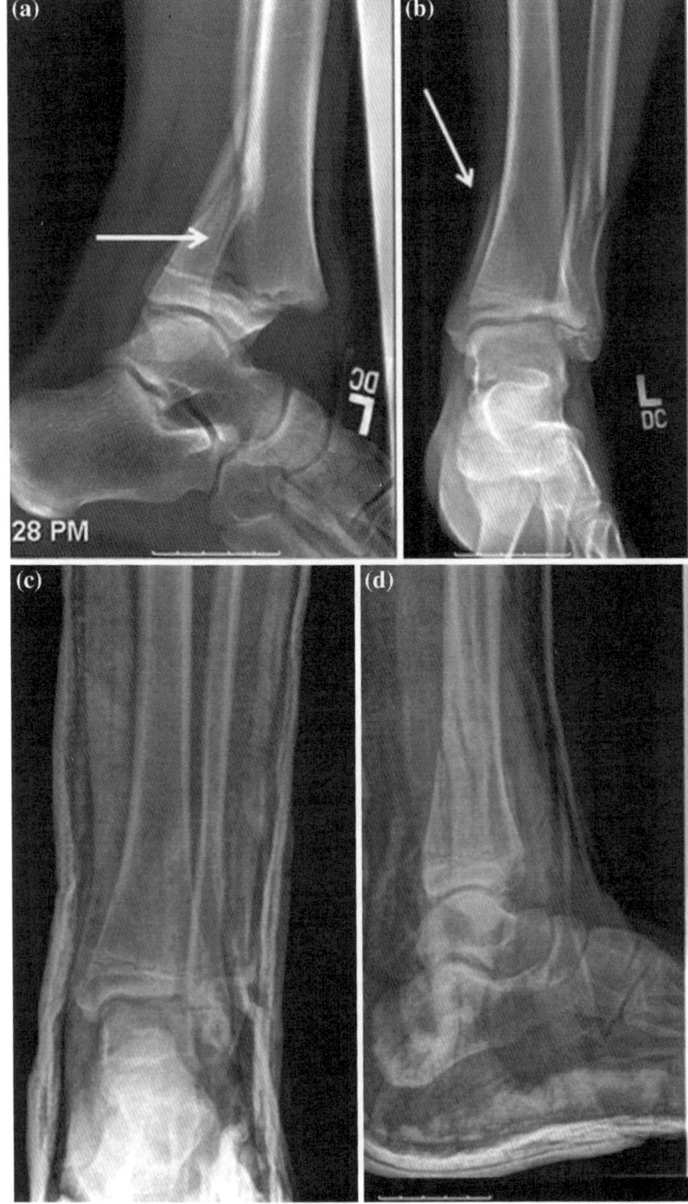
(a)
28 PM
(b)
L
DC
(c)
(d)

◀ **Fig. 16.51** Distal tibial physeal injury (**a**) and (**b**). A 12-year-old with twisting injury to the left ankle presented with pain, swelling, and deformity of the ankle. Radiographs showed type 2 Salter Harris injury of the distal tibial physis (*arrow* points to the metaphyseal part). (**c**) and (**d**) Closed reduction and cast was done

Management:

- Orthopedic referral:
  - surgical intervention may be indicated for markedly compressed fracture with loss of calcaneus height (Fig. 16.52).

FRACTURE BASE OF THE 5TH METATARSAL BONE

Mechanism of injury:

- Twisting injury with avulsion of the base of the 5th metatarsal by the tendon of peroneus brevis and plantar fascia.

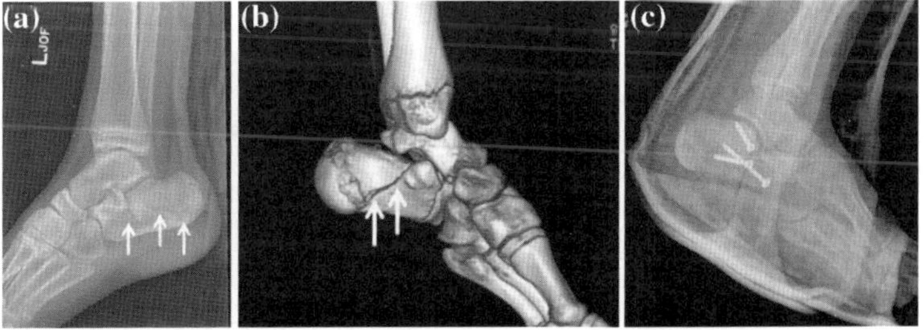

Fig. 16.52 Calcaneus fracture. A 12-year-old boy, jumped from 6 feet high, fell on his heel, complained from foot pain and swelling, Radiograph showed calcaneus fracture with compression of the bone and loss of height (*arrows*) (**a**). 3D CT (**b**) showed the fracture line better (*arrows*). Open reduction was done with restoration of normal contour and anatomy of the calcaneus (**c**)

Types of fracture of the base of 5th metatarsal (Fig. 16.53):

- Avulsion of the apophysis:
  - Widening of the growth plate in the radiographs.
  - Can be treated with immediate weight bearing with no need for immobilization.
- Metaphyseal fractures (pseudo-Johns fracture):
  - These are stable injuries.
  - Can be treated with immediate weight bearing with no need for immobilization.
- Metaphyseo-diaphyseal fractures (true-Johns fracture).
  - Prone to develop non union (watershed area with minimum blood supply to this area).
  - Management:
    - Orthopedic referral:
      - Non weight bearing in a cast.
      - Surgery may be indicated for athletic patients to avoid long periods of immobilization in the cast.

Phalanx fractures:

- Common injuries due to falling of heavy objects on the foot of the child.
- Treatment:
  - Weight bearing as tolerated in hard sole shoe.

Spine injuries

- Spine injuries represent dangerous trauma as they may be complicated with neurological deficits.
- A child with multiple injuries (especially those to pelvis or face) should be assumed to have spinal column injury until this is ruled out by careful physical and radiographic evaluation.
- The head circumference in children is relatively bigger than adults. This leads to flexion of the cervical spine when the child is supine on a standard backboard.

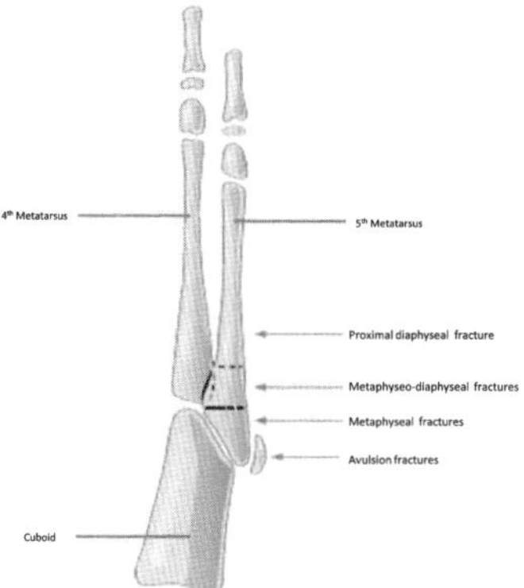

Fig. 16.53 Fracture of the base of the fifth metatarsal

- To allow for adequate transportation of the injured child there should be either a cutout for the head in the transfer board or the body is elevated on a pad to avoid flexion of the cervical spine (Fig. 16.54).

- **Examination:**
  - Careful examination of the spine and assessment of the neurologic condition of the patients should be done.
    - Palpation of each spinous process with attention of tenderness, gaps, or deviation.
    - Detailed neurologic examination is an essential part of the assessment of the child with multiple injuries.

- **Imaging:**
  - Plain radiographs (Anteroposterior and lateral) for the affected side is performed to detect if there subluxation or dislocation of the vertebrae.
  - **'pseudosubluxation"** of the vertebrae is a normal finding that is sometimes found in the pediatric spine: mostly occurs between C2 and C3 and to a lesser extent between C3 and C4 (Fig. 16.55).

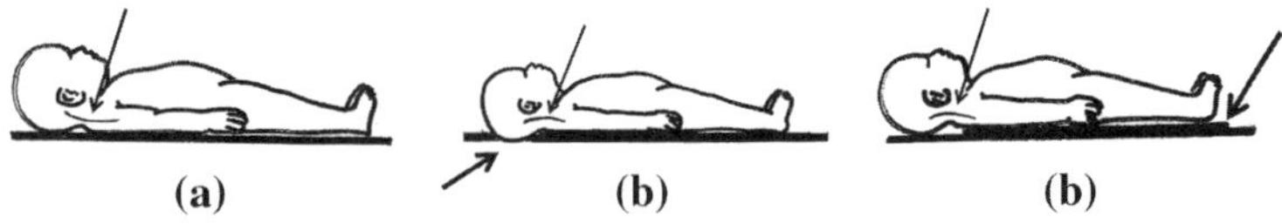

Fig. 16.54 Children have relatively bigger head. **a** Straight board will cause flexion of the cervical spine (*arrow*). **b** A cut in transfer board (*thick arrow*) will maintain cervical lordosis (thin arrow). **c** Raising the child body over a pad (*thick arrow*) will also maintain cervical lordosis (*thin arrow*)

  - It is present in about one-third of lateral views of children less than 10 years old.
  - The finding is more pronounced if the radiographs are taken in flexion.
  - The body of the vertebra above is at an anterior position compared with the vertebra below.
  - The proper alignment of the vertebrae can be assessed using the anterior border of the posterior spinous processes (spinolaminar line or Swischuk line), which should be continuous with no breaks.

- **Clearing the cervical spine in pediatric patients with multiple traumas:**
  - Clearance of the cervical spine in children with multiple injuries may be difficult to achieve as these children are 'distracted' with other injuries and fractures or not responsive (from associated brain injury or high doses of narcotics).
  - In 'distracted patients', **magnetic resonance imaging** of the cervical spine can be used to clear their cervical spine.
  - Most of the cervical spine in young children is cartilaginous and cannot be adequately visualized by CT. In addition, concerns about cancer risk related to CT in pediatric patient are increasing due to high amount of irradiation associated with its use.

Spinal Cord Injury Without Radiographic Abnormality

- Spinal cord injury can sometimes occur in children without radiographic abnormality in the plain radiograph. This is

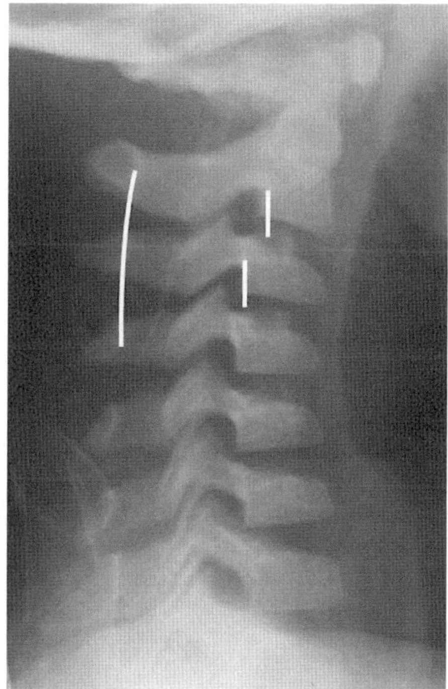

Fig. 16.55 Pseudosubluxation of the vertebra. Radiograph of the lateral cervical spine of a 6-year-old boy who sustained injury to his neck. The body of C2 is anterior to C3; however, the anterior border of the posterior spinous processes of C1–C3 is in line, indicating normal alignment of the cervical spine

called SCIWORA (Spinal Cord Injury Without Radiographic Abnormality).

- It is thought to be caused by distraction mechanism because the spinal cord is the least elastic structure in the spinal column. The vertebrae with the discs in between can be elongated more than what the cord can tolerate. It is more common in children younger than 8 years.

- **Management of cervical injury:**

- All trauma patients should be assumed to have cervical spine injury until their spine is cleared.
  - □ Cervical spine precaution (application of cervical collar) should be applied to all pediatric trauma victims.
- If there is suspicion of cervical trauma:
  - □ Orthopedic, spine, or neurosurgical referral.
- Steroid administration:
  - □ For cases of cervical spinal cord injury.
  - □ The rationale of steroid administration is to decrease the inflammatory response in the spinal cord which occurs with spine trauma.
  - □ Steroid administration is a controversial issue, and no clinical study had assessed its efficacy in the pediatric population. However, high-dose steroid is still a common practice in the United States.

SOFT TISSUE INJURIES

Peripheral Nerve Palsy:

Causes of nerve injuries:

- ■ Fracture of the bone or joint dislocation, e.g.:
  - Humerus fracture can be associated with radial nerve palsy.
  - Supracondylar fracture of the humerus can be associated with anterior interosseus nerve, ulnar nerve, or radial nerve palsies.
  - Elbow dislocation: ulnar nerve palsy
  - Sacral fracture: S1 and S2 roots.
  - Knee dislocation: common peroneal nerve.
- ■ Open nerve injuries:

- Lacerations:
  - Lacerations of the skin (knife, glasses) may be associated with nerve injuries.
- Gunshot wounds.

- Post surgical:
  - Surgical instruments and retraction can cause nerve injuries.
    - Surgeries around the elbow can cause radial, ulnar, or posterior interosseous nerve injuries.
- Medical conditions:
  - Lead toxicity.
  - Charcot Marie Tooth.

Pathological types of nerve injuries (see Chap.5):

- **Neuropraxia**: stretching of the nerve. Recovery is usually complete.
- **Axonotemesis**: injury of the nerve axon with intact neural sheath.
- **Neurotemesis**: injury to both the nerve axon and neural sheath. Worst prognosis (complete severing of the nerve).

CLINICAL PICTURE OF SOME COMMON NERVE INJURIES

Radial nerve injuries:

Motor:

- **Wrist drop** (inability to extend the wrist) (Fig. 16.56)
- Finger drop (inability to extend the fingers at the metacarpo-phalyngeal joint).

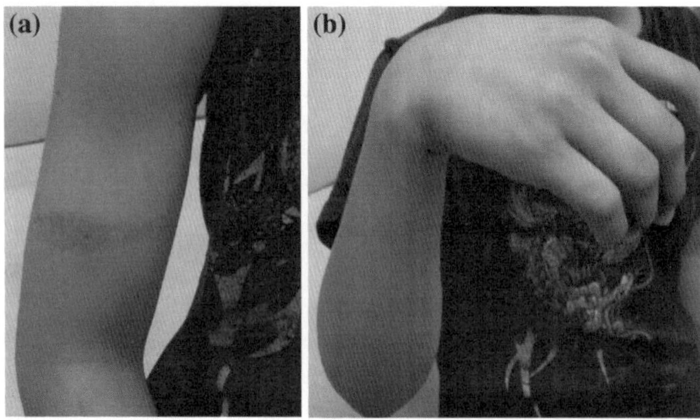

Fig. 16.56 Radial nerve palsy. **a** A 12-year-old male was playing 'tag-of-war' and had wrapped the rope around his arm. **b** Patient developed radial nerve palsy with wrist drop after the game

Sensory:

- Small area of sensation loss at the base of the thumb.

Ulnar Nerve Injury

Motor:

- paralysis of the intrinsic muscles of the hand.
    - Inability to perform finger adduction and abduction (interossei muscle).
    - inability to extend the small and the ring finger at the interphalangeal joint level (interossei and lumbricals) (**partial claw hand**) (Fig. 16.57).

Sensory:

- Loss of sensation from the medial $2\frac{1}{2}$ or $1\frac{1}{2}$ digits.

Median nerve injury:

Motor

- Inability to flex the index (±middle) finger.

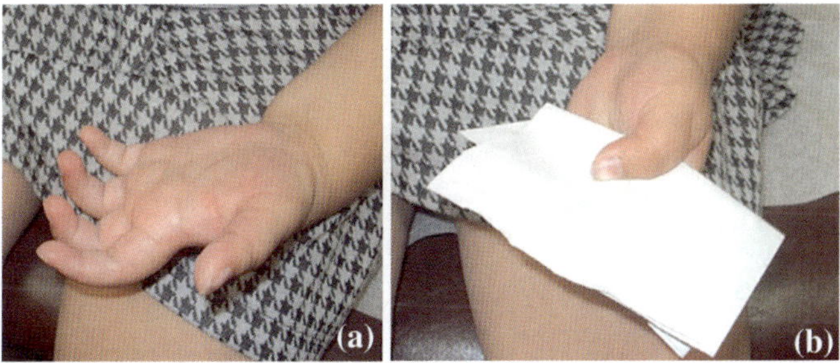

Fig. 16.57 Ulnar nerve palsy. An 8-year-old girl with ulnar nerve palsy after supracondylar fracture of the humerus. **a** Patient has inability to extend the small and the ring finger at the interphalangeal joint level (interossei and lumbricals) (partial claw hand). **b** Because of paralysis of the adductor pollicis, when the patient is asked to hold a paper in between the thumb and the palm, the patient will flex the IP of the thumb to grasp the piece of paper rather that adducting the thumb (Froment's sign)

Sensory:

- Loss of sensation of the palmar aspect of the index and thumb.
- Sensation over this area is very important for hand function.

Posterior interosseus nerve:

Motor:

- **Finger drop**: inability to extend the fingers at the level of the metacarpo-phalyngeal joint.
- Inability to extend the distal phalanx of the thumb

No sensory deficit.

Common Peroneal Nerve

Motor:

- **Ankle drop**: inability to dorsiflex the ankle the toes.
  - The affected child will flex his knee more during gait to clear his foot from the floor **(high stepage gait).**

Sensory:

- Loss of sensation on the dorsum of the foot.

DISLOCATIONS

Shoulder dislocation

- see Chap.11

Acromioclavicular separation

- see Chap.11

Elbow dislocation:

- see Chap.11

NURSEMAID ELBOW (PULLED ELBOW)

Definition:

- Subluxation of the radial head from the annular ligament.
- **Nursemaid elbow is a common condition in young children that needs to be identified by pediatricians and emergency care physicians.**

Pathology

- Slippage of the head of the radius under the annular ligament.

Age

- Nursemaid elbow most commonly occurs in children aged 1–4 years.

History

- Child with no obvious history of trauma suddenly refuses to use his/her arm.

- Common scenarios include the following:
  - A toddler held by his or her hand then the child and adult move in opposite directions.
  - A toddler is pulled by the wrist up and over an obstacle.
  - An arm is pulled through the sleeve of a sweater or coat.
- The condition is usually unilateral but may bilateral.
- **Radiograph should be obtained to exclude fractures or dislocation.**

Treatment

- **Reduction maneuvers:**
  - This can be accomplished by immobilizing the elbow and palpating the region of the radial head with one hand.
  - The other hand applies axial compression at the wrist while fully supinating the forearm then flexing the elbow (Fig. 16.58).
  - As the arm is manipulated, a click or snap can be felt at the radial head.
  - **Another reduction maneuver** is to extend the elbow, one hand palpating the radial head and the other hand is supinating-pronating the wrist while maintaining radial deviation and axial compression of the wrist.
  - If reduction was successful (a click is felt), the child should be observed in the emergency department:
    - Most children will show immediate return of function after about 15–30 min.
  - If reduction was not successful and radiographic findings reveal no fracture, another attempt at reduction is performed.
  - If reduction cannot be obtained, the arm is immobilized in a sling and the child should be followed after few days. Spontaneous reduction usually occurs in the next few days after injury.
  - Post-reduction films are not necessary.
  - Educate the parents about the risk of recurrence.

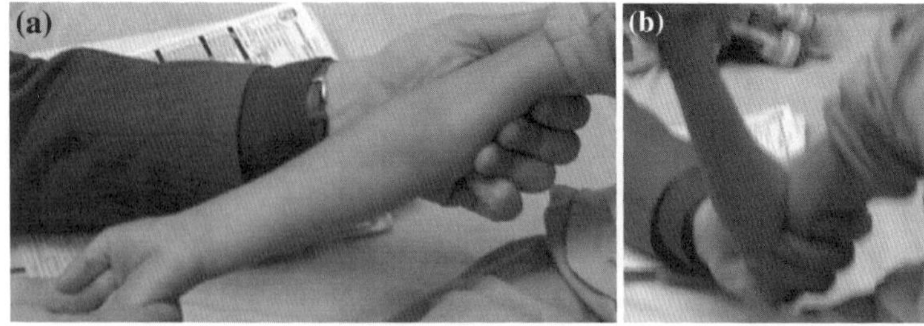

Fig. 16.58 Reduction maneuver for nursemaid elbow. The elbow is extended with the forearm supinated then the elbow is brought to full flexion

- Always make sure that no fracture is missed (e.g., lateral condyle fracture or radial neck fracture).

Indication of orthopedic referral

- With failed reduction in the emergency room and the child is still refusing to use the arm in the follow up visit.

HIP DISLOCATIONS:

- Hip dislocation is rare in children.
- It occurs mainly in adolescent with high energy injuries (motor vehicle collisions).
- It can be **posterior (more common)** or anterior.
- Posterior dislocation can be associated with acetabular fracture.
- Patient will have severe hip pain, deformity of the extremity, and possible sciatic nerve palsy.
- Radiographs will show head of the femur out of the acetabular socket (Fig. 16.59).
- **Management:**
  - Urgent orthopedic consultation:

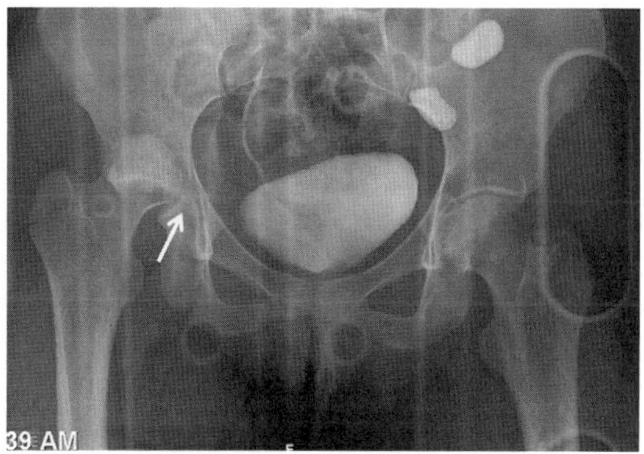

Fig. 16.59 A 16-year-old girl, was a passenger in motor vehicle collision. Patient presented to the emergency room with right hip pain. Radiograph of the pelvis shows right hip dislocation (notice the empty right acetabulum (*arrows*) compared to left hip)

- □ Hip dislocation is an orthopedic emergency as it can lead to disruption of the blood supply to the head of femur.
- □ Closed reduction is attempted, if it fails, open reduction will be needed.

PATHOLOGICAL FRACTURES

■ Background

- Pathological fractures are caused by an underlying disease process that weakens the structural integrity of bone.
- Causes can include neoplastic and non neoplastic conditions.
- non neoplastic:
  - □ Infections such as osteomyelitis, metabolic bone disease such as rickets, renal osteodystrophy, hyperparathyroidism, and osteoporosis due to different reasons.

- neoplastic:
  - Malignant tumors including metastatic tumors (such as neuroblastoma), osteosarcoma, wilm's tumor, Ewing sarcoma, leukemias, and lymphomas (Fig 13.14).
  - Non malignant lesions include eosinophilic granuloma, unicameral bone cyst (Fig 16.18), osteochondroma, fibrous dysplasia, chondroblastoma.

- **Evaluation**
  - Evaluation of patients with possible pathological fracture should include the following:
    - Mechanism of injury can help differentiate between traumatic and pathological fractures.
    - The age of the patient can be helpful in determining the most likely cause.
    - The patient's diet, previous medical conditions as well as evaluation for possible abuse can be helpful.
    - Characterization of pain including duration of pain, exacerbating factors as well as inflammatory and neurological signs should be determined.

- **Diagnosis**
  - Labs should include alkaline phosphatase, phosphorous, calcium, PTH, Vitamin D, BUN/Creatinine.
  - Radiographic studies should be obtained. Common radiographic findings may include osteopenia, metaphyseal cupping, presence of solitary or multiple lesions.
  - Bone scan, CT of chest as well as MRI of affected bone can be helpful in determining extent of bone involvement as well as determine possible metastasis.

CLINICAL SCENARIOS

4-year-old boy falls of while playing on to his right arm, the right elbow was swollen bruised and painful. neurovascular exam of the right upper extremity shows absent radial pulse and intact neural exam. Radiographs show supracondylar fracture type III	Brachial artery injury or spasm Urgent orthopedic consult. Urgent reduction and reassess. If no improvement, open exploration
12-year-old boy was hit by a car. He had fracture of the left tibia. Closed reduction and cast was done and patient was discharged home next day. The following day, the child is brought to the emergency department with severe agonizing pain not controlled by hydrocodone. Radiographs did not show change of the fracture from immediate post reduction films.	Compartment syndrome. The cast and all padding should be completely split and skin exposed. Raise the leg to the heart level. If no improvement, urgent orthopedic consult

REFERENCES

Abdelgawad AA, Kanlic EM. Management of children with multiple injuries. J Orthopedic Trauma. 2011; 70(6).1568–74.

Price CT, Flynn JM, Management of fractures. In: Morrissy RT, Weinstein SL, editors. Lovell & Winter's Pediatric Orthopaedics. 6th ed. New York: Lippincott Williams & Wilkins; 2005. p. 1430–1525.

Staheli LT. Trauma. In: Staheli LT, editor. Practice of Pediatric Orthopedics. 2nd ed. New York: Lippincott Williams & Wilkins; 2006.

McCarthy JJ. Musculoskeletal trauma. In: Song KM, editor. Orthopaedic Knowledge Update: Pediatric. 4th ed. Rosemont, IL: American Academy of Orthopedic Surgeons; 2011.

Chapter 17
Approach to a Limping Child

Amr Abdelgawad and Osama Naga

INTRODUCTION

- The "limping child" is a common complaint in the pediatric clinic.
- Various pathologies can cause limping in children.

HISTORY

- ***Classification of limping according to age, chronicity, and pain condition:***

Age-based approach to limping child:

Toddlers (aged 1–3 year)

- Infectious/inflammatory.
  - Transient synovitis.
  - Septic arthritis.
  - Osteomyelitis.
- Trauma.
  - **Toddler's fracture.**
  - Puncture wounds, lacerations.
  - Contusions.
- Neoplasm.

A. Abdelgawad and O. Naga (eds.), *Pediatric Orthopedics*,
DOI: 10.1007/978-1-4614-7126-4_17,

    - Metastasis.
    - Leukemia.

- **Developmental dysplasia of the hips**.
- Neuromuscular disease.
    - **Cerebral palsy**.
    - Spina bifida.
- Leg length discrepancy.
    - Fibular hemimelia.
    - Hemihypertrophy.

Children (aged 4–10 years)

- **Injuries become more common cause of limping**.
    - Fractures.
    - Laceration.
- **Legg-Calve-Perthes disease (LCP).**
- Infections/inflammatory.
    - Transient synovitis becomes more frequent in this age group.
- Rheumatoid conditions.
- Neoplasm.
    - Leukemia.
    - Ewing sarcoma.

Adolescents (older than 11 years)

- **Slipped capital femoral epiphysis** specially in obese adolescents.
- Arthritis.
    - Gonococcal arthritis (among sexually active adolescent).
    - Rheumatologic causes: juvenile arthritis.
- Trauma.
- Leg length discrepancy.

- Post traumatic or post infectious LLD.

- Neoplasm such as osteosarcoma.
- Foot conditions.
  - Tarsal coalition.
  - Sever's disease (see foot chapter).

"Chronicity of symptoms"-based approach to limping child:

Causes of acute limping:

- **Think in infection, inflammation, or trauma**.
- **Less commonly acute neoplasm (e.g., Leukemia)**.
  - **Infection:**
    - Septic arthritis.
    - Osteomyelitis.
    - Lyme disease.
    - Foot infection (ingrowing toenail, puncture wound infection).
  - **Inflammation:**
    - Transient synovitis.
    - Rheumatoid arthritis.
  - **Trauma:**
    - **Most common cause of acute limping**.
    - Absence of history of trauma does not exclude this category (the child could have fallen when no one was watching him).
      - Fractures.
        - Salter Harris type I of the distal fibula is a common injury in young children (equivalent to adult ankle 'anterior talofibular ligament' sprain).
        - Toddler's fracture (see trauma chapter).
      - Contusions of soft tissues.

- Sprain (rare in young children, more common in adolescent).
- Slipped capital femoral epiphysis (acute type).

- **Neoplasm:**
  - Rare cause of acute limping.
  - Leukemia or very aggressive osteosarcoma or aggressive metastasis to bone.

Causes of chronic limping:

- Bony deformity.
  - Limb length discrepancy.
  - Dislocated hip.
- Neuromuscular conditions.
- Chronic vascular condition.
  - Perthes disease.
  - Osteochondritis dessecans of the knee.
  - Kohler's disease.
- Tumor of the bone.
- Chronic painful conditions: e.g., Tarsal coalition.
- Chronic slipped capital femoral epiphysis.

"Pain-based" approach for limping:

- **Most causes of limping are painful**.
- Painful causes will lead to antalgic gait (see later).

Non painful limping:

- Hip Dysplasia.
- Limp length discrepancy.
- Neuromuscular causes of limping.

Management:

Ask the family about:

- **History of trauma**.
- **Fever, chills, or other constitutional** symptoms.
  - Infections.
  - Malignancies.
  - Rheumatologic conditions.
- **History of travel**.
  - Lyme disease.
- **A history of upper respiratory tract infectious symptoms**.
  - Transient synovitis may occur after recent URI.
  - Post-streptococcal reactive arthritis may occur after streptococcal pharyngitis.
- **History of increased activity**.
  - Stress fracture.

Examination:

Assessment of the child gait.

- The child is asked to walk for about 30 ft.
- The young patient who is reluctant or refusing to walk may be encouraged by having the parent or caregiver stand on the opposite side of the room.
- Abnormal gaits.
  - **Antalgic (Painful) gait.**
    - The child tries to decrease the stance phase (the phase that the child has the foot on the floor) of the affected side because of the pain that occur with bearing weight on that side.
    - It occurs with any painful condition.

- **Trendelenburg (waddling) gait**
  - The child leans toward the involved extremity during the stance phase.
  - Indicates underlying proximal muscle weakness or hip instability.
  - The stance phase is equal between involved and uninvolved sides.
  - Pathophysiology.
    - The hip abductor muscles are not able to support the body weight during the stance phase when the center of the gravity is in the midline between two sides.
    - The trunk swings over the affected leg during the stance phase to decreased the distance between the center of gravity and the affected hip, hence decreasing the required work needed from the abductor muscle.
    - If the condition is bilateral, the trunk swings from side to side.
- **The toe-walking gait**
  - See causes of toe walking in foot chapter.

- **Orthopedic examination:**
  - Examination of the hips, knees and ankles.
    - Range of motion, tenderness, deformity.
  - Examination of the back.
    - Tenderness (fracture or infection).
    - Signs of spina bifida (patchy hair, dimple).

Neurologic examination:

- **Detailed assessment of the following:**
  - Motor function.
  - Sensation.
  - Deep tendon reflexes.
  - Signs of myopathy (Gower's sign).

General examination:

- To identify general manifestations of causes of limping e.g.:
  - General signs of infection.
  - General sings of rheumatologic condition.

Imaging:

Plain radiograph

- **Radiographs of the affected part.**
- If radiograph is normal but the patient is having persistent pain or symptoms, proceed with other imaging studies.

MRI

- MRI is the imaging modality of choice for soft tissue involvement.
- It is sensitive modality for
  - Suspected infections or tumors.
  - Stress fracture.

CT scan

- It provides a detailed visualization of bony anatomy.

Bone scan

- Sensitive for identification of:
  - **Infections.**
    - Early septic arthritis.
    - Osteomyelitis.
    - Discitis.
  - Avascular necrosis of the hip.
  - Tumors (especially **osteoid osteoma**).
  - Stress fractures (MRI is currently used more often for this indication).

Ultrasound

- Indications.

- Joint effusion (especially for the hip joint).
- Suspected foreign body in muscles or sole of the foot.
- Abscess.

Laboratory

Labs are occasionally necessary for evaluation of a child with musculoskeletal disorder

- Markers of infection:
  - CBC with differential count.
  - ESR, and C-reactive protein.
- Labs specific for each disease: e.g.,
  - Lyme disease.
  - Rheumatologic condition.
  - Rheumatic fever.

Treatment:

- Depends on the specific cause of limping.

REFERENCES

Leet AI, Skaggs DL. Evaluation of the acutely limping child. Am Fam Physician. 2000;61(4):1011–8.

Sawyer JR, Kapoor M. The limping child: a systematic approach to diagnosis. Am Fam Physician. 2009;79(3):215–24.

Leung AK, Lemay JF. The limping child. J Pediatr Health Care. 2004;18(5):219–223.

Chapter 18
Casts, Splints, and Braces

Amr Abdelgawad and Osama Naga

CASTS AND SPLINTS

Definition:

- Methods to achieve immobilization of the extremity.
- **Difference between cast and splint:**
  - **The cast:** the casting material is applied all around the extremity (Fig. 18.1).
  - **The splint:** the casting material is applied as a slab on one side of the extremity and then wrapped around the extremity by elastic bandage (Fig. 18.2).
- Choice of splint versus cast depends on multiple variables:
  - Expected swelling: if marked swelling is expected, splint is preferred as it allows more expansion and can accommodate more swelling.
  - Required stability: cast gives more stability than splint.
  - Experience of physician: **for non-experienced physician: splint is a safer option**

Casting material:

- There are two main types of casting material (plaster of Paris (Figs. 18.1 and 18.2) and fiberglass (Fig. 18.3). see Table 18.1.

Indications:

Casts and splints are used to

- Immobilize the extremity e.g.:

A. Abdelgawad and O. Naga (eds.), *Pediatric Orthopedics*,
DOI: 10.1007/978-1-4614-7126-4_18,

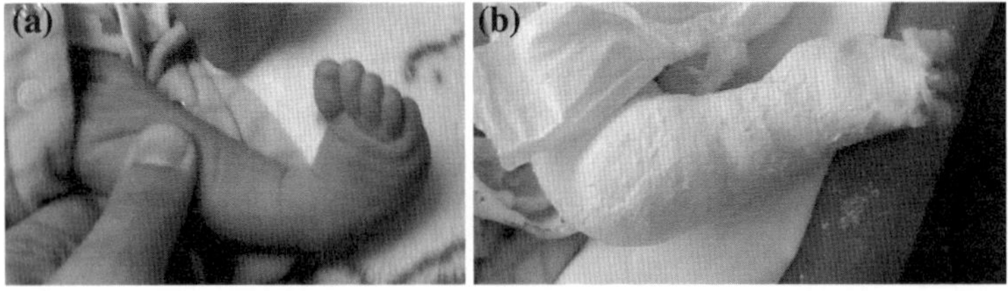

Fig. 18.1 Cast. First cast for Club foot **a**. **b** The casting material is applied all around limb. Plaster of Paris had been used in this case to allow for molding of the cast

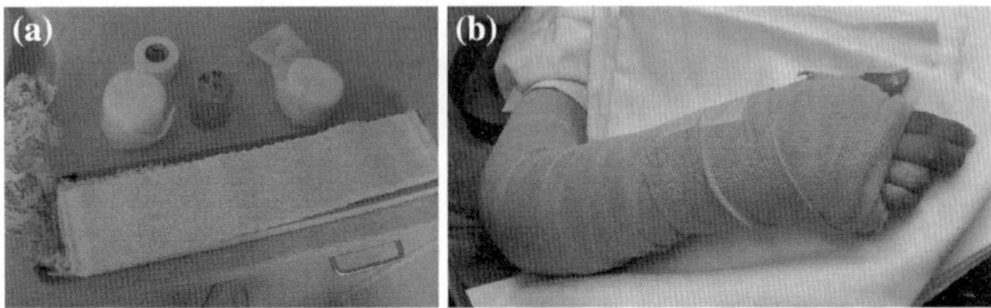

Fig. 18.2 **a** Splint. **b** The slab is applied to one side and wrapped around with bandage

TABLE 18.1 TWO MAIN TYPES OF CASTING MATERIAL

Plaster of Paris	Fiberglass
Heavier	Lighter in weight
Non-water proof	Water-proof
Can be molded easily	Harder to mold
Takes longer time to harden	Takes less time to harden.

- Factures
- Dislocation
- Sprain
- After orthopedic operation.

- Correction of deformity:
  - Serial casting is applied to obtain gradual correction of the deformity (e.g., Ponseti casting of club foot)

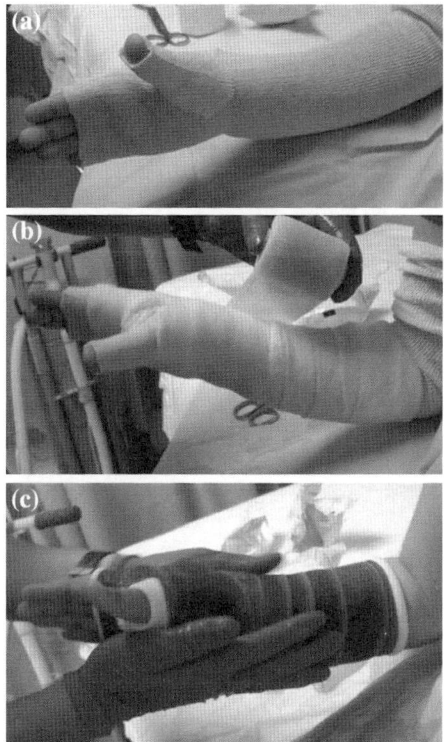

Fig. 18.3 Application of a cast. **a** Stockinet is applied to the extremity, followed by cotton padding. **b** Then the rolls of cast are wetted and applied. The stockinet is reflected to avoid sharp edge of the cast. **c** A color 'of patient choice' is added and molding is done

Technique of application:

- To immobilize part of a limb, the cast and/or the splint should extend across the joints above and below that segment (Fig. 18.3).
    - E.g., Fracture of both bones of the forearm needs a cast or splint that crosses the elbow and the wrist.
- Reduction (if needed) is obtained first.

- Adequate padding (cotton rolls) of all bony prominences is applied.
  - Inadequate padding can lead to pressure necrosis.
- The casting material is wetted to allow it to start the chemical reaction for hardening.
  - Cast is wetted by as rolls
  - Splint is wetted as a slab
- While the casting material is still malleable, apply it to the extremity, then perform the molding.
- **The neurologic and vascular condition of the limb must be examined and documented before and after cast application**.
- Radiographs should be obtained after cast application (if reduction was performed) to ensure and document proper reduction.

Pitfalls of applying cast/splint:

- Too loose: will not give adequate support
- Too tight: can cause swelling, possible compartment syndrome
- Too short (does not cross the joint above): will not give adequate support

Instruction given to families when their children have casts/splints:

- Keep the limb elevated for the first 48 h.
- Keep the cast clean, avoid playing in the dirt.
- Keep the cast dry
  - The only cast that can become wet is fiberglass cast with waterproof inner padding (not commonly used).
  - Wrap the cast with water tight bag before giving shower, or use sponge bath.
- Avoid inserting any object inside the cast
- Not allowing the child to use a ruler or other object to scratch his skin

- Use proper precaution when transporting a child with spica cast by a car: a special car seat able to safely accommodate the child is needed.
    - Please refer to AAP website for current recommendations for the most recent available car seats that can be used with spica cast.

Management of common cast complications

Itching:

- Antihistamines.
- Hitting or rubbing the outside of the cast.
- Spray the talc down the cast.
- Avoid warm areas (more sweating will cause more itching).
- Directing the hair dryer on the cold mode to the opening of the cast.
- **Never to do:**
    - Scratch with a pin or ruler or a knitting needles.

Foreign material accidentally disappears inside the cast:

- Foreign objects can fall inside the cast (usually while the child was using them to scratch his skin), example include: pens, erasers, rulers
- **Management:**
- It is recommended not to leave the objects inside the cast as it may cause pressure necrosis and result in ulcers of the skin
- Orthopedic referral:
    - Changing the cast
    - Removal of the object through a window in the cast.

Tight cast:

- If the cast is tight, it can cause swelling and possible compartment syndrome which can cause permanent damage
- The signs of a tight cast, i.e., the four Ps of ischemia:
    - Pain
    - Pallor

- Paresthesias
- Paralysis or paresis

▪ Management:

- **This is an urgent condition (refer to Emergency room or immediately available orthopedic clinic)**
- The cast has to be split completely, including the padding (making sure that the cast and all padding had been cut and widely separated).

Wet cast/splints:

▪ Happens if children jump in the water (pool/sea/under the shower)
▪ The only cast that can become wet is fiberglass cast with waterproof inner padding (not commonly used).

Management:

- If the cast/splint is only mildly wet: use the hair dryer on the cold mode to dry it.
- If the cast/splint is very wet (soaked): the cast has to be changed.

Removal of the cast:

▪ With special cast cutters. They look like rotating saws but they oscillate (not rotate).
▪ The blade is advanced all the way though the cast material until there is loss of resistance**, then it is pulled out from the cast** and moved to the adjacent area and pushed down again.
▪ Do not advance the cast while it is touching patient skin or through the casting material.
▪ Injury from removal of the cast occurs mainly due to thermal injury (burn) from the hot blade and not from the blade cutting the skin (Fig. 18.4).
▪ How to avoid burns from cast removal:

- Well-padded casts to protect the skin from the blade.
- Using cast saw with built in fan
- Cooling the blade frequently during cutting by a wet cloth.

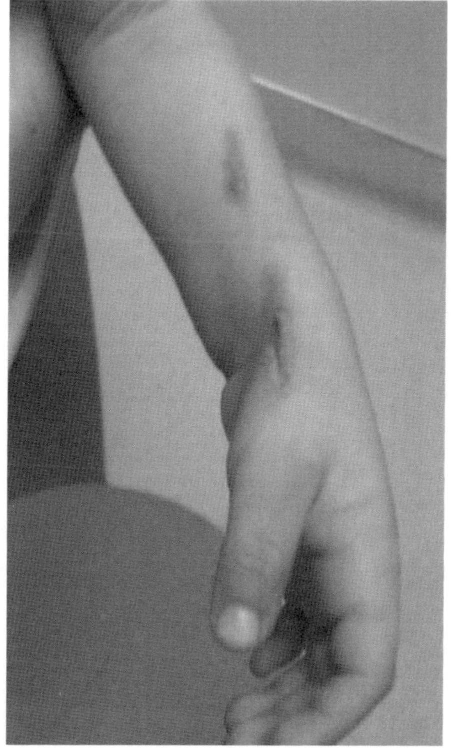

Fig. 18.4 Cast burn. A 6-year old boy who had burns of the hand while removing the cast

BRACES (ORTHOSIS)

Definition:

- Removable splints that are applied to different regions of the body for support or prevention of deformity.
- They are usually fabricated from materials that are light and can tolerate high stresses (e.g., carbon fiber).
- They can be 'over the shelf (pre fabricated)' or custom made.

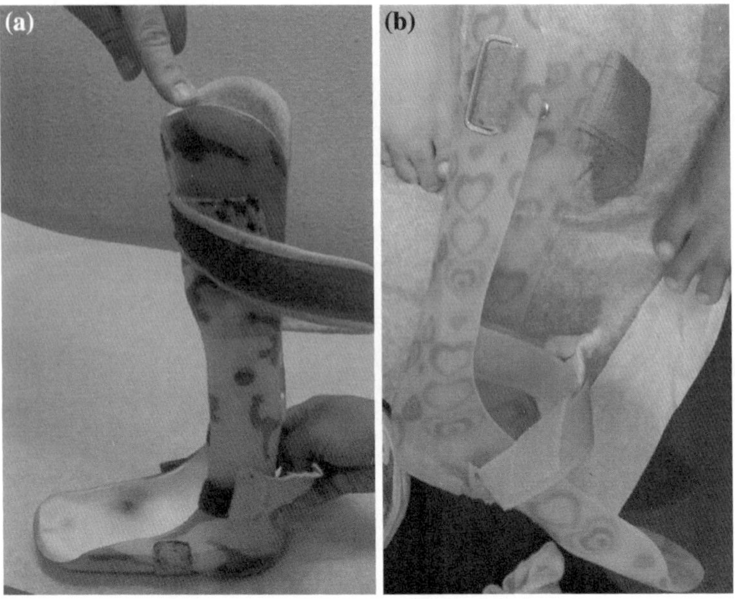

Fig. 18.5 **a** and **b**. Different types and shapes of AFO

Types:

- The braces are usually named according to the part of the body to which they are applied to:
- Commonly used braces:

Ankle foot orthosis (AFO)

- Used to control foot and ankle position and prevent development of deformity (especially ankle equines) (Fig. 18.5).
- **One of the commonest used braces in pediatric population**.
- Can be rigid brace (does not allow any ankle movement) or hinged
    - The hinge will allow movement in one direction (dorsiflexion) and lock the movement of the other direction (plantar flexion) to prevent development of equines while allowing for range of motion of the ankle.

Knee ankle foot orthosis (KAFO)

- Used to control foot, ankle, and knee position.
- Commonly used with spina bifida patients who do not have good control on their quadriceps muscle to help them with controlling the knee joint during gait.

Foot Abduction Orthosis:

- Used after casting in cases of Club foot (Fig. 8.17/foot).

Spinal brace:

- Used to prevent progression of scoliosis (see spine chapter).

REFERENCES

Grant AD, Amir A. Casts. In Staheli LT, Song KM, editors. Secrets of Pediatric Orthopedic. 3rd ed. Philadelphia: Mosby Elsevier; 2007. p. 69–73.

Fisk JR, Supan TJ. Orthoses (Braces and Splints). Staheli LT, Song KM, editors. Secrets of Pediatric Orthopedic. 3rd ed. Philadelphia: Mosby Elsevier; 2007. p. 74–76.

Chapter 19
Pediatric Spine

Amr Abdelgawad and Osama Naga

GROWTH AND DEVELOPMENT OF SPINE

- There are two periods of rapid growth of the spine:
  - The first 5 years in life (about 1.4 cm/year).
  - From the age of 10 years until skeletal maturity (about 1.2 cm/year).
- From 5–10 years old the growth of spine is slowed down (about 0.6 cm/year).

Lung development:

- In the first 8 years of life: the lung develops by increasing the number of alveoli (hyperplasia).
- From 8 to 15 years of age: the lung develops by increasing the size of alveoli (hypertrophy).
- The lung size at the age of 10 years is half its adult size.
- **Early fusion surgery before the age of 9 years will result in poor pulmonary functions later on life.**

Deformity of the spine:

The deformity of the spine can be in the coronal plane (scoliosis) or the sagittal plane (exaggerated kyphosis or lordosis).

A. Abdelgawad and O. Naga (eds.), *Pediatric Orthopedics*,
DOI: 10.1007/978-1-4614-7126-4_19,

SCOLIOSIS

Definition:

- **Lateral** curvature of the spine associated with a rotational element.

Types of scoliosis:

- **Congenital:**
  - Due to **bony deformity** (vertebral column or chest wall) (Fig. 19.1).
- **Neuromuscular:**
  - Due to neuromuscular causes (e.g., cerebral palsy, high level spina bifida, traumatic spinal cord injury, muscular dystrophies) (Figs. 19.2 and 19.3).
- **Syndromic:**
  - Almost all syndromes can be associated with scoliosis (e.g., dysplasias, connective tissue disorders e.g., Marfan syndrome, osteogenesis imerfecta, Prader Willi syndrome, Neurofibromatosis) (Figs. 4.4 and 4.5 in general).
- **Idiopathic:**
  - **Most common cause of scoliosis.**
  - No underlying cause can be identified.

The idiopathic scoliosis is further classified according to the age of onset into:

- **Infantile:** the scoliosis starts in the first 2 years of life (Fig. 19.4).
- **Juvenile:** the scoliosis starts between 3 and 9 years old.
- **Adolescent:** the scoliosis starts at or after the age of 10 years. It is the **most common type** (Fig. 19.5).

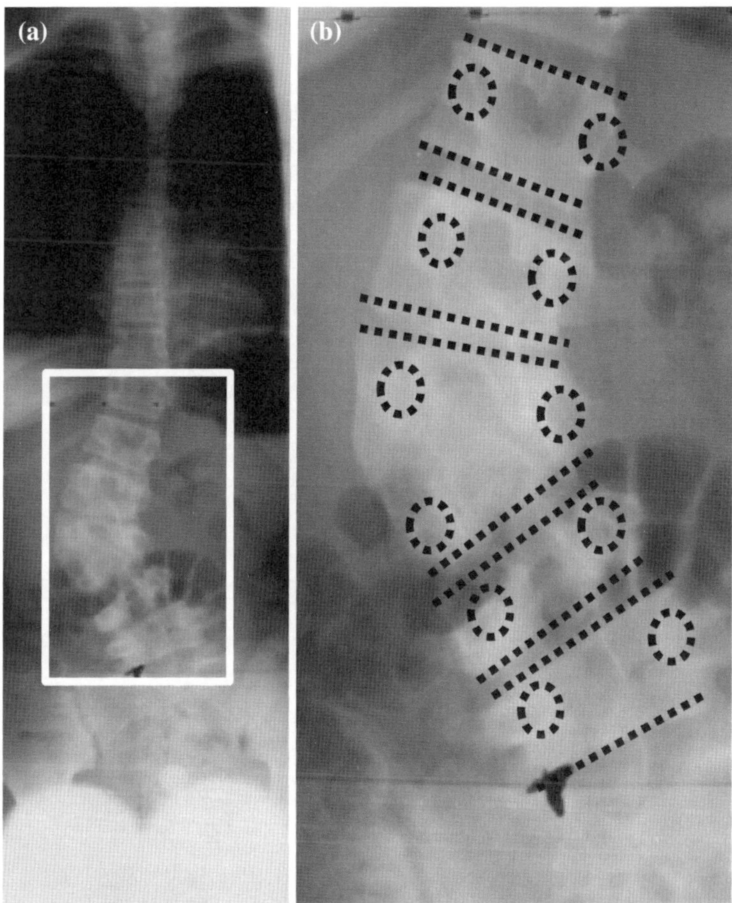

Fig. 19.1 Congenital scoliosis. **a** A 13-year-old girl with congenital scoliosis due to fused hemi-vertebra. **b** Magnified view of the curve shows each vertebra has two pedicles except the block vertebra at the apex of the curve which has 2 pedicle (*dotted circles*) on the convex side and one pedicle on the concave side. This indicates the presence of hemi-vertebra on the convex side that had created the curve

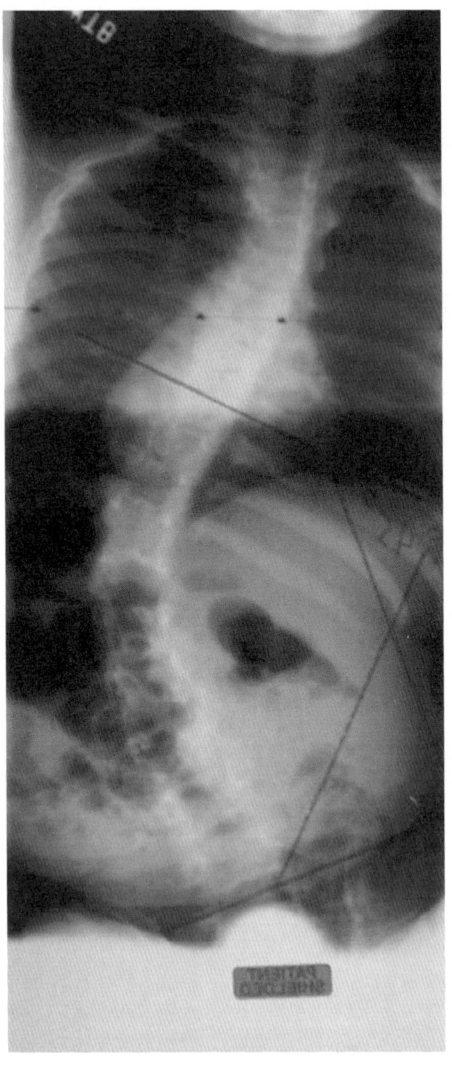

Fig. 19.2 An 8-year-old girl who had motor vehicle collision 3 years earlier which resulted in complete spinal cord lesion at the level of T6. Patient has now 42° thoraco-lumbar curve distal to the injury level

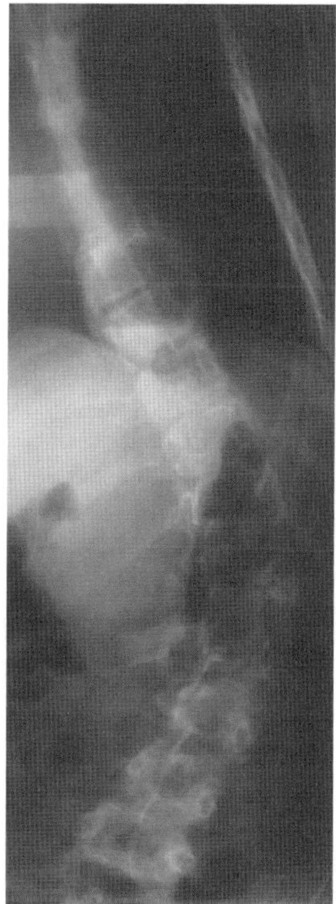

Fig. 19.3 Neuromuscular scoliosis. A 13-year-old boy with quadriplegic cerebral palsy. Patient has long C-shaped scoliosis of the thoraco-lumbar spine

ADOLESCENT IDIOPATHIC SCOLIOSIS

Incidence:

- The condition is more common in girls.
- For curves more than 40°, **girls to boys is 10:1**.

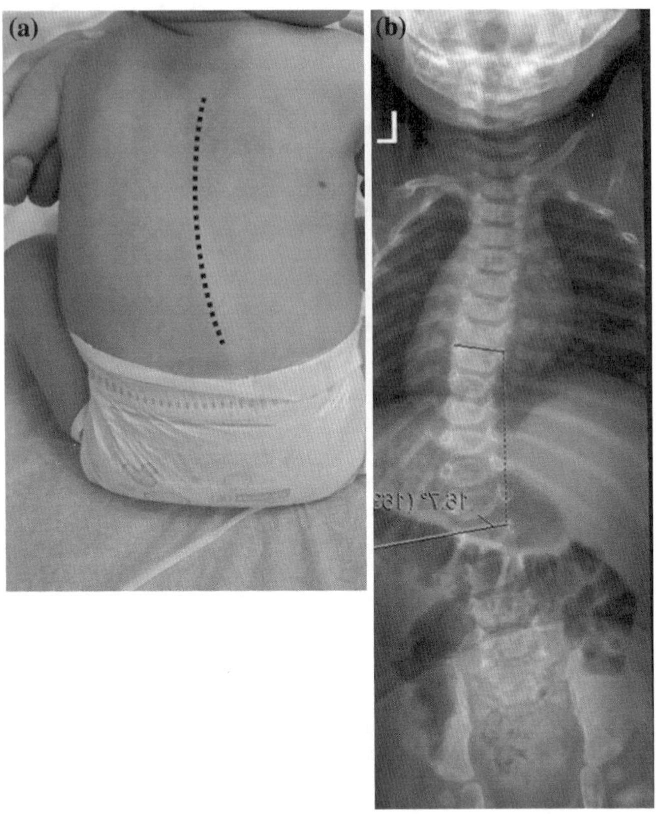

Fig. 19.4 Infantile idiopathic scoliosis. **a** An otherwise healthy 6-month-old boy with scoliosis. **b** Radiograph does not show any bony anomaly. Because of absence of any identifiable cause, this scoliosis is considered idiopathic

- The condition runs in families (genetic predisposition).

Natural progression of adolescent idiopathic scoliosis:

- The curve continues to progress as long as the child is growing.
- At the end of skeletal growth, most curves will stop progression

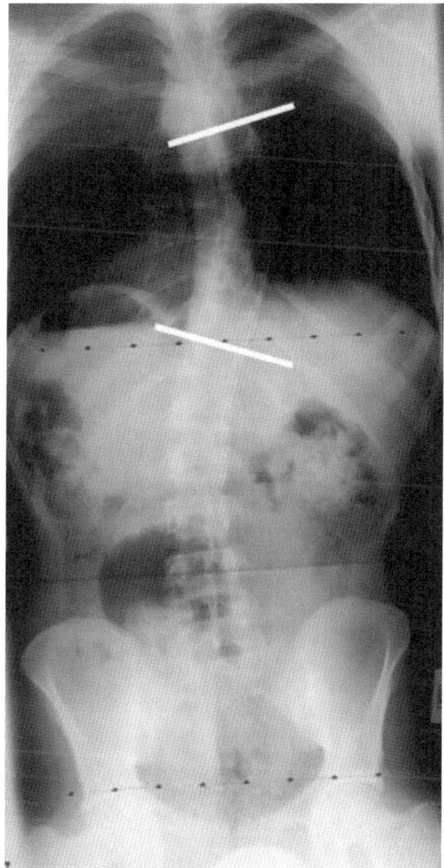

Fig. 19.5 Adolescent idiopathic scoliosis. A 13-year-old girl with mid thoracic curve and no other identifiable cause

- Large curves (thoracic curves more than 50° or lumbar curves more than 35°) may continue to progress even after skeletal maturity.
- The curve of the AIS progress maximally in the period of **"peak height velocity" or "rapid growth phase"**.

- **The rapid growth phase can be identified by:**
  - One year before menarche age in girls.
  - Open tri-radiate cartilage
  - Risser Stage 0 (see later)
- **How to know that the child reached skeletal maturity:**
  - History: 2 years after menarche
  - Radiographs: Risser stage 5
- Careful screening of girls around the age of menarche is very crucial to detect the condition.

Clinical picture:

- The condition is usually **asymptomatic**. This makes the annual screening vital to detect the condition.
- With advanced deformity:
  - Unequal shoulder level.
  - Unequal breast sizes.
  - Leaning towards one side.
- **Pain is NOT a symptom of AIS. If there is pain, MRI is recommended.**

Physical exam:

- Adam forward bending test (Fig. 19.6) will show thoracic hump.
- Thorough neurological exam:
  - Motor, sensory, and reflexes of the lower extremity are normal in AIS.
  - Superficial abdominal reflexes are normal
- Scoliometer (Fig. 19.7):
  - A leveling assessment device used to subjectively assess if one side of the body is higher than the other side with forward bending.

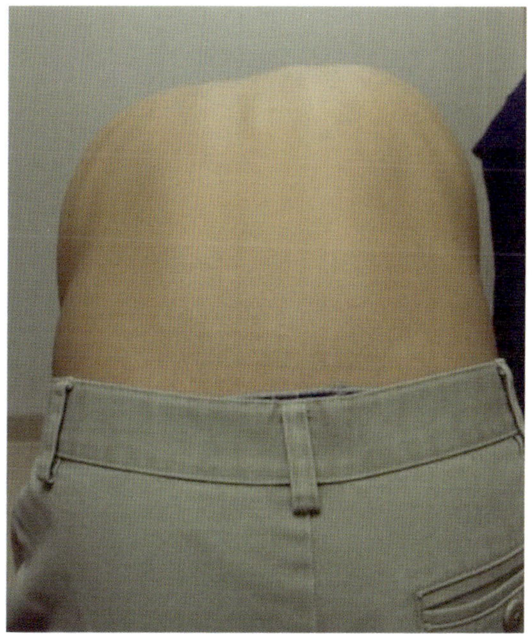

Fig. 19.6 Adam forward bending test. A 14-year-old boy (seen from the back) with right thoracic 'hump' when pending forward

- It assesses the rotational part of the scoliosis (not lateral curvature)
- **7° in rotation by scoliometer is the indication for referral to orthopedic surgeon.**

Radiographs:

- The radiographs are better to be posterior–anterior radiographs and not anteroposterior to decrease the amount of irradiation to the breast tissue (these girls will have repeated radiographs during their growth and all efforts should be done to decrease the amount of irradiation to their breasts to decrease the incidence of breast cancer).

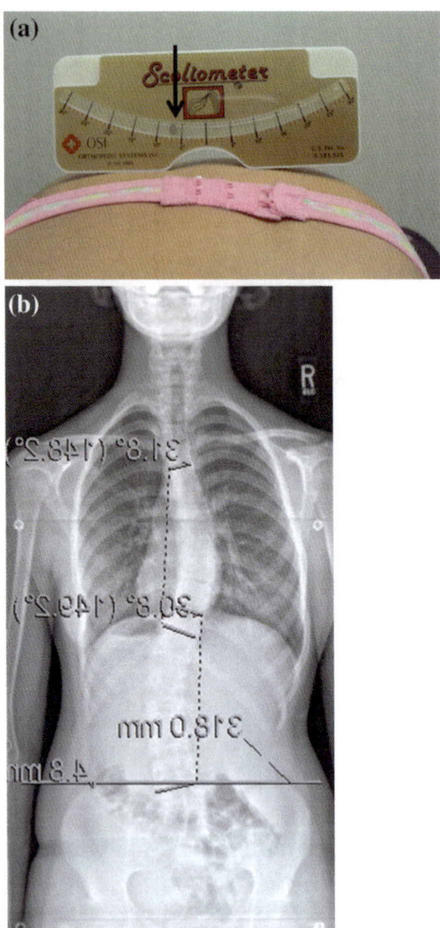

Fig. 19.7 Scoliometer. A 14-year-old girl with adolescent idiopathic scoliosis. **a** Scoliometer shows 7° of unleveling (*arrow*). **b** Radiograph shows 31° of mid thoracic level

- The following is assessed in the radiographs:
    - Cobb's angle.
    - Skeletal maturity (Risser Stage and tri-radiate cartilage).

- Direction of the curve.

- The curve of the scoliosis is measured with **Cobb angle** (Fig. 19.8).
- Cobb angle is the angle between the superior end plate of the most tilted upper vertebral and the inferior end plates of the most tilted lower vertebrae.
- **How to draw the Cobb angle:** see Fig. 19.8.
- **The diagnosis of scoliosis**: the Cobb angle has to be greater than 10°.

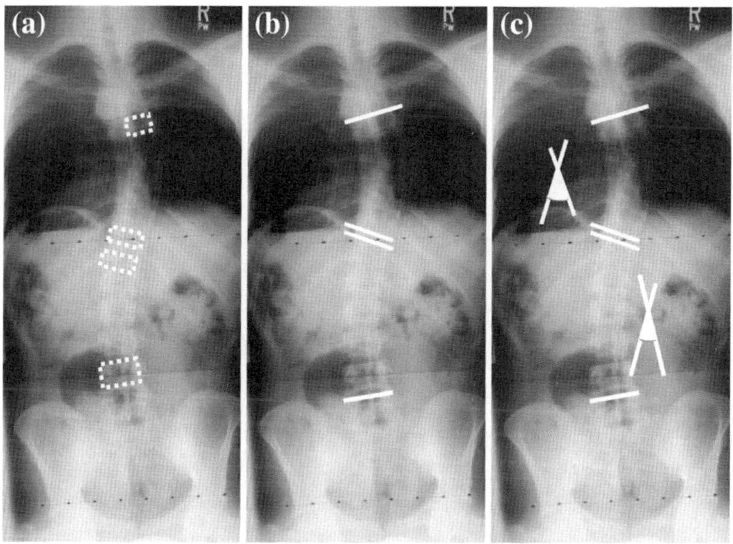

Fig. 19.8 How to draw the Cobb angle. First, for each curve (thoracic and lumbar) decide which is the most tilted upper vertebra and most tilted lower vertebra (eyeballing) (**a**). Second, draw a line across the upper end of the most tilted upper vertebra and the lower border of the most tilted lower vertebra, and draw perpendicular line to these lines [(**b**) repeat that for each curve]. Measure the angle between the two perpendicular lines (**c**). For electronic digital radiographs (e.g., PACS), there is no need to draw perpendicular line as the angles can be measured once the lines are drawn on the upper and lower most tilted vertebra

- **The direction of the curve** is the direction of the convexity (Right sided curve means that the convexity of the curve is towards the right).
- The typical curve of AIS is **right thoracic** curve.
- **Risser stage:**
    - Indicates the stage of skeletal maturity (Fig. 19.9).
    - It depends on the ossification of the iliac apophysis which proceeds from lateral to medial.
    - Fusion of the growth plate will indicate skeletal maturity (Risser stage 5).
    - Risser stages 4 and 5 indicate being close to full skeletal maturity (less chance of curve progression).
- **Tri radiate Cartilage:**
    - Open tri radiate cartilage (in the floor of the acetabulum) indicated that the child still has to go through his/her rapid growth phase (not close to skeletal maturity) which carries more risk of progression of the curve.

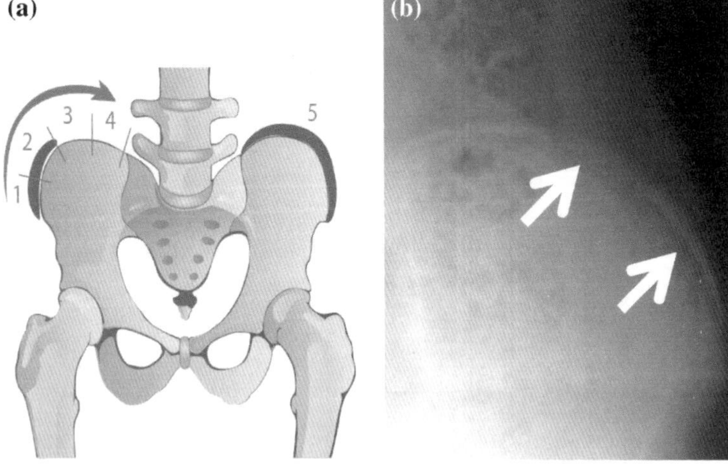

Fig. 19.9 Risser sign. Fusion of the iliac apophysis proceeds from lateral to medial. Complete fusion indicates Risser stage 5. Radiographs shows Risser stage 4 (the apophysis is ossified from medial to lateral but still not fused with the iliac bone (*arrows* pointing to the open growth plate)

Indication for referral to orthopedic surgeon:

- For curves more than 20°.

Indication for obtaining MRI for patient with AIS:

- Pain
- Left thoracic curves
- Abnormal neurological exam
- Infantile and Juvenile scoliosis (curves which develop before the age of 10 years old) (due to high incidence of intrathecal anomalies, e.g., syringomyelia)

Treatment of AIS:

- Follow up for curves less than 25 degrees.
- **Bracing is indicated if there is:**
    - Patients with significant skeletal growth remaining (Risser stage 0, 1, and 2) **and** the following curves:
        - More than 5° of progression (e.g., curve progressed from 18° to 24°)
        - Curves more than 25°.
- Surgery is indicated for:
    - Thoracic curves of more than 50° in skeletally mature children (Risser stage 5) or
    - Thoracic Curves of more than 45° in skeletally immature children (Risser stage 1, 2).
- The standard surgery for scoliosis is fusion of the spine (the vertebrae of the curve are converted to one solid bony mass) to prevent further progression of the disease.

CONGENITAL SCOLIOSIS

- **Definition:**
    - Scoliosis due to bony anomaly of the vertebral column or chest wall (Fig. 19.1).

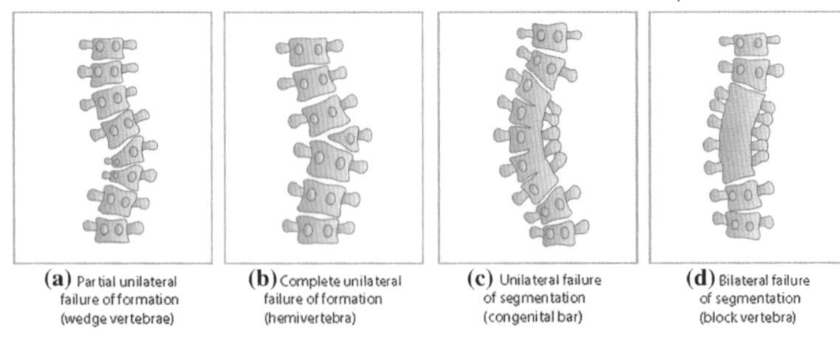

Fig. 19.10 Different pathologies of congenital scoliosis

- **Pathology:**
  - Different vertebral anomalies can lead to scoliosis (Fig. 19.10).
  - Most of the these cases are balanced curves (e.g., two hemi vertebra in the contra lateral sides balancing each other).
  - The progression is maximum if there is a **fully segmented hemivertebra on one side with contra lateral bar on the other side**.
  - Rib fusion on one side will cause the spine to be concave on that side.
  - Congenital scoliosis is associated with other congenital anomalies in more than 50 % of individuals e.g., heart and kidney. Adequate assessment of these systems is required for children presenting with congenital scoliosis.
- **Treatment:**
  - Orthopedic referral if the condition is progressive (or predicted to be progressive e.g., in case of segmented hemivertebra with contra lateral bar).

THORACIC INSUFFICIENCY SYNDROME

Definition:

- A condition in which the thoracic cage cannot support the lung function. The chest volume is highly restricted in these cases.

Cause:

- Early fusion surgery.
  - When part of the spine is fused, it does not grow any more. If the fusion surgery is done in the spine early in life (before 8 years old), the thoracic volume will be restricted.
- Congenital e.g.,
  - Jarcho-Levin Syndrome (bilateral rib fusion and spine shortening.
- Rib fusion (congenital or post surgery).

EARLY ONSET SCOLIOSIS

Definition:

- Any type of scoliosis (congenital, neuromuscular, idiopathic, syndromic) that develop early in life (before the age of 8 years old) (see lung development).
- MRI is usually indicated in congenital and idiopathic cases due to high incidence of intrathecal anomalies (e.g., syringomyelia)
- All efforts are done to delay fusion surgery in these patients as this will lead to thoracic insufficiency syndrome.
  - New 'fusionless' techniques have been developed recently (e.g., growing rods or casting (Fig. 19.11)

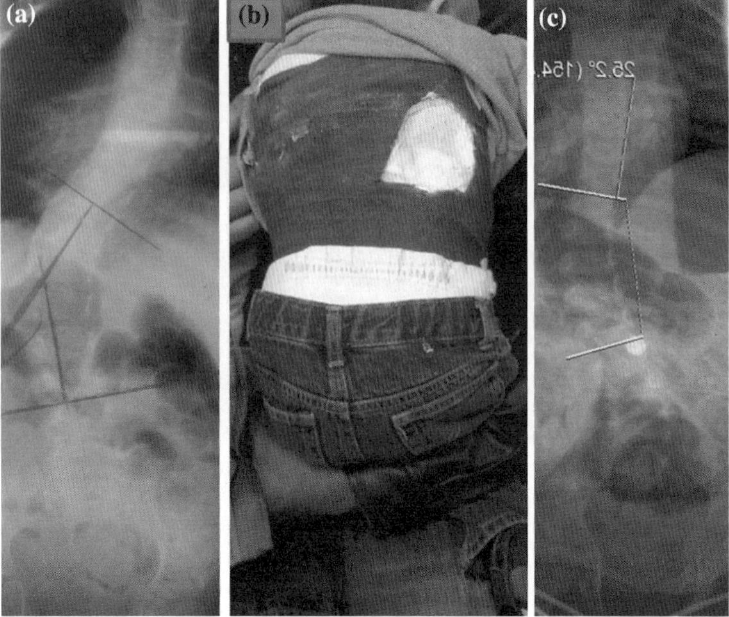

Fig. 19.11 Casting for early onset scoliosis. **a** A 2 year-old boy with infantile idiopathic scoliosis that had been progressing over one year (from 30° at the age of one year to 48° at the age of two years). **b** Casting of the trunk was done to control the curve while allowing the child to grow. **c** The cast controlled the curve to 25°

KYPHOSIS

Definition:

- Increase in the sagittal (lateral) convexity of the spine more than the normal values.
- Normal thoracic spine lateral curvature (kyphosis) is 30–45°.

Causes of Kyphosis:

- Postural kyphosis.

- Scheueremann Kyphosis: The most common cause of pathological kyphosis.
- Congenital kyphosis (wedge vertebra).
- Infection (TB spine).
- Trauma (compression fracture).

POSTURAL KYPHOSIS

Definition:

- Flexible kyphosis that is related to the posture that the child acquires during various positions (setting, standing, or walking).

Clinical presentation:

- Mild kyphosis with no sharp angle.
- The curve is easily corrected with pulling the shoulder back or lying prone.

Radiographs:

- No anterior wedging or end plate irregularities (characteristics of Scheuermann kyphosis).

Management:

- Physical therapy and postural exercises.

SCHEUEREMANN KYPHOSIS

Definition:

- Juvenile developmental disease with increase thoracic or thoraco-lumbar kyphosis due to **structural** deformity of the spine with increased anterior wedging of the vertebrae.

Pathology:

- Osteochondritis of the growth plate of the vertebra. This will cause abnormal growth of the vertebra with anterior wedging.
- Usually in adolescent boys.

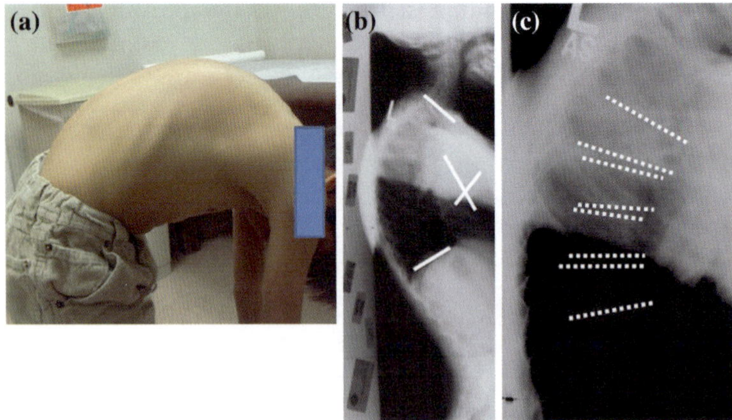

Fig. 19.12 Scheuermann Kyphosis. **a** A 14 year-old boy with increased thoracic kyphosis. **b** Lateral thoracic radiograph shows thoracic kyphosis between T1 and T12 67°. **c** Close view of the vertebrae shows anterior wedging of the vertebra (anterior part of the vertebra narrower than the posterior part). The vertebral end plates are outlined by the dotted lines.

Clinical presentation:

- Deformity (bent back deformity) (Fig. 19.12)
- The deformity is **fixed and cannot be corrected by straightening the back** (in contrast to postural kyphosis).
- Sometimes, the condition is associated with mid-back pain (50 % of patients).
- On exam: increased thoracic hump with forward bending.
- Neurological exam of the lower extremity: usually normal (rarely with advancing disease neurological deficits can occur in lower extremities).

Lateral radiograph of the spine shows:

- **For the diagnosis of Scheuermann kyphosis: presence of 3 consecutive vertebrae with more than 5° anterior wedging** (Fig. 19.12).

- **Anterior wedging** of the vertebra (anterior part of the vertebra is narrower than the posterior part).
- Increase thoracic kyphosis more than 50°.
- Narrowing of the disk space.
- Schmorl nodes, which is a herniation of the disk material (nucleus pulposus) in the body of the vertebrae.

Treatment:

- Physical therapy:
    - Aggressive thoracic extensor strengthening and hamstring stretching exercises.
- Referral for orthopedics:
    - Bracing for curves less than 70 degree if the child still has more than 2 years of skeletal growth
    - For curves more than 70 degrees: possible surgical treatment to correct the deformity. Most important surgical indication is unacceptable esthetic appearance. Persistence back pain and neurological manifestation are other indications for surgery.

INFECTION OF THE SPINE

Definitions:

- **Diskitis**:
    - Inflammation of the intervertebral disk usually seen in toddlers.
    - The most common location is lumbar vertebrae
- **Vertebral body osteomyelitis:**
    - Inflammation of vertebral body.
    - Usually starts at the vertebral end plates

- **The distinction between diskitis and vertebral osteomyelitis is hard** and most cases will have some affection of both the inter-vertebral disk and the vertebral body.

Etiology:

- Hematogenous spread
- ***Staphylococcus aureus*** **is the most common organism isolated**
- Other organisms include: *Kingella kingae, group A streptococcus, and E Coli*

Clinical presentation:

- Limping
- Back pain
- Refusal to walk
- Most patients will have mild or no fever
- Spinal motion is voluntarily reduced to alleviate the pain
    - Paraspinal muscle spasm is common
    - Flexion of the spine compresses the anterior element and causes discomfort (*the child will refuse to pick up an object from the ground)*
- Older children might have **fever and abdominal pain**

Laboratory:

- Complete blood count may remain normal
- ESR and CRP are usually elevated.
- Blood cultures.
- Image guided biopsy from the affected area.

Radiographs:

- A PA and lateral radiograph of the thoracolumbar spine is the first image to be ordered when the condition is suspected (Fig. 19.13).
- Characteristic finding; often takes 2-3 weeks to show these changes:
    - Narrowing of the disk space
    - Irregularities of the adjacent vertebral end plates

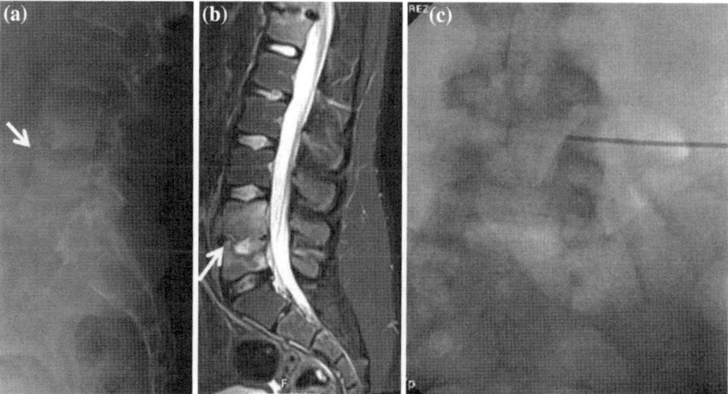

Fig. 19.13 A 12-year-old boy with 3 months history of back pain, patient has been treated for 'mechanical back pain.' **a** Radiographs showed severe narrowing of the L4–L5 intervertebral disk with irregularities of the adjacent vertebral end plates. **b** MRI showed destruction of intervertebral disk at the L4–L5 level and increased T2 signal within the L4–L5 vertebral segments. **c** Fluoroscopic guided specimen for culture was done that resulted in growth of *S aureus*

- Osteopenia.

- Technetium bone scan:
  - Hot spot in the affected disk

MRI:

- Most sensitive imaging study (Fig. 19.13).
- Becomes positive early in the disease process (in contrast to plain radiograph).
- Can identify abscess formation (which is an indication of surgical interference).

Treatment:

- Start antibiotics covering for *Staph Aureus*.
- Length of therapy is 4–6 weeks.
- 1–2 weeks of IV antibiotics, followed by oral antibiotic.
- The treatment protocol varies according the response (clinical response and ESR).

- Rest, analgesic, and immobilization in spinal orthosis.
- Surgical treatment is rarely required.
  - Indications are:
    - No improvement after appropriate antibiotic treatment.
    - Abscess formation.
    - Marked deformity (kyphosis)

SPONDYLOLYSIS AND SPONDYLOLISTHESIS

SPONDYLOLYSIS

Definitions:

Spondylolysis is a bone defect in pars interarticularis of the vertebra (Fig. 19.14).

Pathology and incidence:

- This condition may represent stress fractures, associated with sports that involve repeated extension position of the spine (football, gymnastics, and divers).
- The condition is present in about 7 % in adolescents and up to 20 % in participants of sports that involve repeated extension of the back.
- Most common in Alaskan Eskimos males (50 %).
- The condition is asymptomatic in the majority of cases.
- It is the most common cause of nonmuscluar back pain in adolescents.
- Most commonly affected vertebra is L5, less common in L4.

Clinical presentation:

- Patient will complain of low back pain that increase with extension of the spine during sports activity.
- Limited flexion of the lumbar spine.
- Extension of the spine will cause severe back pain in the lower lumbar area radiating to the back of the thighs.

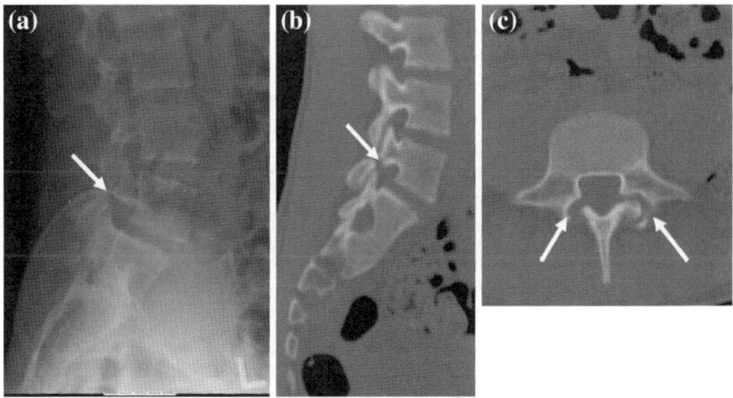

Fig. 19.14 A 14-year-old boy complains of low back pain. a and **b** Radiograph shows defect of L5 pars interartcularis (compare L5 with L4). **c** CT scan shows the defect more precisely (*arrows*)

- Straight leg raising test: pain in the posterior thigh, but usually does not extend distal to the knee (hamstring tightness).

Imaging:

- Spondylolysis can be found in the radiograph as an accidental finding.
- The defect can be seen in the lateral view of the lumbar spine but it is more obvious in the oblique view (Scotty dog with a collar appearance) (Figs. 19.14 and 19.15).
- Chronic lesion usually shows osteolysis around the defect. Acute lesion will have sharp edges of the fracture.
- CT scan will show the defect in the pars interarticularis (Fig. 19.14).
- Bone scan with single-photon emission CT (SPECT) will help differentiate between acute and chronic lesion (hot lesion in acute cases and cold in chronic cases)

Treatment:

- **NSAIDs, and rest from the sport** until the pain decreases.
- Adolescent can resume sport activity when they are pain free.
- Brace (lumbar corset), if the pain does not improve with rest.

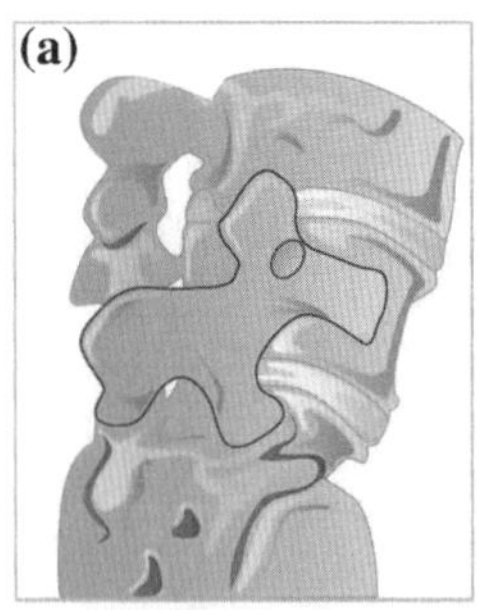

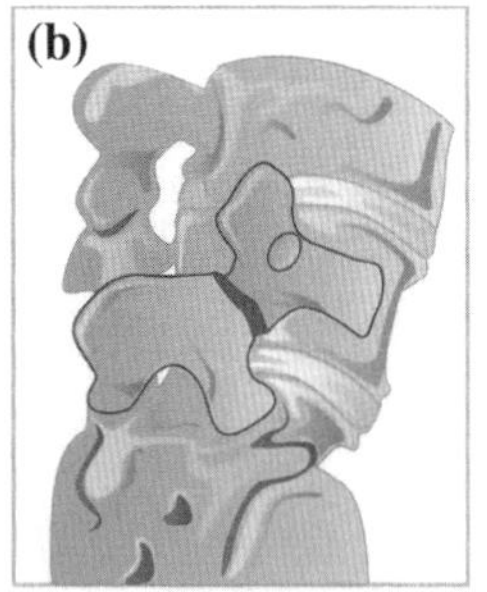

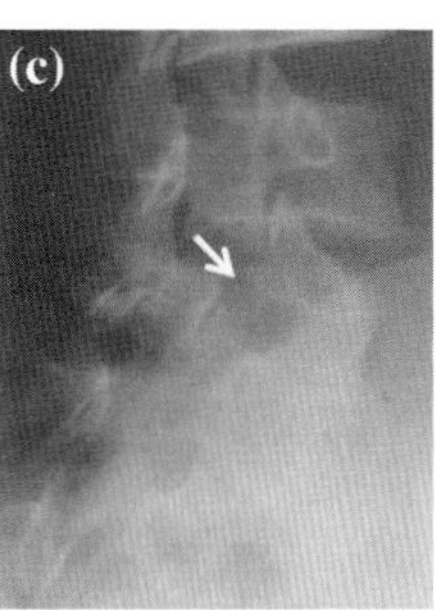

Fig. 19.15 Scotty dog collar sign. **a** Oblique view of the lumbar vertebrae has the shade of Scotty dog. **b** With spondylolysis, the defect in the pars interarticularis give the appearance of collar in the neck **c** Oblique radiographs showing the defect in the pars interarticularis and Scotty dog collar sign. (*arrow*)

- Acute lesion can be treated with more aggressive immobilization (Thoraco-lumbar-sacral orthosis (TLSO))
- Orthopedic referral if no improvement (Surgery is rarely indicated in Spondylolysis).

SPONDYLOLISTHESIS

Definition:

- Forward slippage of upper vertebra in relation to the vertebra below Fig. 19.16.

Pathology:

- There are two types of spondylolisthesis in children and adolescent:
  - Dysplastic:
    - Due to dysplastic lumbosacral articulation.
    - About 15 % of cases of spondylolisthesis.
  - Ischemic:
    - Due to pars defect (Spondylolysis).
    - Most common type (about 85 %).

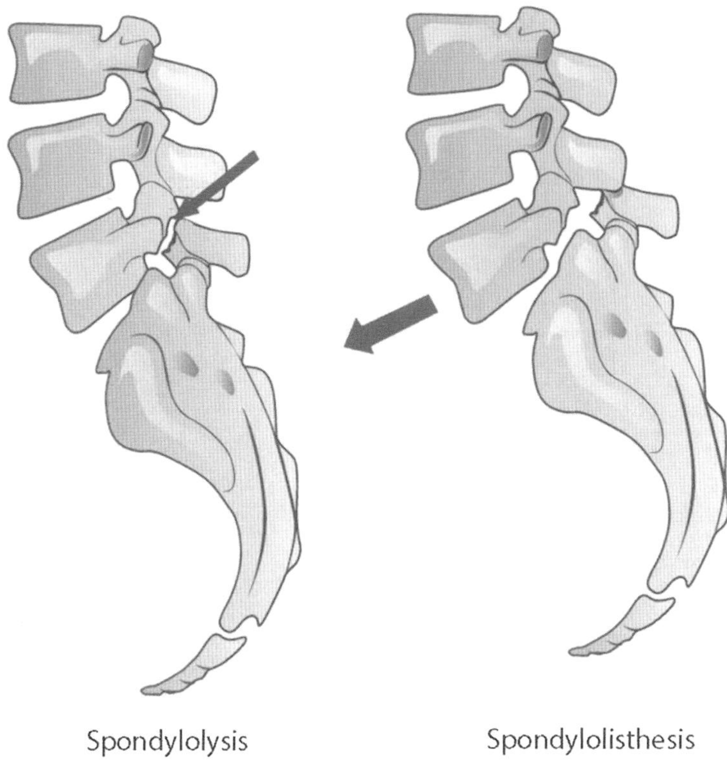

Fig. 19.16 Spondylolysis is the presence of defect in the pars of the vertebra. Spondylolisthesis is the 'slippage' of the vertebra above in relation to the vertebra below

- □ Only about 5 % of cases of spondylolysis progress to symptomatic spondylolisthesis.
- □ Despite spondylolysis being more common in boys, high grade spondylolisthesis is more common in girls.

Risk of progression:

- Growth spurt
- Females

- Dysplastic spondylolisthesis.
- Slippage progression is more common in a child or adolescent with initial slippage of more than 50 %.

Clinical picture:

- Low back pain with extension activities.
- Hamstring tightness

Radiographs:

- Forward slippage of L5 over S1.
- The degree of slippage is expressed as a percentage of the vertebral width.

Treatment:

- Orthopedic referral.
  - Surgical treatment is usually needed for high slip
- No contact sports if the slippage is more than 50 % of the vertebral width.

TORTICOLLIS

Definition:

- It is the clinical finding of tilting the head to one side in combination with rotation of head to the opposite side.
- The child will have one ear close to the ipsilateral shoulder while the chin and the face are pointing to the other shoulder (Fig. 19.17).

Orthopedic causes of torticollis:

- Congenital torticollis (most common type)
- C1, C2 subluxation
- Atlantoaxial rotator displacement
- Upper cervical spine anomalies (Fig. 19.18)

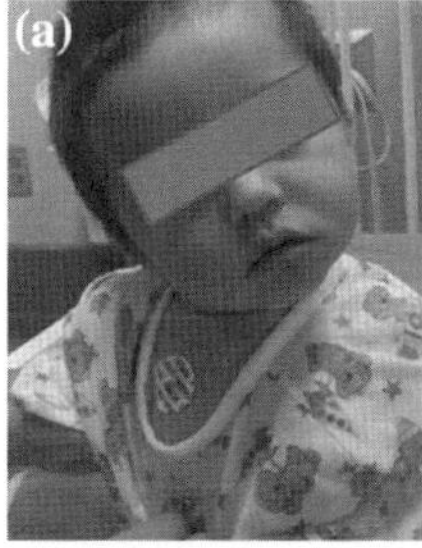

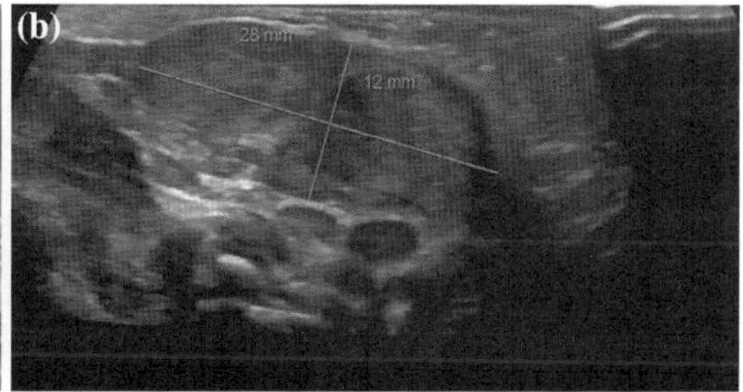

Fig. 19.17 Torticollis. A 1-year-old boy with congenital muscular torticollis. **a** Note the child head is tilted to the right (the right ear is close to the right shoulder) with the face and chin are directed to the left side. Patient has tight sternomastoid on the right side. **b** Ultrasound showed fibrotic mass in the sternomastoid (2.8 × 1.2 cm)

- Vertebral osteomyelitis
- Basilar impression

Non orthopedic causes

- Sandifer syndrome (gastroesophageal reflux, hiatal hernia)
- Neoplasm
  - Posterior fossa tumor
  - Soft tissue tumor
- Infection
  - Retropharyngeal abscess
- Ocular
  - Visual disturbance
  - Oculogyric crisis
  - Spasmus nutans (nystagmus, head bobbing, head tilting)
- Neurological
  - Syringomyelia
  - Alnord-Chirari malformation

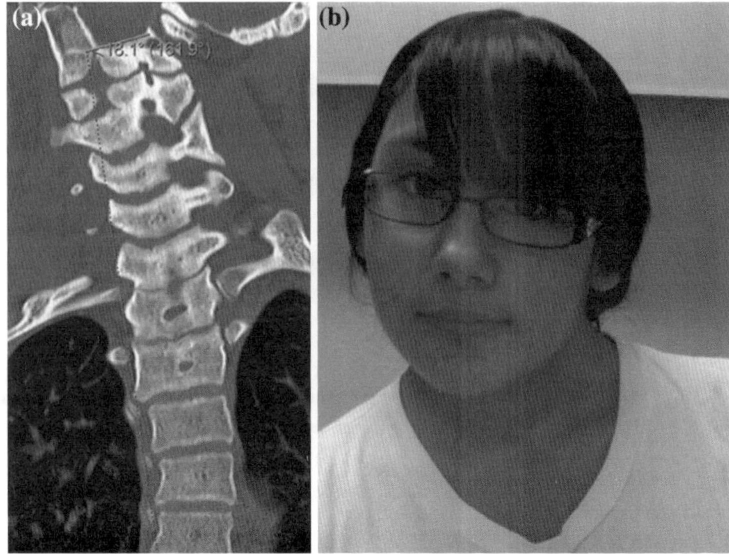

Fig. 19.18 A 16-year-old girl with torticollis due to upper cervical vertebral anomalies. **a** CT scan shows the vertebral malformation (notice the fusion of the upper cervical vertebrae). **b** The patient has Facial asymmetry (*right side* slightly bigger than *left side*)

- Paroxysmal torticollis of infancy
- Wilson disease
- Dystonic drug reaction e.g., metoclopramide

Congenital muscular torticollis:

- The most common causes of torticollis (Fig. 19.17).
- It is due to fibrosis of the sternomastoid muscle.
- The tight sternomastoid is on the side where the ear is closer to the shoulder (opposite to the side where he is facing).
- May be related to birth injury or malformation within the muscle.

Treatment

- **Aggressive physical therapy for stretching** sternocleidomastoid muscle.
- If no improvement: orthopedic referral (release of muscle is indicated if no improvement with physical therapy).

Paroxysmal torticollis of infancy

- Unknown etiology (maybe due to vestibular dysfunction).
- Gross and fine motor delays are indentified in about half of patients.
- Episodes can last for less than a week and the side of deformity can alternate.
- The condition is self limited and usually resolve by 3 years of age.

Atlantoaxial Rotary Instability

Definition:

- Fixed rotation of C1 on C2.
- One of the common causes **of torticollis in children.**

Causes:

- Retropharyngeal irritation (Grisel's disease)
  - Caused by upper respiratory infection or retropharyngeal abscess
- Trauma
- Down's syndrome

Imaging:

- Dynamic CT
  - CT with head straight forward, and then rotated to right and left.
  - Will show fixed rotation of C1 on C2 that does not change with head position.

Treatment:

- If subluxation is less than one week:
    - NSAIDs, soft collar, and stretching exercises program
    - Most cases will improve
- If subluxation is more than one week:
    - Orthopedic referral:
    - Possible need for traction (if subluxation is 1 week to one month duration) or fusion of the upper cervical spine (for subluxation more than one month).

General approach to torticollis

- History:
    - History of birth trauma, reflux, fever.
- Examination:
    - Examination of the sternomastoid for tightness and swellings.
    - Neurological and eye examination.
    - Facial asymmetry indicates long duration of affection. These changes are usually permanent and fixing the torticollis may not reverse the changes (Fig. 19.18).
- Imaging:
    - Radiograph of the cervical spine:
        - Usually cannot identify the bony lesion because of the overlap and cartilaginous nature of most the spine in the young age.
    - CT spine: will show bony anomaly in most cases (Fig. 19.18).
    - MRI: if neurological cause is suspected.
- Ophthalmology and neurology consult may be needed if no identifiable cause could be found.

KLIPPEL-FEIL SYNDROME

Definition:

- It is a congenital fusion of cervical vertebrae (failure of segmentation)

Clinical Presentation:

- **Clinical Triad** (Fig. 19.19)
  - Short-webbed neck
  - Low hair line
  - Restriction of neck motion: this may expose the child to increased risk of neck injuries due to decrease flexibility.
- In adult, patients may develop neck pain or neurological disorders as result of disk degeneration, spinal stenosis.
- **Associated anomalies**
  - Sprengel deformity (High scapula).
  - Cervical scoliosis.

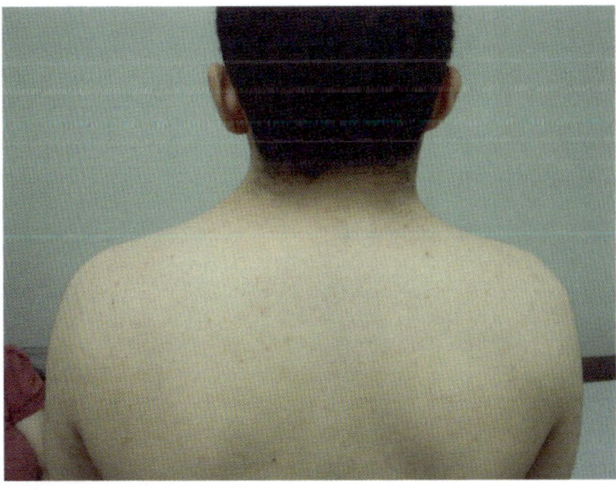

Fig. 19.19 Klippel-Feil Syndrome. A 12-year-old boy with Klippel-Feil syndrome. Notice the short-webbed neck and low hair line

- Genitourinary system anomalies (unilateral renal agenesis, duplicating renal collecting system, horseshoe kidney).
- Auditory system anomalies.
- Heart and neural axis anomalies.

■ **Diagnosis**

- Flexion and extension cervical radiograph
- MRI

■ **Treatment**

- Most cases have near normal function, need no treatment.
- If neurological or musculoskeletal problems: orthopedic referral.

SPRENGEL DEFORMITY

Definition:

- Upward position of the scapula due to failure of normal scapular descent during fetal life (Fig. 19.20).

Clinical presentation:

- Unequal scapular level: scapula on one side is higher than the scapula on the other side.
- Decrease range of motion of the affected shoulder.
- May be associated with congenital scoliosis, Klippel-Feil syndrome, and renal anomalies.

Treatment:

- Most cases have normal function, need no treatment.
- If there is a decrease shoulder range of motion: orthopedic referral.

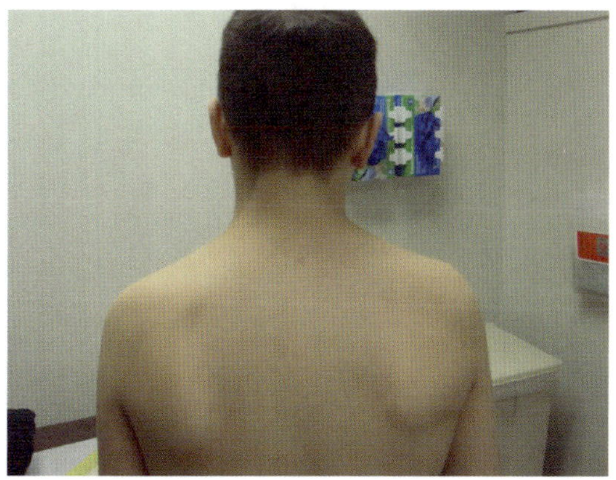

Fig. 19.20 Sprengel deformity. A 13-year-old boy with Sprengel deformity. Notice the right scapula is higher than the left side

CHILDHOOD BACK PAIN

Cause of back pain in children:

- Mechanical back pain (muscle strain)
- Deformity:
  - Sheuremann kyphosis.
- Infection
  - Diskitis
  - Vertebral body osteomyelitis
  - TB spine
- Trauma to spine:
  - Vertebral fracture.
  - Osteoporotic compression fracture.

- Spondylosis and spondylolisthesis
- Tumor
  - Osteoid osteoma (painful scoliosis).
  - Leukemia
- Disk prolapse (Herniated nucleus pulposus)
- Sacroiliac (SI) joint pain:
  - mechanical (muscle strain).
  - limb length discrepancy.
  - septic arthritis.
  - inflammatory arthritis (Ankylosis spondylitis or Rieter).

GENERAL APPROACH TO A CHILD WITH BACK PAIN

- **History:**
  - Assessment of the pain (when, where, onset, course, what decrease, what increase, **radiation to the lower extremity**, relation to activity, if it prevents the child from doing his/her activity).
  - History of one of the red flags (see later)
- **Examination:**
  - Assessment of deformity (kyphosis, scoliosis)
  - Assessment of the range of motion of the back:
    - Pain with extension of the spine, possible spondylosis or spondylolisthesis
    - Pain with flexion, possible vertebral body or disk disease
    - A child with diskitis or osteomyelitis will bend his hips and his knees (not his back) to pick up an object from the floor.
- **Assessment of the sacroiliac (SI) joint**
  - Palpation of the SI joint.
  - Compression of the iliac wings.
  - FABER test (Flexion, Abduction, External Rotation) of the hip will cause pain over the SI joint.

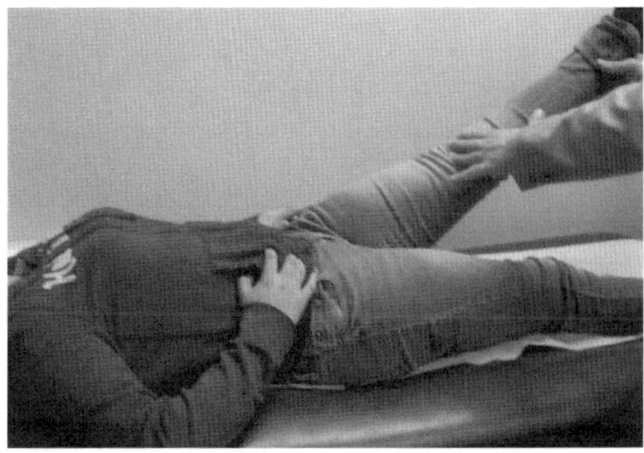

Fig. 19.21 Straight leg raising test to assess for radiculopathy of the lower lumbar and sacral root. The patient lies supine with elevation of the leg while knee extended

- **Straight leg raising test:**
  - Patient lies supine (Fig. 19.21).
  - The test is performed by raising up one leg (flexing the hip) while the knee is extended.
  - Positive results requires shooting pain in the back of the lower extremity radiating **distal to the knee level.**
  - Positive result indicates radiculopathy (nerve root compression).
  - Causes of radiculopathy:
    - Disk prolapsed (herniated nucleus pulposus).
    - High grade spondylolisthesis.
- **Neurological exam of the lower extremity:**
  - Motor: assessment of the motor power of main muscle groups.
  - Sensory (Fig. 19.22).
  - Reflexes (knee and ankle reflexes).

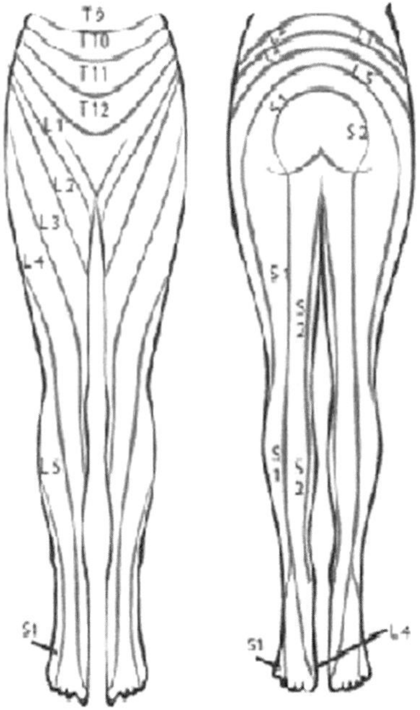

Fig. 19.22 Sensory dermatomes. Sensory innervations of the lower extremity

Red flag in history or exam for child with back pain (warrant more work up to identify the cause):

- Weight loss or fever
- Weakness or numbness of lower extremities
- Bowel or bladder problems
- Trouble walking (or inability to walk in small children)
- Pain that prevents the child from sleeping.
- Age less than 5 years.

Radiographic Diagnosis:

Plain radiograph of the spine:

- Start always with plain radiographs.
- Will assess bony lesion and the alignment of the spine.
- Two views (Anteroposterior and lateral) centered over the painful part of the spine
- If suspecting spondylolysis, add oblique views (Scottish dog collar appearance)

Bone Scan and SPECT (Single-photon emission computed tomography):

- Helpful in detecting bone tumor and infections.
- Can differentiate between acute and chronic spondylolysis.

CT spine:

- Better assessment of the bony structure.
- Coronal, sagittal, and 3D reconstruction can show the deformities of the vertebra better that plain radiographs.

MRI:

- Better assessment of the soft tissues (herniated disk, infection, intra thecal tumors).

Indication for MRI of the spine:

- Presence of any signs of the red flags.
- Severe low back pain not responding to medical treatment.

Laboratory studies:

- Markers of infection (CBC with diff, ESR, and C-reactive protein).
- Markers of seronegative spondyloarthropathy (HLA B-27).

MECHANICAL (MUSCULAR) BACK PAIN

Definition:

- Back pain due to muscle strain.

Clinical presentation:

- This diagnosis can only be given after exclusion of all other pathology by clinical exam and negative radiographs.
- More common in adolescent, very rare in young children less than 10 years old.
- **Currently is the most common cause of back pain in adolescent.**

Treatment:

- **Local heat, NSAID medication.**
- Therapy for strengthening of **abdominal a**nd back muscles
- Decease physical activities (sports) until pain improves.
- Short term use of back brace (controversial)
- If condition persists: proceed with more imaging studies (bone scan or MRI) (Fig. 19.13).

Septic sacroiliitis:

- The child will present with back/hip pain with general signs of infection.
- Blood culture may be positive in about 50 % of cases.
- MRI and Bone scan will show the condition.
- *S aureus* is the most common organism.
- The condition can be treated medically without surgical interference in most cases.

HIGH YIELD FACTS

- Congenital scoliosis is associated with other congenital anomalies in more than 50 % of individuals e.g., heart and kidney
- Indication for referral to orthopedic surgeon in scoliosis is curves more than 20° (or 7° of rotation in scoliometer).
- Surgery is generally indicated for patients with scoliosis if the thoracic curves is more than 50° in skeletally mature children.
- For AIS: bracing is indicated for patients with significant skeletal growth remaining (Risser stage 0, 1, and 2) and the following curves:

  - More than 5° of progression (e.g., curve progressed from 18° to 24°).
  - Curves more than 25°

- Sheuermann kyphosis, the deformity is fixed and cannot be corrected by straightening the back (in contrast to postural kyphosis). Most important surgical indication is unacceptable aesthetic appearance.
- Mechanical (muscular) pain is the most common cause of adolescent back pain, while spondylolysis is the most common cause of nonmuscluar back pain in adolescents.
- Most cases of spondylolysis are asymptomatic (7 % of the population after skeletal maturity have radiological evidence of spondylolysis).
- Two types of spondylolisthesis are present in adolescent: dysplastic and isthmic.
- Congenital muscular torticollis is the most common cause of torticollis and it is due to fibrosis of the sternomastoid. First treatment is by aggressive therapy.
- Klippel-Feil syndrome involves fusion of cervical vertebrae, the affected individual is at risk of neck injuries due to decrease cervical flexibility.

CLINICAL SCENARIOS

The presenting patient	The most probable diagnosis and plan of action
17-year-old boy with thoracic kyphosis which cannot be corrected by straightening of the back; radiograph showed wedging of three consecutive anterior vertebral bodies at the apex of the curve.	Sheuermann kyphosis • Therapy for postural exercises • The child is 17 years old, so bracing is not an option for him (near skeletal maturity) • Referral for orthopedics for curves more than 70°: possible surgical treatment to correct the deformity
5-year-old boy with back pain, fever, physical examination showed tenderness in the midline of the lumbar area and spasm in the paraspinal muscles, WBC is 15,000 and ESR is 45.	Diskitis • MRI of the spine • Anti staph Antibiotic
13-year-old female (one year post menarcheal) in her yearly exam found to have right thoracic hump. She has no complaint. Exam is normal apart from the back deformity. Radiographs show right thoracic curve of 27°. No other anomalies of the spine.	Adolescent idiopathic scoliosis • Bracing is indicated in this case
14-year-old boy, plays football, coming to the office with history of 6 months of worsening back pain. On exam, patient has hamstring tightness but intact neurological exam of the lower extremity. Radiographs shows anterior slippage of L5 over the sacrum	Ischemic spondylolisthesis • NSAID, therapy, rest • If the slippage is more than 50 % of the width of the vertebra (grade III or IV), patient will need to quit football

REFERENCES

Fucs PM, Meves R, Yamada HH. Spinal infections in children: a review. Int Orthop. 2012 Feb;36(2):387–95. Epub 2011 Oct 28.

Garg S, Johnston CE. Early onset scoliosis. In Song KM, editor. Orthopedaedic Knowledge Update: Pediatrics. 4th ed. Rosemont, IL: American Academy of Orthopaedic Surgeons; 2011. P. 243–257.

Harvey J, Tanner S. Low back pain in young athletes. A practical approach. Sports Med. 1991 Dec;12(6):394–406.

Glancy GL. The diagnosis and treatment of back pain in children and adolescents: an update. Adv Pediatr. 2006;53:227–40.

Hedequist D, Emans J. Congenital scoliosis: a review and update. J Pediatr Orthop. 2007 Jan-Feb;27(1):106–16.

Lonstein JE. Spondylolisthesis in children. Cause, natural history, and management. Spine (Phila Pa 1976). 1999 Dec 15;24(24):2640–8.

Campbell RM Jr, Smith MD, Mayes TC, Mangos JA, Willey-Courand DB, Kose N, Pinero RF, Alder ME, Duong HL, Surber JL. The characteristics off thoracic insufficiency syndrome associated with fused ribs and congenital scoliosis. J Bone Joint Surg Am. 2003 Mar;85-A(3):399–408.

Tracy MR, Dormans JP, Kusumi K. Klippel-Feil syndrome: clinical features and current understanding of etiology. Clin Orthop Relat Res. 2004 Jul;(424):183–90.

Chapter 20
Neuromuscular Conditions

Amr Abdelgawad and Osama Naga

INTRODUCTION

- Children can suffer from different neurological conditions that can affect their musculoskeletal system.
- These conditions are best treated by multi dispensary approach which includes pediatrician, pediatric orthopods, physiatrists, neurologist or neurosurgeon and possibly urologist.

CEREBRAL PALSY

Definition:

- Non progressive (static) injury to the growing brain. This injury has to cause postural or movement disorder
- The insult has to occur early in the development of the child's brain (prenatal-natal or early post natal).
- Despite that the injury to the brain is non progressive, the musculoskeletal manifestation of cerebral palsy may progress with time.

Etiology:

- In most cases the exact cause is unknown
- Prenatal factors include
  - Intrauterine infections e.g., TORCH
  - Maternal thyroid abnormalities
  - Prenatal strokes.

A. Abdelgawad and O. Naga (eds.), *Pediatric Orthopedics*,
DOI: 10.1007/978-1-4614-7126-4_20,

- Perinatal factors include:
  - Birth asphyxia
- Post natal factors include:
  - Infections (e.g., neonatal sepsis)
  - Ischemia (near drawing)
  - Trauma (shaken baby syndrome).

PATHOLOGY, CLASSIFICATION, MANAGEMENT

See Chap. 14.

MYELODYSPLASIA (SPINA BIFIDA)

Definition:

- Neurological conditions due to congenital abnormality of the posterior spinal elements.

Spina bidifa is classified:

- **Spina bifida occulta:**
  - Absence of the posterior component of the vertebral column **with no neurological affection**.
  - Usually discovered as accidental finding the radiographs
  - Affects about 7.5 % of population.

- **Meningocele:**
  - Absence of the posterior component of the vertebral column **with abnormal development of the meninges.**
  - The neural element inside the meninges stays intact, however patients may suffer from:
    - **lipomeningocele:** lipoma associated with meningocele.
    - **Tethered cord syndrome:** tethering of the filum terminale connecting the lower end of the dura to the sacrum. This can cause motor and sensory manifestations.
- **Myelomeningocele:**
  - Absence of the posterior component of the vertebral column **with abnormal development of the meninges and neural element**.
  - More common than meningocele
  - Patients will suffer from motor, sensory and autonomic defects distal to the area of affection.
  - **Neurological affection is more severe than meningocele or lipomeningocele**.
- **Caudal regression syndrome:**
  - Partial or complete absence of the sacrum with its neurological elements.

Functional Classification

The spina bifida patients are classified according to **the level of the most distal working functional level** (usually this level of affection is not very clear and not similar on both sides).

- **Thoracic:** these children will be wheel chair bound, also will develop spinal column complication (scoliosis or kyphosis/lordosis).
- **High lumber (L1,2):** minimal walking.
- **Low lumber (L3,4):** They can walk with braces. When they grow up and their weights become heavier, they will prefer to use the wheel chair for faster and more energy-efficient ambulation.
- **Sacral:** they can walk near normal. They can develop high arched foot (cavus foot).

Associated conditions:

- **Arnold Chiari malformations and hydrocephalus.**
- **Congenital foot deformities.**
- ***Children with spina bifida have high prevalence of latex allergy (about 40 %). This is the highest percentage in any population. Any child with the spina bifida should be treated with "latex precautions".***

Orthopedic problems in the spina bifida patients
Hip dysplasia:
Because of weak muscles (especially hip abductors), the femoral head starts to subluxate out to the hip joint (Fig. 20.1).

- For the potential walker (L4-5) patients: orthopedic referral for possible intervention.
- If the patient is not potential walker (L2 or higher): dislocation will not be painful and will not affect his function. No treatment is required.

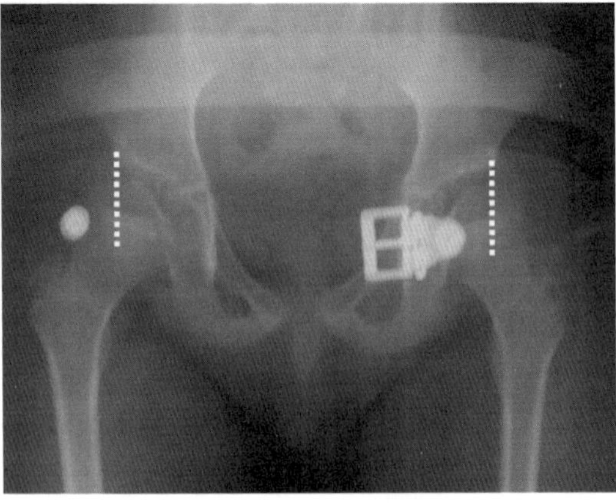

Fig. 20.1 A 7-year-old spina bifida patient with L3 level. The patient is able to walk using *HKAFO* (Hip-Knee-Ankle–Foot Orthosis) (notice the *shadow* of the hip part of the prosthesis in the upper part of the radiograph). Patient has bilateral hip dysplasia as approximately one third of the femoral head is not covered by acetabulum (lateral to the *dotted line* which is the lateral edge of the acetabulum)

Spine deformity:

- Children with spina bifida (especially thoracic level) can develop spinal deformities.
- Most common spinal deformities are:
  - **Scoliosis**
  - **Lumbar kyphosis:** the child will have "kyphos" or "gibbus deformity" of his lower back. This condition can lead to skin ulcers.
  - **Lumbar hyperlordosis:** exaggerated lumbar lordosis (Fig. 20.2).

Management of spinal deformities:

- Bracing (can be effective for scoliotic curves, not used for kyphosis as it may cause skin problems).

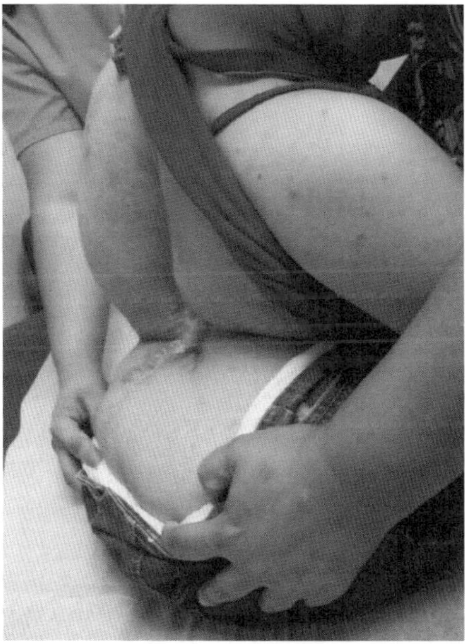

Fig. 20.2 A 16-year-old girl with spina bifida. Patient has hyperlordosis of her lower spine. The picture shows the scar of the previous surgery on the spine

- Wheel chair modification.
- Orthopedic referral for surgical treatment. Because of possible anomalies of the meninges and tethered cord syndrome, this is better to be coordinated with a neurosurgeon.

Foot deformity:

- Some of the foot deformities are due to muscle imbalance and some are due to associated congenital anomalies.
- Multiple foot deformities can be present in patients with spina bifida:
  - Congenital clubfoot.
  - Valgus deformity
    - With valgus deformity, patients can develop pressure ulcers over their talar head as this part will be more prominent during weight bearing and the patient does not have protective sensation (Fig. 20.3).
  - Cavus foot

Treatment:

- See Chap. 8.

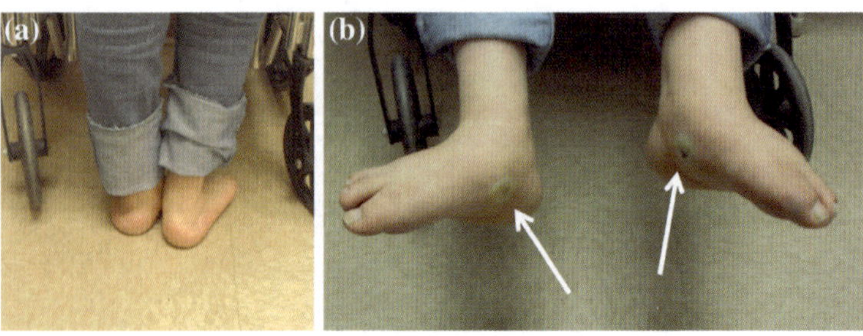

Fig. 20.3 A 15-year-old girl with spina bifida. (**a**) The patient has bilateral valgus feet. (**b**) When this patient stands, she puts more pressure on the talar head which lead to bilateral ulcers over her talar heads (arrows)

MUSCULAR DYSTROPHIES

Definition:

- Muscular dystrophy (MD) is a collective group of inherited noninflammatory progressive muscle disorders without a central or peripheral nerve abnormality.

Heritable MDs include the following:

- Sex-linked MDs
  - Duchenne muscular dystrophy
  - Becker muscular dystrophy
  - Emery-Dreifuss muscular dystrophy
- **Autosomal dominant MDs**
  - Facioscapulohumeral muscular dystrpohy
- **Autosomal recessive MD**
  - Limb-girdle muscular dystrophy

Duchenne Muscular dystrophy (DMD) and Becker Muscular Dystrophy (BMD)
Incidence:

- 1:3500 in DMD
- 1:30,000 in BMD

Genetics:

- The defective gene product is dystrophin gene
- In DMD, the dystrophin is absent.
- In BMD, the dystrophin is reduced in amount (milder form of the disease than DMD).
- Locus of the involved gene is Xp21.

Clinical presentation:

- Children with DMD typically present at age of 2 years:

  - Apparent clumsiness
  - Bilateral limping (waddling gait, see Chap. 17)
  - Excessive falling
  - Toe walking
  - Difficulty climbing stairs

- Examination reveals:

  - Calf hypertrophy (Pseudohypertrophy)
  - Proximal muscle weakness
  - Difficulty getting up from the floor (Positive Gower maneuver) (Fig. 20.4)
  - Hyporeflexia.

- Children are non-ambulatroy by age of 10–14 years.
- Spinal deformities (scoliosis) develop once the patient becomes non ambulatory.
- Fractures of the bones of the lower extremity due to osteoporosis from disuse atrophy (Fig. 20.5).
- Children with DMD has higher incidence of malignant hyperthermia.
- Premature death occurs in early twenties:

  - from cardio respiratory failure.

- BMD is a milder form and patient tend to live past the fourth or fifth decades.

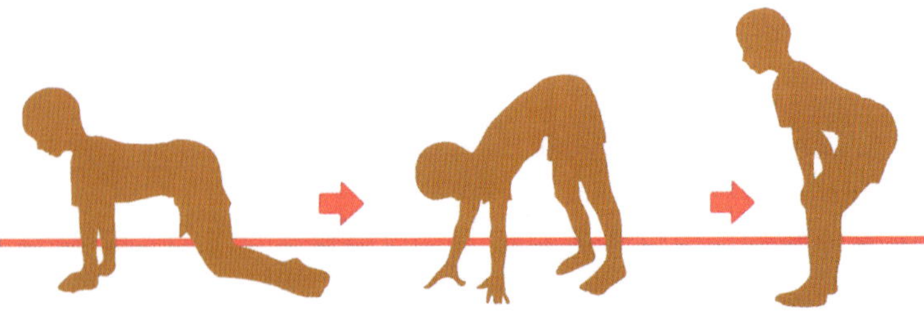

Fig. 20.4 Positive Gower maneuver. When a child is asked to stand up from a squatting position, he uses his hands to push up on his knees and thighs due to lack of hip and knee muscle strength

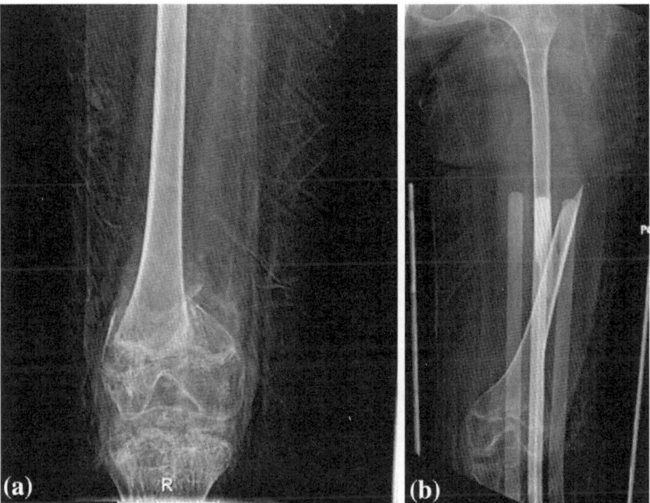

Fig. 20.5 A 13-year-old boy with DMD who fell down while his father was transferring him from bed to chair. The patient sustained bilateral femur fracture (distal femur in the *right* (**a**) and spiral fracture on the *left* side (**b**)). Notice the severe osteopenia and thin cortices

- In BMD, cardiomyopathy often develops earlier and must be monitored closely.

Laboratory:

- The creatin kinase is typically markedly elevated
- Muscle biopsy show dystrophic changes
- PCR for dystrophin gene mutation
- Echocardiogram, EKG
- Electromyography: low amplitude waves.

Orthopedic manifestation of DMD and BMD:

- Equinus deformity:
  - Early, the condition is treated with brace. When the deformity becomes fixed, lengthening of the Achilles tendon is indicated.

- Scoliosis:
  - Scoliosis is the natural history of all non ambulatory patients.
  - Better to treat the condition early before it progress to severe form.
  - **Patients with DMD has tendency to bleed excessively intra-operatively**.
  - The treatment is by spinal fusion to avoid progression of the deformity.
- Hip and knee flexion contracture:
  - Due to prolonged wheel chair setting.
  - For mild deformities: no treatment needed.
  - For severe deformities interfering with setting: muscle release.
- Repeated fractures:
  - Fractures of the bones of the lower extremity due to osteoporosis from disuse atrophy (Fig. 20.5)
  - Orthopedic referral for surgery or casting depending on the fracture type.

SPINAL MUSCULAR ATROPHY

Definition:

- The spinal muscular atrophies (SMAs) comprise a group of autosomal-recessive disorders characterized by progressive weakness of the lower motor neurons.
- This condition can affect the child at different stages in his growth.

Incidence:

- The spinal muscular atrophies are the second most common autosomal-recessive inherited disorders after cystic fibrosis

Clinical Presentation:

- **SMA acute infantile (type I or Werdnig-Hoffman disease)**
    - Patients present before 6 months of age
    - Severe, progressive muscle weakness with flaccid or reduced muscle tone (hypotonia).
    - Bulbar dysfunction includes poor sucking ability, reduced swallowing, and respiratory failure
- **SMA Chronic infantile form**
    - Most children present between the ages of 6 and 18 months.
    - The most common manifestation is developmental motor delay.
    - Failure to stand by 1 year of age.
    - Scoliosis becomes a major complication in many patients with long survival.
- **SMA juvenile form, (Kugelberg-Welander disease or SMA type 3)**
    - Present around the age of 2 years.
    - Longevity can extend well into middle adult life.
    - Progressive muscle weakness is proximal in distribution.

Diagnosis:

- Genetic testing
- EMG:
    - Fasicular pattern of degeneration.

Orthopedic manifestations SMA:

- similar to DMD and BMD.

CHARCOT MARIE TOOTH SYNDROME

Definition:

- Charcot-Marie-Tooth (CMT) disease is the most common inherited neurologic disorder.
- CMT is characterized by inherited neuropathies without known metabolic derangements.

Incidence:

- The prevalence of CMT disease is 1 person per 2,500 population.
- Most common cause of congenital peripheral neuropathy.

Etiology:

- Autosomal dominant is the most common but can be autosomal recessive.

Clinical Presentation:

- General manifestations:
  - Sensation of pain and temperature is usually intact.
  - Deep tendon reflexes (DTRs) are markedly diminished or absent.
  - Vibration sensation and proprioception are significantly decreased.
  - Patients may have sensory gait ataxia, and Romberg test is usually positive.
  - Essential tremor is present in 30–50 % of patients with CMT disease.
  - Enlarged and palpable peripheral nerves are common.
- Musculoskeletal manifestations:
  - Patients initially may complain of difficulty walking and frequent tripping.

- due to foot and distal leg weakness.

- Frequent ankle sprains and falls are characteristic.
- Pes cavus due to weakness and denervation of the intrinsic muscle of the foot [the disease affect tibialis anterior muscle more than peroneus longus resulting in plantar flexion of the first ray (see Chap. 8)].
- Hand weakness results in clumsiness in manipulating small objects.
- Muscle cramping
- Distal muscle wasting may be noted in the legs resulting in the characteristic stork leg **or inverted champagne bottle appearance.**
- Spinal deformities (e.g., thoracic scoliosis).

Diagnosis
Genetic tests:

- The definitive molecular genetic diagnosis can be done by blood sample.

Laboratory:

- All routine laboratory tests are normal in individuals with CMT disease.

Electromyography/nerve conduction study:

- Perform these studies first if CMT disease is suggested.
- Findings vary depending on the type of CMT disease.

Orthopedic manifestations:

- Cavus foot:
  - see Chap. 8.
- Wrist and foot contracture:
  - Treated early by bracing. When the condition becomes fixed, surgical release may be needed.
- Scoliosis:
  - Orthopedic referral.

HIGH YIELD FACTS

- Cerebral palsy has to be due to non progressive lesion early in the child development.
- The higher the defect in patient with spina bifida, the worse the disability.
- About half of spina bifida patients have latex allergy.
- DMD present at the age of 3 years old, becomes non ambulatory at the age of 12–13.
- Child with CMT disease initially may complain of difficulty walking and frequent tripping
- CMT is the most common cause of cavus foot in the developed world.
- Fasciculations are a specific sign of denervation in patients with SMA (Table 20.1).

CLINICAL SCENARIOS

The presenting patient	The most probable diagnosis and plan of action
6 months old male infant brought by his mother to your clinic for regular check up, part of the history the baby is not able to turn from front to back. On physical examination, he is alert, and smiling, but cannot hold the head up when pulled to the sitting position, and he slips through your hands when held vertically. There is a fasciculation noticed in the tongue, all the metabolic labs came back normal, what is the most likely cause.	SMA type II
3 years old boy noticed by his the mother that he became clumsy, and frequent falling, and swollen lower leg, and stand up in different way than other kids, on physical examination, there is a proximal muscle weakness, and hypertrophy of calf muscles, what is the best lab to order to assist in the diagnosis:	The most likely cause is muscular dystrophy ■ CPK is usually 30–300 greater than normal level

REFERENCES

Emery AE. Duchenne's muscular dystrophy. In: Oxford Monographs on Medical Genetics Series #24. 2nd ed. Oxford, United Kingdom: Oxford University Press; 1993.

Emery AE. Population frequencies of inherited neuromuscular diseases–a world survey. Neuromuscul Disord. 1991;1:19–29.

Bradley WG, Daroff RB, Fenichel GM, Jankovic J, editors. Neurology in clinical practice. 2nd ed. Boston: Butterworth-Heinemann; 1996. p. 1829–43.

Pearn J. Classification of spinal muscular atrophies. Lancet. 1980;1:919–22.

Larson AN, Richards BS. Myelomeningocele. In: Song KM, editor. Orthopedaedic Knowledge Update, Pediatrics.105-114. 4th ed. AAOS.

Chapter 21
Musculoskeletal Infections

Amr Abdelgawad and Osama Naga

ACUTE HEMATOGENOUS OSTEOMYELITIS

Definition:

- Acute infections of the bone and the bone marrow.
- The infection spreads from a distant focus to the bone by blood seeding (bacteremia).

Incidence:

- More common in boys.
- Common around the age of 4–6 years.

Predisposing factors:

- Decreased immunity of the child (e.g., HIV, renal failure).
- Sickle cell anemia.

Pathology:

- Usually affects the **metaphysis** of the bone.
  - The metaphysis has sluggish blood supply (Chap. 1 Fig. 1.3).
  - Bacteria from distant focus (skin, teeth, nose, etc.) will be carried by blood (**hence the name Hematogenous**) and then settle in the metaphysis with its slow circulation.
  - Once a bacterial focus is established, phagocytes migrates to the site and produce inflammatory exudates (**metaphyseal abscess**).
- In later childhood, the growth plate fuses with the surrounding bone and the osteomyelitis commonly occurs in the diaphysis.

A. Abdelgawad and O. Naga (eds.), *Pediatric Orthopedics*,
DOI: 10.1007/978-1-4614-7126-4_21,

Microbiology:

- *Staphylococcus aureus* is the most common pathogen in all age groups.
- Group B *Streptococcus and E. coli* are prominent pathogens in neonates (neonatal osteomyelitis).
- *Pseudomonas aeruginosa* is characteristic of the puncture wound to the foot through the shoe.
- *Salmonella and Staphylococcal aureus* are the most common causes of osteomyelitis in children with sickle cell anemia.
- *Strept Pneumoniae* is a common cause of osteomyelitis in children less than 24 months of age.
- *Kingella Kingae* is a common cause of musculoskeletal infections (arthritis and osteomyelitis) in some parts of the world, it should be suspected in children younger than 2 years with osteomyelitis especially if not responding to routine antibiotics.

Clinical picture:

- General signs of infection (fever, vomiting, chills, ill looking).
- Local manifestation of infection (redness, hotness, tenderness, and swelling).
- **Inability to bear weight** in cases of lower extremity osteomyelitis.
- **Laboratories.**
  - Elevated markers of infection, however, these labs may be normal in the first few days.
    - Leukocytes.
    - ESR.
    - C-reactive protein.
- **Imaging:**
  - **Radiograph:**
    - Negative for the first 10–14 days of the disease process.
    - After 10–14 days: periosteal reaction can be seen (Fig. 21.1).
    - Chronic radiographic changes can be seen in cases of chronic osteomyelitis (see later).
    - Helpful to exclude other causes of pain and swelling (e.g., tumor).
  - **Bone scan:**
    - Tri-phasic bone scan will show increased uptake (hotspot) at the infection site.

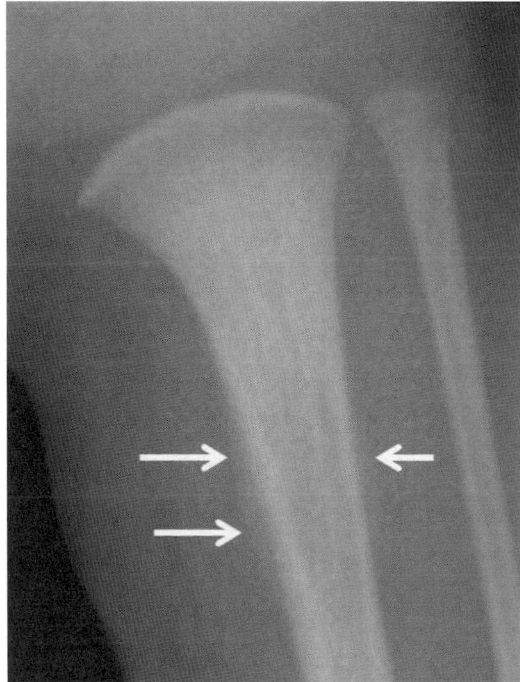

Fig. 21.1 A 6-month-old boy with 10 days history of fever and leg swelling. Radiograph shows periosteal reaction (*arrow*)

  - Useful if suspecting **multiple sites of affection** (neonatal osteomyelitis) because it scans the whole body.
- **MRI:**
  - **Most sensitive method to diagnose osteomyelitis.**
  - Will show enhancement of the medulla at the affected site (increased signal on T2) (Fig. 21.2).
  - Becomes positive very early in the disease process.
  - Can show sub-periosteal abscess (indication for surgical interference).
  - Will show nearby joint affection in cases of combined osteomyelitis with septic arthritis.

▪ **Identify the causative organism** by:
- Blood culture (3 daily consecutive samples).
- Aspiration of the affected part of the bone (image-guided biopsy).

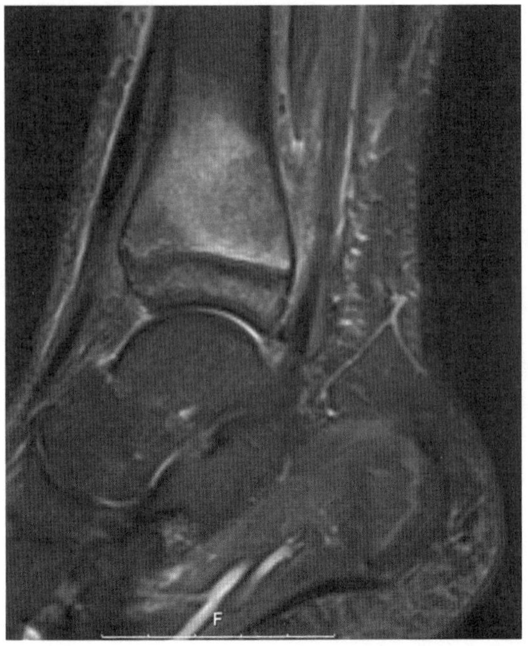

Fig. 21.2 An 8-year-old boy with 4 days history of fever, right leg pain, and inability to bear weight. MRI shows increased T2 signal and enhancement within the distal tibial metaphysis

Differential Diagnosis:

- Ewing Sarcoma:
  - Present with pain and swelling of the affected extremity.
  - Can have elevated markers of infection.
  - Radiographs: will show the characteristics of Ewing sarcoma (see tumor and tumor-like conditions).
- Septic Arthritis:
  - Pain is mainly related to the joint.
  - Both septic arthritis and osteomyelitis can occur simultaneously (especially proximal femur osteomyelitis with septic hip arthritis).
  - MRI will show the area of affection (joint versus metaphysis versus both).

Treatment:

- **Osteomyelitis is a medical condition, with possible need of surgical intervention in certain indications.**
- The main treatment of osteomyelitis is: *delivery of* ***correct*** *antibiotic in the* ***appropriate*** *dose for an* ***adequate*** *period of time.*
- **The choice of antibiotic:**
  - Depends on the causative organism.
  - Identification of the causative bacteria is either by culture results or knowledge of the most prevalent bacterial pathogens at various ages in the area that the patient lives in.
  - **Organism-sensitive antibiotic administration for a total of 6 weeks.**
    - **Two weeks of parenteral antibiotic followed by 4 weeks of oral antibiotic.**
  - Start with IV Clindamycin or other broad spectrum antibiotic in communities with low prevalence of MRSA and then shift to culture-specific antibiotic.
  - Vancomycin (60 mg/kg/24 h) IV divided every 6 h can be used in suspecting MRSA infection.
  - Monitor the response of the patient to treatment by:
    - CRP.
    - Clinically (fever and pain).
    - ESR (takes longer time to return to normal).

INDICATIONS OF SURGICAL INTERFERENCE IN CASES OF OSTEOMYELITIS (INDICATIONS FOR ORTHOPEDIC CONSULTS)

- Sub-periosteal abscess.
- No response to medical treatment after 36 h.
- Extension to nearby joint.

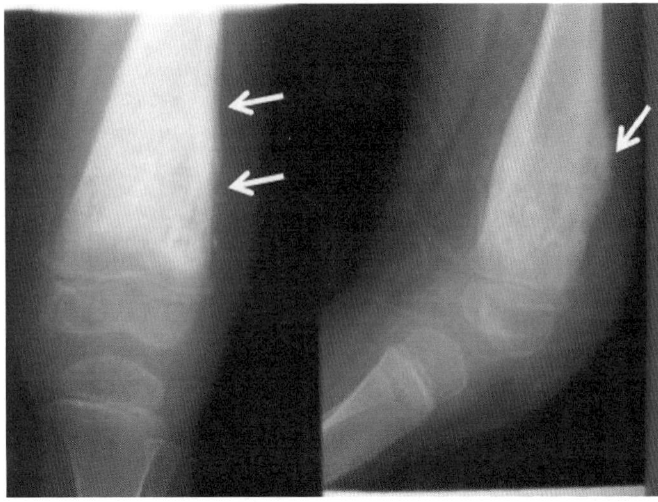

Fig. 21.3 Chronic osteomyelitis. A 6-year-old girl with 5 months history of chronic osteomyelitis of distal femur. Notice the new bone formation (involucrum) of the distal femur (*arrow*)

COMPLICATIONS OF ACUTE HEMATOGENOUS OSTEOMYELITIS

- Extension of infections:
  - Locally to nearby structures as joints.
  - Systemic spread e.g., endocarditis.
- Chronic infections: if acute hematogenous osteomyelitis is not adequately treated the condition becomes chronic osteomyelitis (Fig. 21.3).

NON-HEMATOGENOUS OSTEOMYELITIS

Causes:

- Posttraumatic osteomyelitis:
  - Open fracture.
  - Penetrating trauma.
  - Puncture wounds (see later).
- Postsurgical:
  - After orthopedic surgeries.
- Human and animal bites.
- Decubitus ulcer:
  - e.g., osteomyelitis of the sacrum.
- Local spread of infection:
  - e.g., ingrown toe nail.

Management:

- **Antibiotic treatment:**
  - Similar to hematogenous osteomyelitis.
- **Orthopedic consultation:**
  - Most non-hematogenous osteomyelitis will require surgical debridement.

OSTEOMYELITIS OF THE SPINE

See Chap. 19.

CHRONIC OSTEOMYELITIS

Definition:

- Osteomyelitis with chronic changes of the affected bone.

Pathology:

- If acute osteomyelitis is not cleared completely from the affected bone, chronic osteomyelitis changes will occur in the bone (Fig. 21.3).
  - **Sequestrum**:
    - Dead infected bone becomes separated from the surrounding tissues.
    - The sequestrum shows up as dense more opaque structure in the radiographs.
  - Periosteal new bone formation (**Involucrum**):
    - Multiple layers of new bone formation by the periosteum.
    - This is a reparative process from the bone to strengthen the bone structure.

Management:

- Imaging studies:
  - Radiographs will show the characteristic pathological signs (Fig. 21.3).
  - CT scan: more sensitive for detection of the sequestrum.
- Antibiotic treatment:
  - No need for antibiotic treatment EXCEPT:
    - Acute exacerbation of infection (new onset of local pain, swelling, or fever).
    - After surgical interference to clear infection.
- Orthopedic consultation:
  - Chronic osteomyelitis cannot be cured medically.
  - If there is a sequestrum, it has to be removed surgically, otherwise recurrent infection will occur.

SEPTIC ARTHRITIS

Definition:

- Bacterial infection of the joint.

Pathology:

- Most affected joints are: hip, shoulder, and knee.
- Spread of infection:
  - Septic arthritis occurs as a result of hematogenous seeding of the synovial tissue by the causative organism.
  - Less often, the organism enters the joint space by direct inoculation or extension from nearby site.
- The bacterial products produce cytokines in the joint space.
- Cytokines trigger inflammatory cascade and stimulate chemotaxis of neutrophils into the joint space.
- Neutrophils release proteolytic enzymes and elastase enzymes which have a destructive effect on the articular cartilage.
- Septic arthritis should be treated urgently to avoid destruction of the articular cartilage.
- Microbiology:
  - Most common organism is *Staph Aureus*.
  - Salmonella infection characteristically occurs in patients with sickle cell disease.
  - In sexually active adolescents, *gonococcus* is a common cause of septic arthritis.
  - *Group B streptococcus* is an important cause of septic arthritis in neonates.
  - *Kingella kingae* is recognized as relatively common etiology in children less than 5 years of age. Isolation of the organism had increased with improved culture and PCR method.
  - Candida arthritis infection can complicate systemic infection in neonates with indwelling catheter.
  - Fungal infection can occur as part of multisystem disseminated disease.

Clinical picture:

- General signs of infection (fever, vomiting, ill looking).
- **Refusal to move the joint** (the affected joint is fixed in a flexed position).
  - Marked decrease in the ROM of the joint.
- Inability to bear weight in cases of septic arthritis of lower extremity.

- For superficial joint (e.g., knee):
  - Local signs of infection (swelling, redness, and local tenderness) can be appreciated.
- For deep joints (e.g., hip and shoulders):
  - Local signs may be hard to detect.

Diagnosis

- Elevated markers of infection:
  - ESR.
  - C-reactive protein.
  - WBCs.
- Blood culture: usually positive in cases of septic arthritis.
- **Arthrocentesis:**
  - Aspiration of the joint fluid is done in cases of suspected septic arthritis.
  - **It is the mainstay of diagnosis of septic arthritis**.
  - The fluid is sent for **cell count**, gram stain, crystals, culture, and sensitivity.
  - In cases of infection: the joint aspiration will show:
    - □ WBCs count more than 50,000/ml.
    - □ Organism may be seen by gram stain.
    - □ Positive culture from the joint fluid.
  - Special media is used when suspecting atypical bacteria (e.g., gonococcus, Kingella kingae, or fungal infection).
  - Joint aspirate culture is highly positive in nongonococcal septic arthritis and 25–50 % positive in gonococcal septic arthritis.
- Ultrasound: will show thick joint effusion.
- MRI:
  - Joint effusion (increased signal in T2) (Fig. 21.4).
  - Will show if there is extension to nearby bony tissues (osteomyelitis).
- In sexually active adolescents:
  - Cultures of the genital secretions for possible gonococcal infection.

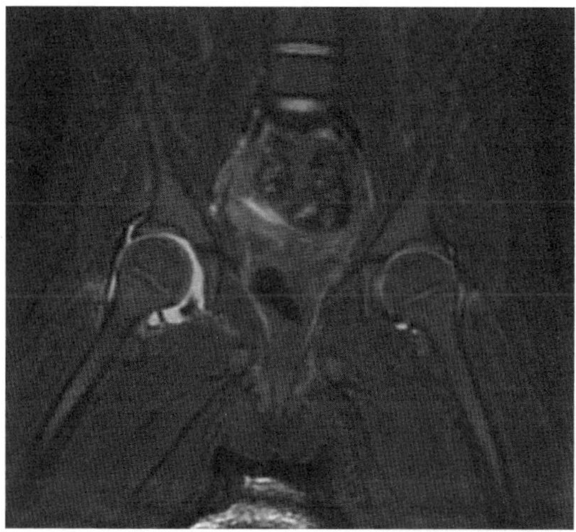

Fig. 21.4 A 5-year-old girl with fever, right hip pain, and inability to bear weight for 3 days. MRI of the pelvis shows right hip effusion with no affection of the proximal femur

Treatment:

- ***Septic arthritis is a surgical condition:***
  - Orthopedic consultation for surgical debridement.
  - ***Urgent consultation to avoid permanent destruction of the cartilage by proteolytic enzymes.***
  - Gonococcal septic arthritis can be treated medically with repeated aspiration. Rarely open drainage is indicated.
- **Antibiotic treatment:**
  - Initial treatment based on the knowledge of the most likely pathogen at various age and the gram stain result of aspirated material.
  - Antistaphylococcal penicillin, e.g., Nafcillin or oxacillin 150–200 mg/kg/day divided every 6 h IV and broad spectrum cephalosporin, e.g., cefotaxime 150–225 mg/kg/day divided every 8 h IV provide coverage for *S. aureus*, *group B. streptococcus* and *Gram negative bacilli*.
  - If MRSA is a concern vancomycin preferred rather than nafcillin or oxacillin.

- □ Vancomycin (60 mg/kg/24 h) IV divided every 6 h is the gold standard for invasive MRSA infection.
- **Organism-sensitive antibiotic administration for a total of 6 weeks.**
  - **Two weeks of parenteral antibiotic followed by 4 weeks of oral antibiotic.**

COMPLICATION OF SEPTIC ARTHRITIS

- Extension of infection to adjacent metaphysis causing osteomyelitis. This occurs most commonly in:
  - The shoulder (through the long head of biceps which pierce the shoulder capsule).
  - The hip (proximal femur metaphysis is intra-articular structure).
- Destruction of the articular cartilage with development of early arthritis.
- Destruction of the capsule and ligaments with dislocation of the joint in cases of hip septic arthritis.

GONOCOCCAL ARTHRITIS

- **Most common cause of septic arthritis is sexually active adolescent**.
- It occurs as a manifestation of disseminated gonococcal infection (DGI).
- Two Pathological types:
  - **Localized septic arthritis** of a large joint.
  - **Arthritis–dermatitis syndrome**: includes the classic triad:
    - □ Dermatitis: small vesicles or pustules.
    - □ Tenosynovitis (inflammation of the tendons) mainly of the tendons on the dorsum of the hand and ankle.
    - □ Migratory polyarthralgia: multiple joints are affected. Tend to involve the upper extremities more than the lower extremities. The wrist, elbows, ankles, and knees are most commonly affected.

- Synovial fluid culture:
  - Synovial fluid cultures are positive for *N gonorrhoeae* in about 25–50 % of cases.
  - Culture: synovial fluid should be cultured on pre-warmed chocolate agar for highest yield.
- Culture from mucosal surfaces (e.g. vaginal, rectal, throat, urethra)
  - Yield is highest if the culture is obtained from the primary infection site.
  - Mucosal surface cultures should be placed on pre-warmed selective plates, e.g., Thayer-Martin.
- Blood culture.
- Patient should also be tested for other STDs, including HIV, hepatitis B, chlamydia, and syphilis.

Treatment:

- Parenteral antibiotics:
  - Ceftriaxone 1 g intramuscularly (IM) or intravenously (IV) every 24 h.
  - Alternatives include ceftizoxime 1 g IV every 8 h or cefotaxime 1 g IV every 8 h.
  - The transition to oral antibiotics can usually be made 24–48 h after clinical improvement.
- **Oral Antibiotics:**
  - Cefixime 400 mg PO bid.
  - Patients should continue oral antibiotics for at least 1 week.
- **Treatment of *Chlamydia*:**
  - 30–50 % of patients are co-infected with *Chlamydia*.
  - All patients should be tested and treated with azithromycin (1 g PO as a single dose) or doxycycline (100 mg PO bid for 7 days).
- **Joint aspiration:**
  - Affected joints should be aspirated to remove purulent material. This may have to be repeated.
    - □ Surgical or arthroscopic drainage is rarely indicated. It should be considered if no improvement occurs within a few days.

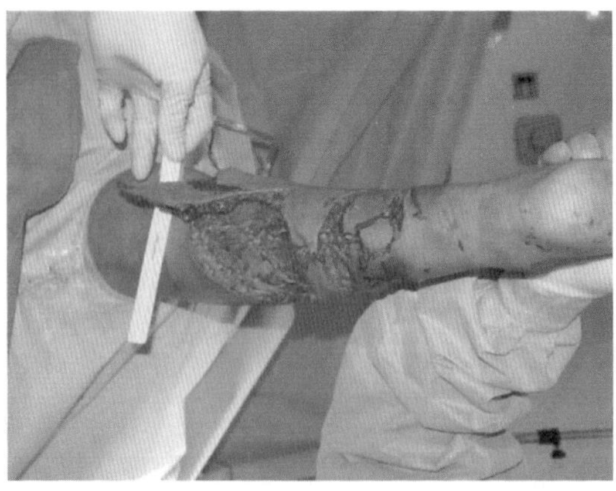

Fig. 21.5 A 13-year-old boy who was attacked by a dog resulting in extensive skin and soft tissue damage in his right calf (courtesy of Dr. E. Kanlic)

SEPTIC ARTHRITIS OF THE HIP

See Chap. 6.

ANIMAL AND HUMAN BITES

Incidence:

- 3–6 million animal bites per year in the United States.

Dog Bites:

- Typically causes a **crushing-type** wound because of their rounded teeth and strong jaws.
- Because of the high energy associated with these bites, it may damage deeper structures such as bones, vessels, tendons, muscle, and nerves (Fig. 21.5).

Cat Bites:

- The sharp pointed teeth of cats usually cause **puncture wounds.**
- This may inoculate bacteria into deep tissues.
  - Cat bites are **more prone to become infected than dog bites**.
  - Infections caused by cat bites generally develop faster than those of dogs.

Human Bites:

- Human bite should be treated aggressively (especially in the hand).
- It is common in children who live in institutions for mentally delayed persons (a method to attack others or defend self).
- **Closed fist injury**:
  - The child (adolescent) uses a closed fist to hit another person in the mouth.
  - The teeth will cause this "human bite" type injury.
  - This injury usually looks very superficial and minimal, however, in most cases, it extends deep in the tissues up to the metacarpophalangeal joint.
  - The bite site when examined will be more proximal than the level of the metacarpophalangeal joint.
    - This is because of during the position of closed fist; the skin over the metacarpophalangeal joint is pulled distally. When the fist is released, the injury site will move proximal.
  - This type of human bite can cause **septic arthritis** of the metacarpophalangeal joint.

Other Animals:

- The bites of foxes, raccoons, skunks, bats, dogs, and cats have been clearly linked to rabies exposure.
- Bites from large herbivores, e.g., horses; generally have a significant crush element because of the force involved.

Microbiology:

- Common bacteria involved in bite wound infections include the following:
  - **Dog bites**:
    - ☐ ***Pasteurella species (Pasteurella canis)***
    - ☐ *Staphylococcus* species.
    - ☐ *Streptococcus* species.
  - **Cat bites**:
    - ☐ ***Pasteurella species (Pasteurella multocida)***
    - ☐ *Actinomyces* species.
    - ☐ *Propionibacterium* species.
    - ☐ *Bacteroides* species.
  - **Human bites**:
    - ☐ ***Eikenella corrodens***
    - ☐ *Staphylococcus, Streptococcus.*
    - ☐ *Corynebacterium* species.
    - ☐ *Staphylococcus aureus*.
    - ☐ Blood-borne diseases (HIV, hepatitis).
- **History**:
  - Identify if the animal is known or stray animal.
  - If it is known animal, identification of its vaccination status.
  - Vaccination history of the patient specially tetanus.
  - Pattern of the attack, e.g., was the dog aggravated or the dog attacked without aggravation.
  - Behavior of the animal.
  - Prevalence of rabies in this area.
- **Physical exam:**
  - Assess the following:
    - ☐ Amount of soft tissue crushing, and the depth of invasion.
    - ☐ Signs of infection (redness and tenderness around the area of the bite) (Fig. 21.6).
    - ☐ Tendon or tendon sheath involvement (ask the child to flex and extend all the distal joints).
    - ☐ Deformity of the limb indicates possible bone injury.
    - ☐ Joint space violation. If there is septic arthritis, movement of the joint will cause severe pain.
    - ☐ Foreign bodies (e.g., teeth) in the wound.

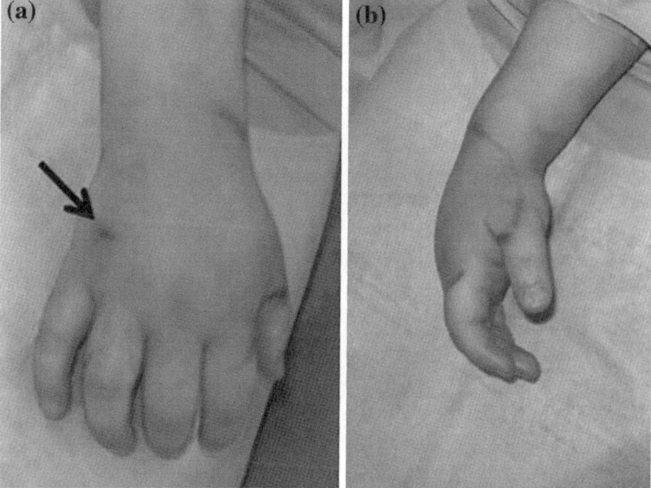

Fig. 21.6 A 3-year-old boy with an infected dog bit. The child was bitten by a dog 4 days before development of redness and swelling around the bite site (*arrow*)

Imaging Studies:

- Radiography assessment for presence of:
  - Foreign body.
  - Fractures.
- MRI:
  - Needed in cases of development of complications from the bite.
  - Can detect deep abscess or bone infection.

MANAGEMENT OF HUMAN AND ANIMAL BITES

- **General:**
  - Fresh bite wounds without signs of infection do not need to be cultured.

- Infected bite wounds should be cultured to help guide future antibiotic therapy.
- Local public health authorities should be notified of all bites and may help with recommendations for rabies prophylaxis.
- Consider tetanus and rabies prophylaxis for all wounds.

■ **Antibiotic therapy:**

- All human and animal bites should be treated with antibiotics.
- The choice between oral and parenteral antimicrobial agents should be based on the severity of the wound and on the clinical status of the the child.
- Oral Amoxicillin–Clavulanate is an excellent choice for empirical oral therapy for human and animal bite injuries.
- Parenteral Ampicillin–Sulbactam is the drug of choice in severe cases.
- If patient is allergic to penicillin, Azithromycin, or Clindamycin in combination with Trimethoprim–Sulfamethoxazole can be given.

■ **Antirabies treatment may be indicated for the following bites**:

- Dogs; if stray dog, not captured or captured dog with proved rabies.
- Cats whose rabies status cannot be obtained.
- Foxes
- Bats
- Raccoons
- Skunks.

■ **Irrigation and Debridement:**

- An effective means of preventing infection.
- Can be done in Emergency department.
  - □ **Debridement**: removing devitalized tissue.
  - □ **Irrigation**: copious irrigation (about 1,000 ml of normal saline or other non-sugar containing fluids).
- For extensive tissue damage, irrigation, and debridement should be done in the operating room (Fig 21.5).

■ **Immediate Primary closure** of the wound is better to be avoided (can cause an abscess later).

- The wounds are better left open for either delayed primary closure (after 3–5 days) or secondary closure by granulation tissue.
- Facial wounds, because of the good blood supply, are at low risk for infection, even if closed primarily. Facial wounds can be closed primarily to obtain better cosmetic results.

- Rest and elevation of the extremity.
- **Orthopedic surgery consultation:**
  - Development of an abscess.
  - Bone, joint, or tendon injury.
  - Presence of deep foreign body.
  - Closed fist injuries (most of these have to be explored to identify joint affection).
- Plastic surgery consultation:
  - Extensive wounds, involving tissue loss.
  - Facial wounds.

PUNCTURE WOUND

- Most of the puncture wound can be treated successfully in the emergency department.
- Deep infection is uncommon and may be associated with septic arthritis or osteomyelitis.
- Most common organisms are *S. aureus* and *Pseudomonas*.
- **Imaging:**
  - If there are suspicions for retained foreign body.
    - □ Radiographs:
      - ○ Will show radio-opaque retained foreign body (Fig. 21.7).
      - ○ Will show the signs of osteomyelitis of the foot (Fig. 21.8).
    - □ Ultrasound:
      - ○ Ultrasound has high sensitivity for foreign bodies in the sole.
    - □ MRI:
      - ○ If suspecting deep abscess or bone infection or deep foreign body that did not show up in other imaging studies.

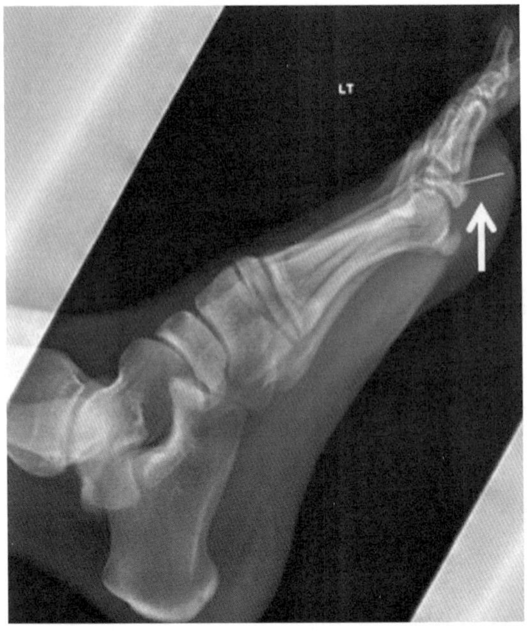

Fig. 21.7 A 16-year-old boy who stepped bare footed over a nail (*arrow*)

- **Treatment**:
  - Irrigation with saline and betadine.
  - Tetanus booster.
  - Antibiotic therapy:
    - □ For simple puncture wounds presenting within 24 h: No prophylactic antibiotic is needed.
    - □ If the patient is presenting after 24 h: anti-Staph antibiotic.
    - □ **Close follow-up is very important to assess development of deep infection.**
    - □ If the patient is presenting after 72 h with signs of infection (swelling, erythema, drainage):
      - ○ Admit for intravenous antibiotics covering both staph and pseudomonas infection.
    - □ Indication for orthopedic consultation:
      - ○ Deep foreign body.
      - ○ Suspected osteomyelitis.

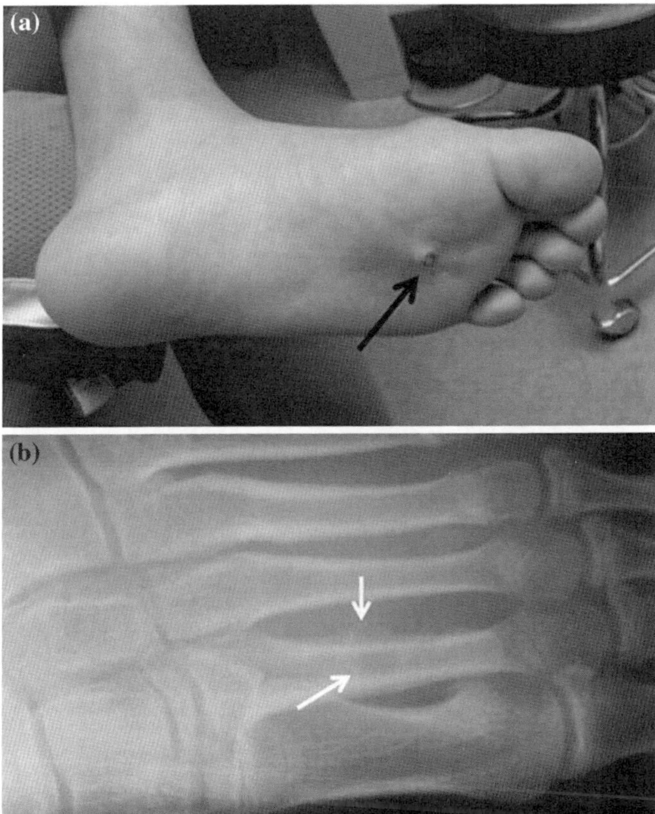

Fig. 21.8 A 14-year-old boy who had a puncture wound to his left foot while wearing his tennis shoes (**a**). The patient continued to have left foot pain and discharge from his puncture wound in the left foot for 6 weeks (*arrow*). Radiographs of the foot (**b**) show signs of chronic osteomyelitis of the second metatarsus (osteolytic lesion with surrounding periosteal new bone formation)

- **Special situations:**
  - Old tennis shoes penetrated by old nails are a high risk of pseudomonal infection:
    - □ Thorough irrigation and surgical debridement under anesthesia followed by oral antibiotic for 10–14 days should be considered in these cases.

HIGH YIELD FACTS

- The most common organisms of osteomyelitis in healthy children are *Staphylococcus aureus* and *beta-hemolytic streptococci.*
- Osteomyelitis spreads mainly hematogenous in children (unlike adult it is local infection).
- *Pseudomonas aeruginosa* is a characteristic causative organism in children with puncture wound through the shoe.
- Bone changes on radiographs may not occur in acute osteomyelitis for 10–15 days.
- In two-thirds of cases of osteomyelitis, the total WBC count is normal.
- Osteomyelitis is a medical condition, with some possible surgical indication.
- Septic arthritis is a surgical condition. Urgent consultation is needed to protect the joint.
- Transient synovitis is usually preceded by upper respiratory infection with or without fever.
- Range of motion of the joint is more affected in cases of septic arthritis than in osteomyelitis.
- ESR is more elevated in septic joint than osteomyelitis.
- Leukocytosis with shift to the left is more common with septic joint than osteomyelitis.
- Marked clinical improvement to short course of NSAID is indicative of transient synovitis.

Pitfalls:

- Normal ESR and total WBC count does not rule out septic joint or osteomyelitis, you may need to repeat.
- Absence of fever does not rule out septic hip or osteomyelitis.
- Child refusal to walk or use one limb is not normal and should be carefully investigated.

CLINICAL SCENARIO

The presenting patient	The most probable diagnosis and plan of action
5-year-old boy presents to the emergency room with swollen red hot tender right knee. Mother denied history of trauma. Child has fever of 39.2. On examination the child refuses to move the right knee. The plain radiographs are negative	Septic arthritis of the knee; urgent orthopedic consult in needed for irrigation and debridement: ■ Aspiration of the knee ■ Cell count, Gram stain, and culture of the fluid ■ Start antibiotic with IV Vancomycin (if living in area with high predominance of MRSA) then change the antibiotic according to culture and sensitivity
7-year-old boy presents with severe left hip pain. He has two days' history of limping with no prior history to trauma. His temperature is 38.2. He is able to weight bear on the affected side with marked discomfort	Septic arthritis of the hip or transient synovitis Proceed with markers of infection ■ If normal, most probably transient synovitis. NSAID, admit for observation or very close follow-up. If no improvement after 24 h treat as septic arthritis ■ If elevated, most probably septic arthritis. Ultrasound-guided aspiration and send fluid for cell count and culture. Orthopedic consult
14-year-old boy presents with swollen tender right index finger for the last 24 h. Had a fight with one of his classmates 3 days ago. He describes that he "punched	Close fist injury with possible septic arthritis of the metacarpophalangeal joint ■ Plain radiograph of the hand for foreign body (tooth)

(continued)

him in the face." On examination; the index finger is swollen with small laceration (5 mm) proximal to the metacarpophalangeal joint. Small amount of drainage can be seen from the wound. Movement of the metacarpophalangeal joint is extremely limited	■ Urgent orthopedic consult

REFERENCES

Kaplan SL. Septic arthritis. In: Kliegman RM, Stanton BF, St. Geme JW, Schor NF, Behrman RE, editors. Nelson textbook of pediatrics, 19th ed. Philadelphia: Elsevier; 2011. p. 2398–400.

Arnold SR, Elias D, Buckingham SC, Thomas ED, Novais E, Arkader A, Howard C. Changing patterns of acute hematogenous osteomyelitis and septic arthritis. Emergence of community-associated methicillin-resistant Staphylococcus aureus. J Pediatr Orthop. 2006;26:703–8.

Bonhoeffer J, Haeberle B, Schaad UB, Heininger U. Diagnosis of hematogenous osteomyelitis and septic arthritis: 20 years experience at the University Children's Hospital Basel. Swiss Med Wkly. 2001;131:575–81.

Taekema HC, Landham PR, Maconochie I. Towards evidence based medicine for paediatricians. Distinguishing between transient synovitis and septic arthritis in the limping child: how useful are clinical prediction tools? Arch Dis Child. 2009;94:167–8.

Weber EJ. Mammalian bites. In: Marx JA, Hockberger RS, Walls RM, editors. Rosen's emergency medicine: concepts and clinical practice. 6th ed. Philadelphia: Mosby; 2006. p. 906–21.

Chachad S, Kamat D. Management of plantar puncture wounds in children. Clin Pediatr (Phila). 2004;43(3):213–6.

Talan DA, Citron DM, Abrahamian FM, Moran GJ, Goldstein EJ. Emergency medicine animal bite infection study group. Bacteriologic analysis of infected dog and cat bites. N Engl J Med. 1999;340(2):85–92.

Index

A. Abdelgawad and O. Naga (eds.), *Pediatric Orthopedics*,
DOI: 10.1007/978-1-4614-7126-4,

Printed by Printforce, the Netherlands